LABELING THE MENTALLY RETARDED

Labeling the Mentally Retarded

Clinical and Social System Perspectives on Mental Retardation

by

JANE R. MERCER

University of California Press
Berkeley, Los Angeles, London

University of California Press
Berkeley and Los Angeles, California

University of California Press, Ltd.
London, England

ISBN: 0-520-02183-5 (cloth)
ISBN: 0-520-02428-1 (paperback)
Library of Congress
Catalog Card Number: 70-182795

Printed in the United States of America

3 4 5 6 7 8 9 0

TO

Harvey F. Dingman
Teacher, Colleague,
and Friend

CONTENTS

Foreword ix
Preface xi

Part I
ORIENTATIONS

1 *The Clinical Perspective* 1
2 *The Social System Perspective* 20
3 *The Research Setting: Riverside, California* 38

Part II
THE SOCIAL SYSTEM EPIDEMIOLOGY

4 *Who Labels Whom?* 53
5 *Who Are Labeled by Clinicians?* 67
6 *The Situationally Retarded* 83
7 *The Labeling Process in the Public Schools* 96

Part III
THE CLINICAL EPIDEMIOLOGY

8	*Defining Mental Retardation for the Clinical Epidemiology*	127
9	*Operationalizing the Mental Retardation Construct*	141
10	*Characteristics of Persons Failing the Adaptive Behavior Scales*	155
11	*Characteristics of Persons Failing the Intellectual Dimension*	165
12	*Characteristics of the Clinically Retarded—the Eligibles*	171

Part IV
CURRENT ISSUES IN THE CLINICAL PERSPECTIVE

13	*A One- or a Two-dimensional Definition?*	185
14	*Which Criterion?*	197
15	*Which Taxonomy?*	222
16	*Sociocultural Modality*	235
17	*Sociocultural Pluralism: Convergence of the Clinical and Social System Perspectives*	255
	Appendix A. Methodological Notes	273
	Appendix B. Items Used for Measuring the Adaptive Behavior of Persons of Various Ages	287
	Appendix C. Items Used for Measuring the Physical Disability of Persons of Various Ages	305
	Bibliography	308
	Index	315

FOREWORD

Harvey F. Dingman, Ph.D.

The history of ideas is very difficult to document. Even the development of a single research project is almost impossible to recapture as persons change and the goals become more varied.

About 1954, Morton Kramer of the National Institute of Mental Health, and George Tarjan, Superintendent of Pacific State Hospital, began a study of the differential patient release rates at the hospital. With the assistance of Stanley W. Wright, Earl S. Pollock, and Philip H. Person, Jr., they showed that mildly retarded patients had a significantly higher rate of return to the community than severely retarded patients. In order to continue and enlarge this study, a special grant was developed with the assistance of Leonard Duhl and Anna M. Shotwell and was subsequently awarded by NIMH.[1] As time went on, it became obvious that the data collected for the study were valuable for planning institutional programs and that it was important to maintain permanent hospital files in such a way as to provide ready access to data concerning patient movement.[2]

As research continued, the importance of the community aspects of mental retardation became evident. Charles Windle and Richard K. Eyman joined the project as regular staff. C. Edward Meyers, Robert B. Edgerton, and George Sabagh were recruited to do research while on special leave from their academic positions, and Jane R. Mercer joined the staff to study the families of the mentally retarded. With the assistance of these investigators plans were made to conduct community research on the problems of the mentally retarded responding to the stress and normal crises of life in a community setting.[3]

It became apparent that a major problem in such a study would be

[1] Population Movement of Mental Defectives and Related Physical, Behavioral, Social and Cultural Factors, 3M-9130.

[2] Data Processing in Mental Deficiency, OM-469.

[3] Mental Retardation in a Community, MH-5687; Computer Aid for Mental Retardation Research, MH-06616.

finding the mentally retarded in the community who had not come into contact with social agencies. To meet this problem, Raymond J. Jessen assisted in developing the two-pronged design for studying the epidemiology of retardation, a field survey and an agency survey, that was adopted for the Riverside research project.

The city of Riverside, California, was selected for study, and support was secured from NIMH.[4] Jane R. Mercer was assigned as field director and with the assistance of Edgar W. Butler developed the interview schedules, the screening procedures, and the sampling schemes which were pretested in the city of Pomona and later used in the survey in Riverside.

Eventually the grants supporting the hospital and community research were combined and funded through NIMH as a program-project grant with the assistance of Philip Sapir, Louis A. Wienckowski, and Howard R. Davis.[5]

This account of the development of a research program in an area where little had been done in a systematic and organized fashion cannot do justice to the conceptual schemes which have been produced by particular individuals in the process of carrying on the project in Riverside. Nonetheless, a word of deep appreciation is in order for the contributions made to the research effort by the group of consultants who have met with us almost monthly over a period of nine years, and particularly to those persons from Riverside in the public schools, the municipal government, civic organizations, and the private sector who were so helpful in giving us assistance.

4 Ibid.

5 Socio-Behavioral Study Center for Mental Retardation, MH-08667.

PREFACE

Our study of mental retardation in the community has been much like starting a journey to a vaguely defined destination with a compass but no road map. The general direction was specified in the original project proposal, but the detailed map had to be drawn en route. As the map was drawn and redrawn at critical junctures, our destination was clarified and proved to be in a direction somewhat different than that anticipated at the beginning of the journey. Thus, the history of the research project is, in large measure, a history of the intellectual evolution of those who participated. We did not begin and end our venture at the same place intellectually, and do not wish to leave the impression that we started this endeavor fully aware of our destination.

The movement in the study has been from a traditional, clinical view of the nature of mental retardation to a more relativistic social system perspective. These changes have resulted, primarily, as a consequence of working back and forth between empirical data and theoretical constructs. In this process, two models have been generated: a pluralistic clinical perspective and a social system perspective.

It is not possible to recognize individually every person who contributed directly or indirectly to a research effort of this magnitude. The two persons most responsible for initiating the study of mental retardation in the community are George Tarjan, M.D., and the late Harvey F. Dingman, Ph.D. As coprincipal investigators, they assumed administrative and scientific responsibility for recruiting key staff and overseeing the general progress of the study.

We are very grateful to the Applied Research Branch of the National Institute of Mental Health for their funding and continued support.[1] Howard Davis, Louis Wienckowski, and Philip Sapir from the NIMH staff have been particularly helpful and supportive over the years. The Health Sciences Computing Facility at the University of California,

[1] This investigation was supported by Public Health Service Research Grant No. MH-08667 from the National Institute of Mental Health, Department of Health, Education, and Welfare, and Public Health Service General Research Support Grant No. 1-SO1-FR-05632-02, from the Department of Health, Education, and Welfare.

Los Angeles, directed by Wilfrid Dixon, has provided computer support for much of the data analysis.[2]

There are many who have been generous with their advice and critical comments. We especially appreciate the efforts of those who have maintained a continuing interest in the study: C. E. Meyers, Georges Sabagh, Richard Eyman, Raymond Jessen, Neil Warren, Robert Edgerton, Robert Greenfield, Sidney Justice, Robert Nisbet, Rosemarie McCartin, Charles V. Keeran, and Curtis R. Miller. They have provided ready consultation at every critical decision point from questions on sampling design to statistical analysis of the data.

There are many others who took time to serve as members of our advisory board and contributed valuable insights and criticisms as we developed the research plan. Many will find that their suggestions were followed. Others may disagree heartily with what we have done. They represent a variety of disciplines and an even greater variety of perspectives. We have been grateful for the diversity and feel it contributed immeasurably to the vitality of the research effort: Craig MacAndrew, Jan Hajda, Harvey J. Locke, James A. Peterson, Troy S. Duster, Aaron Cicourel, Lindsey Churchill, Joseph A. Gengerelli, Daniel M. Milner, Harold M. Skeels, Robert B. McIntyre, Malcolm B. Stinson, M. Hamovitch, Walter R. Goldschmidt, Harold Garfinkel, Edgar Winans, F. N. David, P. John Kim.

Without the support and counsel of key persons from the city of Riverside we might never have survived the first summer of fieldwork. We wish especially to thank then City Manager, H. K. Hunter; Chief Probation Officer, Bert Van Horn; and Probation Officer, Eleanor Chapman; Superintendent of the Riverside Unified School District, Bruce Miller; and his Director of Pupil Personnel Services, Richard Robbins; the three men who have served as Directors of the Special Education Program of the Riverside Unified School District during our study, John Whiteman, Donald Ashurst, and Albert Marley; Director of Psychological Services and Special Education, Riverside County Schools, George Fox; Leah Bond, Shirley Flogerzi, and Ada Crilly of the Retarded Children's Association; Everett Stone and Mildred Parks, Riverside County Health Department; Milford L. Hill, Department of Vocational Rehabilitation; and Paul Wiley, Riverside County Department of Public Welfare.

Edgar Butler provided administrative skills and technical competence which greatly facilitated the fieldwork for the pretest and the household survey. George Sitkei, Charles Watts, Donald O'Brien, Douglas Dewar, and Liv Eklund conducted the psychometric testing in the

[2] Computing Assistance was obtained from the Health Sciences Computing Facility, UCLA, sponsored by NIH Grant FR-3.

homes. The enthusiastic response and dedicated interviewing done by the teachers of Riverside and surrounding communities during the household survey and the agency survey provided a major portion of the data. We thank Laurence Pleas, Royce Bell, Ann Brucker, and Philip Laney for serving as survey supervisors and the following for serving as interviewers: John Blanchard, Diana Boyce, George Schipper, Helen Hernandez, Tony Hernandez, Harold Carr, William O'Leary, Ernest Robles, June Simms, Feliciana Velasquez, Murlene Bigelow, Elizabeth Coleman, Merly Haga, Linda Hunter, Christine Jerpe, Arthur Friese, Gerd Pollitz, Carol Porter, Gayle Wolf, Anthony Purpero, Charles Harvey, Albert Montgomery, Kathleen Park, Dorothy Sirrine, Ronald Youngs, Nellie Clay, James Ervin, Gaynell Fraley, Evelyn Hale, Eleanor Jennings, Gretchen Nunamaker, Jerry Perkins, Andrew Gordon, Martha Sondrup, Barbara Wheelock.

Students from the University of California, Riverside, provided a steady flow of assistance in every aspect of the study. We especially wish to thank William Blischke, Edward D. Bryan, T. C. Weir, Sharon Blischke, Judith Baughman, Lynn Adamson, George Boutin, Wayne Brown, John Kalin, Randall Nelson, George Lightburn, Sally McCuish, Patricia Webber, and Jolly O'Hare for their contributions. Cathy Kalin, Enid Bondar, Sandra McGann, Ada Bewley, Rosa Linhart, and Sharon Monthony shared the burden of typing numerous versions and revisions of the manuscript.

The support and counsel of key personnel of the Socio-Behavioral Laboratory at Pacific State Hospital sustained the project from beginning to end. We especially wish to thank Richard K. Butkus, John M. Cassidy, Maurine Paulsen, June Nakatani, Werner Lohmann, Janet Stotz, Audrey Burghardt, Yuvetta J. Powell, Thelma Fraser, and Philip Kalm from the data processing staff; June Lindley, Mary Bennett, Lynn Whitlinger, and Janet Palmer of the office staff.

Finally, there has been one person who, more than any other individual, has made this manuscript possible. She began on the project as an undergraduate, remained to do graduate work, and has since become the central figure directing data collection, coordinating data analysis, and supervising the editing and typing of this manuscript—June F. Lewis. Without her tenacity, devotion, and good humor this book would never have been completed.

To all of these persons, I am deeply grateful. Any deficiencies in this product, however, are solely my responsibility.

If the names selected to represent the persons described in the case studies bear any similarity to those of actual persons, the similarity is purely fortuitous.

J. R. M.

Part I

ORIENTATIONS

Chapter 1

THE CLINICAL PERSPECTIVE

The question, "What is it really?" "What is its right name?" is a nonsense question . . . one that is not capable of being answered. . . . The individual object or event we are naming, of course, has no name and belongs to no class until we put it in one. . . . What we call things and where we draw the line between one class of things and another depend upon the interest we have and the purposes of the classification.
Most intellectual problems are, ultimately, problems of classification and nomenclature.
S. I. Hayakawa, *Language in Action*

The questions "Who are the persons in a community who are really mentally retarded? What is the right prevalence rate?" are nonsense questions, questions that are not capable of being answered. Persons have no names and belong to no class until we put them in one. Whom we call mentally retarded, and where we draw the line between the mentally retarded and the normal, depend upon our interest and the purpose of our classification. The intellectual problem of mental retardation in the community is, ultimately, a problem of classification and nomenclature.

The perspective from which human behavior is viewed determines its meaning. What things are called and where the line is drawn between one class of things and another is socially arbitrated and then validated through common usage. Most definitions we use to interpret the world are learned from others and are sufficiently imbedded in the cultural heritage to make it difficult to extract and objectify them for analysis. This difficulty arises because traditional ways of classifying reality and cataloging behavior are structured by our language and thought systems. Thus, it can be an arduous, even painful task to identify the fundamental elements of a traditional frame of reference and explore its basic assumptions. However, this intellectual task is essential if we are to recognize the extent to which accepted postures influence our perceptions and may conceal fruitful, alternative ways of structuring reality.

We have identified two contrasting perspectives from which mental retardation may be viewed: the clinical perspective and the social system perspective (Mercer, 1965; Mercer, 1972). The clinical perspective classifies mental retardation as a handicapping condition, which exists in the individual and can be diagnosed by clinically trained professionals using properly standardized assessment techniques. The social system perspective classifies mental retardation as an acquired social status. Like any social status, that of mental retardate is defined by its location in the social system vis-à-vis other statuses, and by the role prescriptions that define the type of performance expected of persons holding the status.

The clinical perspective is the familiar frame of reference which forms the intellectual basis for the academic disciplines that train persons in the field of mental retardation. It is the perspective that directs community action programs and guides research. Because of its pervasive influence, the assumptions of the clinical perspective are seldom examined and its implications are rarely explored.

Who Is Normal?

The clinical perspective is the frame of reference commonly adopted by persons in the helping professions—those in the field of medicine, psychology, social work, and education. Within this general perspective, there are two contrasting definitions of "normal": the pathological model contributed by medicine and the statistical model advanced by psychology and education. The two approaches are used interchangeably by clinicians. The widely accepted clinical definition of mental retardation adopted by the American Association for Mental Deficiency incorporates both models (Heber, 1961).

The pathological model of normal was developed in medicine as a conceptual tool for comprehending and controlling disease processes and organic malfunctioning. Medical concern is aroused when conditions occur which interfere with the physiological functions of the organism. Consequently, the focus of the medical model is on pathology and the symptoms of pathology. Diseases are defined by the biological symptoms which characterize them. Emphasis is on defining the nature of the abnormal, and normal tends to be treated as a residual category containing organisms that do not have abnormal symptoms. That is, normal = absence of pathological symptoms; abnormal = presence of pathological symptoms.

How does one recognize a pathological symptom? In medicine, this question is ordinarily answered through functional analysis. Pathological processes are identified by the fact that they tend to destroy the biological organism as a living system. Any biological manifestation can be evaluated against this universal standard. Those processes which interfere with system preservation are "bad," i.e., pathological, while those which enhance the life of the organism are "good," i.e., healthy. Because members of the same species are very similar biologically, findings based on manifestations of biological processes operating in one human organism can be generalized with a high level of validity to other human organisms. Although inductive logic is implied, it is less crucial than in the statistical model. For this reason, findings generated within a pathological model frequently transcend societal boundaries. Stable patterns of biological pathology manifest themselves in roughly comparable forms in many different societies. The disease model is a universal model. Differences in prevalence rates for biological dysfunctions are accepted as real differences in the amount of pathology in the populations being studied.

A clinician diagnosing an individual, using a medical model, begins with an abstract construct of the nature of the symptoms that constitute a particular disease entity and determines whether these pathological symptoms are present in a particular case. If they are present, the person is sick. The pathological model is conceptually a bipolar construct. At one pole is normal, which is equated with health and the absence of pathological symptoms. At the other pole is abnormal, defined as the presence of pathological signs and equated with disease, illness, "unhealth." Persons may be ranged along the continuum. It is assumed that it is best to fall close to the normal pole. To be abnormal, i.e., unhealthy, is bad, and should be prevented or alleviated. Thus, the pathological model is essentially evaluative. The clinician is constantly involved in making judgments about the biological state of his clients in terms of a health-pathology dimension which is readily translated into a good-bad polarity. Clinician and client usually agree that health is better than illness and that action should be taken to remove all pathological symptoms. Because the pathological model concentrates on symptoms, persons viewed from this vantage point are likely to be described in terms of what is wrong with them.

The statistical model for normal is familiar to anyone who has been introduced to the concept of the normal curve. Since Francis Galton first realized that an individual's attributes can be described by his relative position in a frequency distribution of other persons, the normal curve has been used to establish norms for populations.

Unlike the pathological model, which defines the symptoms of pathology by a functional analysis, the statistical model defines abnormality according to the extent to which an individual varies from the average of the population on a particular trait. Establishing the statistically normal is a straightforward process. The investigator specifies the population of persons on which the norms will be based and then measures the entire population or a representative sample of the population on the attribute being normed. Scores on the measure are organized into a frequency distribution, and the average score, i.e., the statistical mean, is calculated. The mean is accepted as the norm. Customarily, persons with scores that deviate not more than one standard deviation above or below the mean are regarded as falling in the "normal range," and comprise approximately 68% of the population. Therefore, in the statistical definition, normal = statistical mean plus or minus one standard deviation from the mean.

Those whose scores fall more than one standard deviation above the mean, but less than two standard deviations above the mean, are classified as "high normals" (approximately 13.6% of the population), and those whose scores fall more than one standard deviation below the mean, but less than two standard deviations, are labeled as "low normals" (approximately 13.6% of the population). Those whose scores are more than two standard deviations above the mean are "abnormally high" (approximately 2.3% of the population), and those with scores more than two standard deviations below the mean are "abnormally low" (approximately 2.3% of the population).

In establishing a statistical norm, the investigator uses the characteristics of the particular population being studied to establish the boundaries of normal. Unlike the bipolar pathological model, the statistical model defines two types of abnormals: those who have abnormally large amounts of the characteristic measured and those who have abnormally small amounts. In the pathological model, it is always "bad" to have pathological signs. However, the statistical model, as a model, is evaluatively neutral. It depends on the attribute being measured whether it is "good" to be high or "good" to be low. In measuring some characteristics, it is "bad" for an individual to be located in either extreme; for example, it is "bad" to be either extremely heavy or extremely thin. In other cases, it is "good" to be abnormally low and "bad" to be abnormally high. In the case of IQ it is "good" to be abnormally high and "bad" to be abnormally low.

The use of a statistical model to define normal-abnormal appears in nearly pure form in the American Association on Mental Deficiency definition of the various levels of mental retardation (Heber, 1961). In this definition, IQs reported in standard deviation units are the major criteria for determining the level of mental retardation, and each level has its own diagnostic designation. An IQ of 100 is set as the statistical mean. A standard deviation on the Wechsler Intelligence Scales and the Stanford-Binet LM Form has been established as 15 points. Therefore, a person whose score is plus or minus one standard deviation (15 IQ points) from the mean of 100 is "normal" (IQ 85–115). A person whose score is between one and two standard deviations below the mean (IQ 70–84) is "borderline"; those with scores between two and three standard deviations below the mean are "mildly retarded" (IQ 55–69); those with scores between three and four standard deviations below the mean are "moderately retarded" (IQ 40–54); those with scores between four and five standard deviations below the mean are "severely retarded" (IQ 25–39); and those with scores more than five standard deviations below the mean are "profoundly retarded" (IQ under 25).

The statistical model may be used to establish norms for biological characteristics such as body temperature, height, and weight, but, unlike the pathological model, it is not limited to the description of biological characteristics. It can just as readily be used to establish norms for behavior. This helps to explain the uneasy marriage of the two dissimilar definitions of "normal" which appear in the official nomenclature. In the American Association on Mental Deficiency nomenclature, the statistical definition parallels the pathological definition and no attempt is made to integrate the disparate conceptual models from which the two are generated.

The pathological model is used to assess biological manifestations. The statistical model is used to assess behavioral manifestations not readily comprehended within a pathological model. Thus, the clinical definition of mental retardation presented in the official nomenclature is based on a dual standard of "normal"—a pathological model for biological manifestations and a statistical model for behavioral manifestations (Heber, 1961).

When evaluations using a statistical model are conducted in conjunction with evaluations using the pathological model—as is true in the case of mental retardation—there is a tendency to think in terms of one model while operating with the other. Behavioral patterns are translated into pathological signs. The implicit logic that underlies this transformation is as follows: Low IQ = "bad" in American society: a social evaluation. "Bad" = pathology in the pathological model. Therefore, low IQ = pathology. Thus, IQ, which is not a biological manifestation but is a behavioral score based on responses to a series of questions, becomes conceptually transposed into a pathological sign carrying all the implications of the pathological model. Statistical abnormality is equated with biological pathology without any evidence based on functional analysis that this statistical sign is related to the biology of the organism or that it has any functional relationship to system maintenance.

When a statistical model is used to define normal performance, the norms emerging from measurements taken on one population cannot be safely generalized beyond that population. Unlike the pathological model, statistical definitions of "normal" are neither trans-societal nor universal. Statistical norms, even for biological characteristics such as skin color, head circumference, height, or weight, that have been established on the population of the United States are obviously not valid for the population of Mexico. This is even more true of characteristics such as perceptual skills, motor coordination, competence in the verbal use of a particular language, information about a particular culture, abstract reasoning, or IQ.

The statistical model requires that the characteristic being measured be distributed normally. If this is not true, a statistically defined "normal" is misleading. Should the distribution be skewed, the mean will tend to move in the direction of the skew. Even more serious, if the distribution is bimodal or trimodal but is treated as unimodal, distinct distortions appear.

Suppose, for example, we are interested in establishing "normal" height for the population of the United States, but ignore the fact that the distribution is bimodal and that the average female is shorter than the average male. Of course, we can calculate a "normal" height for the combined sexes—but what is its value? The average is too small to tell us much about males and too large to tell us much about females. When a population is split evenly into two different groups, as with sex, and the means are sufficiently different, bimodality is obvious and not likely to be ignored. However, when the subgroup is small relative to the total population, its impact on the distribution may be miniscule and easily overlooked. Members of the subgroups remain in the combined distribution defined as "abnormals." For instance, a statistical norm based on a population consisting of 20% females and 80% males would define most of the females as "abnormally" short. These simple statistical propositions place severe restrictions on the statistical model as a frame of reference for defining normality.

Even within a single society, the normal range established on the basis of testing a representative sample of the entire society will reflect the characteristics of the most numerous group in that society and automatically will categorize the characteristics of less numerous groups as abnormal if they vary systematically from the general population on the characteristic being studied. For example, a normal curve of skin pigmentation based on the total population of the United States would classify the Black minority as abnormal, just as a test of English-language usage would classify children of Mexican and Puerto Rican heritage from Spanish-speaking homes as abnormal. When a statistical model is used, small numbers with a particular characteristic = abnormality. With this model, there will always be abnormals in a population because there are always two extreme tails to any distribution. Abnormality is intrinsic to the model.

Pathology as an Attribute of the Individual

The clinical perspective regards mental retardation as an attribute of the individual. Clinicians describe a person by saying that he is mentally retarded or is not mentally retarded in much the same sense that they would say he is tubercular or is not tubercular, is feverish or is not feverish, and so forth. Implicit in these statements is the assumption that the condition characterizes the individual and that the condition exists as an entity regardless of whether the person is aware of its presence or whether others recognize his pathology. Thus, from a clinical perspective, a case of mental retardation can exist undiagnosed in much the same sense that a case of rheumatic fever can exist undiagnosed and unrecognized. The symptomatology exists as an entity quite apart from whether it has been identified and labeled.

Mental Retardation as a Syndrome

The clinical perspective regards mental retardation as a pathological condition, which can be identified by characteristic patterns of symptoms. These configurations of biological symptoms are organized into syndromes, which are given specific labels—Down's syndrome, Klinefelter's syndrome, and so forth. However, there are syndromes that do not involve any biological signs. In such instances, the statistical model is used, and a low score on an intelligence test tends to be accepted as a symptom of pathology. Although organic involvement cannot be established in cases classified as undifferentiated, familial, or sociocultural, there is a distinct tendency to assume that "minimal brain dysfunction" exists but cannot be detected because of the inadequacy of present diagnostic tools. When more-sensitive measures are devised, it is presumed that some kind of organic dysfunction will be discovered. Until then, the statistical rather than the medical norm must suffice.

Mental Retardation as Suprasocietal

We noted earlier that biological norms based on functional analyses using a pathological model can frequently be generalized to the entire human species. Surgeons face essentially the same problems in human heart transplants whether they are operating in South Africa, Denmark, or California. It is valid to assume that there are stable patterns of biological pathology that transcend any particular cultural system and the society which bears that culture. Biological malfunctions will manifest themselves in roughly comparable forms in many different societies, and the cultural differences between those societies are irrelevant. In these instances, the culture-blind pathological model can be transferred readily from one society to another and still retain its power to predict and to illuminate. Because it transcends cultural differences, i.e., is supracultural, the pathological model is also suprasocietal. The clinician diagnosing a case of pneumonia does not have to take into account the culture of his patient or the society in which he lives. However, this is not true of statistically established norms, except when they deal with strictly delimited biological functions. When the characteristics being normed are culturally determined, cultural differences are not irrelevant. A pathological model in mental retardation is most efficient when applied to conditions that show clear evidence of biological dysfunction, and it becomes progressively less useful as biological factors become more obscure. At this point, a statistical model is likely to be used, but definitions of normal behavior based on a statistical model are not suprasocietal and, hence, cannot be treated as supracultural.

Both models for normal are used simultaneously in the clinical perspective, but the difference in their generalizability creates a critical discontinuity. This hiatus is usually resolved by the logical transformation described earlier—a low IQ is interpreted as a pathological sign and treated as if it had been identified as a symptom by functional analysis. The pathological model, with its wider applicability, prevails. In this context, prevalence rates for all types of mental retardation in Taiwan are compared with those from Sweden, Norway, or the Eastern Health District of Baltimore. Investigators recognize the variability in cultural milieu and realize that different societies reward and promote different kinds of behavior. However, recognition of these differences has not precluded cross-societal comparisons. The pathological model takes precedence over the statistical model. Differences in prevalence rates for mental retardation in various societies and various subcultures of the same society are accepted as real differences in the rate of pathology in the populations being studied.

The suprasocietal nature of the assumptions of the clinical perspective become especially critical in a complex, industrial society such as urban America. Within contemporary American society there are numerous intrasocietal segments—both socioeconomic and ethnic—which have their own distinctive cultures. Some of these groups form identifiable social systems within the larger society and have cultural characteristics that differentiate them from the core culture. Each of these intrasocietal social systems has a characteristic configuration of statuses, roles, and norms. Adults and children in such societal segments are reinforced for behaviors that conform to the role expectations of that group and, consequently, may develop patterns of response which are rewarded in that societal segment but which may not be valued and rewarded in the larger society. In some cases, behavior patterns inappropriate to roles in certain segments of the larger society are devalued and may result in an individual's being labeled as deviant, even mentally retarded, when he is operating outside of his cultural group. Thus, studies of prevalence and incidence, even when conducted within the same society, encounter many of the same issues that arise in cross-societal comparisons, if the society being studied is multicultural and pluralistic.

Mental Retardation and the Logic of Cause and Effect

The pathological model promotes cause-and-effect reasoning. Biological dysfunctions are explained by locating those factors, internal or external, that can be shown to produce the dysfunction. Research conducted from a pathological model focuses almost exclusively on causal hypotheses. Social action concentrates either on preventing causal factors from producing the dysfunction or on removing the causes in order to produce a cure once those factors have begun to operate. The primary justification for epidemiological studies is that a knowledge of the distribution of handicapping conditions in the population may provide clues to etiology.

When mental retardation is conceptualized from a pathological model, the logical framework is that of cause and effect. Distinctions have been made between endogenous or "primary" retardates whose retardation is believed to be caused by inherited factors, and exogenous or "secondary" retardates whose retardation is believed to be acquired. Detailed clinical classification systems for codifying types of retardation, such as those of the American Association for Mental Deficiency (Heber, 1961) and the International Index of Diseases (1962) have been organized around causal ideas. Explorations of the causes of mental retardation run the full range from genetic studies to investigation of cultural factors as possible causal agents.

The clinical perspective has influenced the types of research questions that have been posed in mental retardation research. Typical questions are "What is the etiology of mental retardation? What can be done to prevent this condition? What can be done to cure this condition? How can we develop more reliable and more valid diagnostic instruments? How many people are afflicted by mental retardation?" All of these questions are identical to those which might be asked about contagious diseases. They are questions suggested by the very nature of the clinical perspective and illustrate how the frame of reference used in describing a phenomenon will predispose an investigator to explore certain kinds of research hypotheses.

Mental Retardation and Biological Emphasis of the Pathological Model

The pathological model encourages biological explanatory systems, and research tends to center around the study of individuals as isolated organisms rather than as persons functioning in a social network. The social context in which individuals live is viewed as irrelevant, except when there is some hypothesized relationship between certain environmental factors and physiological changes in the organism. Frequently, organic involvement is inferred even when it cannot be empirically established. The tendency to think in biological terms even when there is little or no evidence of organic pathology has been a particularly noticeable aspect of writing and thinking in the field of mental retardation. The focus of much research has been on trying to determine the exact nature of the biological concomitants of environmental factors.

"What is the nature of the organic damage produced by living in disadvantaged circumstances, which might account for higher rates of mild mental retardation in these populations? Is it inadequate diet? Is it inadequate prenatal and postnatal care? Could lack of environmental complexity permanently impair brain function?" and so forth. The biological bias of the medical model also encourages concentration on developing diagnostic tools that will be sensitive to minimal brain damage and other types of obscure organic pathologies that are presumed to exist. Detection of organic lesions would help verify the cause-and-effect linkage and validate the pathological model.

Because the pathological model is particularly effective when we are dealing with biological variables, those hypotheses most effectively handled by the model are likely to be selected for testing—hypotheses concerning biological factors in etiology. The possible effect of this biological bias on mental retardation research was explored. All etiological studies reported in papers abstracted in *Mental Retardation Abstracts* for the four-year period 1964–1967 (National Institute of Mental Health, 1964–1967) were reviewed and organized by etiological groupings.

Apparently, there has been little or no interest in exploring etiological hypotheses for those types of mental retardation which have "functional reaction alone manifest," i.e., which have no observable biological component. Although over half of the persons labeled as mentally retarded would fall in this category, only 0.1% of the 2,013 etiological reports appearing during this four-year period studied this group of individuals. There were only three papers in 1964 and no papers in subsequent years covering the etiology of mental retardation in normal-bodied persons. Instead, etiological studies centered almost exclusively on biological questions, which the pathological model can handle readily. The most popular etiological research area was "disorders of metabolism, growth, or nutrition," with 34.2% of the total papers. This is followed by "infectations or intoxications," having 22.8% of the papers, and reports on "general genetics," with 14.9% of the papers.

The Diagnostic Emphasis: Is He "Really" Retarded?

Accurate diagnosis is a fundamental value in the clinical tradition. If one assumes that retardation exists as a pathology that can be identified by diagnostic instruments, then accurate diagnosis is essential in the search for this assumed clinical reality. Consequently, the clinical perspective has led to a heavy emphasis on the development of valid and reliable diagnostic tools so that persons will not be misdiagnosed. This quest has led to a proliferation of tests of intelligence. *The Sixth Mental Measurements Yearbook* describes 80 group tests of intelligence, 28 individual tests of intelligence, 20 tests of specific aspects of intelligence, and 15 multi-aptitude batteries. Even more are currently in print but not described (Buros, 1965). Work is under way to develop and eventually standardize a scale to measure adaptive behavior, which may be used in conjunction with intelligence tests in diagnosing mental retardation (Leland et al., 1966).

Scheff has argued that there is a pervasive and fundamental code in medical decision-making which holds that it is much worse for a physician to dismiss an ill patient than it is for him to retain a well one. This code is based on a deterministic medical model, which sees disease as an unfolding process which, if untreated, may eventually endanger life itself. Within this framework, retaining a well patient may do little harm, but releasing a sick one could have serious consequences. Therefore, when in doubt, a conscientious practitioner will continue to suspect pathology (Scheff, 1966). It is reasonable to suppose that those diagnosticians of mental retardation who believe that treatment and training programs benefit participants will share the values of this medical code. On the other hand, there is also abundant evidence that clinicians are ambivalent about this unwritten code and quite sensitive to the social implications of the diagnosis of mental retardation. If there has been any systematic, historical bias in diagnosing mental retardation, it seems to be in favor of considering a person "normal" until conclusively proven to be otherwise. More serious apprehension has centered around the possibility of labeling someone as retarded who is not "really" retarded than around the alternative possibility of not labeling a person who could qualify as retarded. Binet expressed his concern with "mislabeling" as early as 1905. "It will never be to one's credit to have attended a special school. We should at the least spare from this mark those who do not deserve it. Mistakes are excusable, especially at the beginning. But if they become too gross, they could injure the name of these new institutions" (Binet, 1905).

This apprehension is revealed in the literature on diagnostic procedures and problems of differentiating "pseudoretardation" from "real" retardation (Arthur, 1947, 1950; Cassel, 1949; Guertin, 1950; Kanner, 1949*b*; Waskowitz, 1948).

Codification of "Core Cultural" Behavioral Expectations

The formalization and codification of behavioral norms into standardized measures establishes the role expectations and norms of the dominant society as the legitimate canon of acceptable behavior because this group is the overwhelming majority in the population on which tests are normed.[1] Binet tried to choose content for his tests with which all persons would be familiar. However, in a complex, pluralistic society, this is an impossible task. Items and procedures used in intelligence tests have inevitably come to reflect the abilities and skills valued by the American "core culture." This "core culture" consists mainly of the cultural patterns of that segment consisting of white, Anglo-Saxon Protestants whose social status today is predominantly middle and upper class. This cultural domination dates back to colonial times and has never been seriously threatened (Gordon, 1964).

What kinds of abilities and skills does the "core culture" value? Of the 128 intelligence tests listed in Buros, 58 were measures of general intelligence with no subtests. Measures of general intelligence are all highly loaded with verbal skills and knowledge. Of the 70 tests that have subtests, 77% have subtests entitled vocabulary, language, or verbal. Fifty-one percent have subtests entitled arithmetic, quantitative, or numerical, and 53% have subtests entitled reasoning, logic, or conceptual thinking (Buros, 1965). The number of subtests in intelligence tests that measure skills such as manual dexterity or mechanical ability is negligible. To score as intelligent in American society one must be

[1] In norming the Wechsler-Bellevue I and the Wechsler Adult Intelligence Scale (WAIS), the factors of subcultural differences in performance were not taken into account. Nonwhite subjects were not included in the original Wechsler-Bellevue standardization. In the 1955 WAIS standardization, some 10% of the total sample of 1,686 were nonwhite, a percentage roughly representing the proportion of nonwhites in the population of the United States in the 1950 census. According to Wechsler, "No attempt was made to establish separate norms for different racial (or national) groups in either the W-B I or the WAIS. The norms as they stand, particularly on the WAIS, seem to be reasonably representative of the country as a whole, and to this extent may be said to represent a fair cross-section of what may be called 'American intelligence' as of the time of standardization" (Wechsler, 1958, p. 90–91).

The final 1937 standardization group for the Stanford-Binet Intelligence Test "consisted of 3,184 native-born white subjects, including approximately 100 subjects at each half-year interval from 1½ to 5½ years, 200 at each age from 6 to 14, and 100 at each age from 15 to 18. Every age group was equally divided between sexes." Testing was done in 17 communities in 11 states distributed between urban, suburban and rural schools. The final sample contained no Blacks, was slightly higher in socioeconomic level than the census population, and had disproportionately more urban than rural subjects. The 1960 revision did not involve a restandardization. Over 4,000 subjects were used to determine the selection of items to be retained and to determine present item difficulty. These children "were not chosen to constitute a representative sample of American school children," although care was taken to avoid special, selective factors. Thus, the "native-born white subjects" of the 1937 standardization remain the basis for Stanford-Binet norms (Terman and Merrill, 1960).

highly verbal in English, adept with mathematical concepts, and facile in abstract conceptualization. One receives little official credit for musical, artistic, or mechanical abilities. The ability to live amicably with other human beings counts not at all in the psychometric test situation.

The Anglocentrism inherent in the mental tests most frequently used for diagnosing intelligence has been thoroughly documented (Altus, 1949; Darcy, 1953; Eells et al., 1951). We must conclude that the evaluations that produce the definition "mental retardate," for the most part, embody the values of the core culture. Because diagnosticians themselves have usually internalized the values of the core culture, they tend to accept these values as given and to perceive any individual who deviates markedly from these values as abnormal. Groups in the social structure sharing the values of the core culture tend to accept the labels attached as a consequence of the application of these values without serious questioning. For example, it seems self-evident to a member of a middle-class American family that there is something seriously wrong with an adult who cannot read or write in English. This opinion might not be so widely shared by persons in peripheral social systems who speak other languages. Different skills are required in different social settings. We can only speculate what forms an intelligence test designed for Harlem Blacks, barrio Mexican-Americans, or Hopi Indians might take. It is easy to imagine that linguistic and numerical skills would have considerably less salience.

Elaboration of the Diagnostic Nomenclature for Mental Retardation

The clinical perspective leads to an expansion and elaboration of the diagnostic nomenclature, which results in ever greater specification of subvarieties of mental retardation. The refinement of instruments for differential diagnosis has made this elaboration of the nomenclature of mental retardation possible. Today, instead of the simple distinction between "amentia" and "dementia" made by Esquirol, we have various gradations of retardation specified in terms of intelligence test scores. Not only are individuals labeled deviant or nondeviant, but the degree and variety of deviance can be specified. Just as the refinement of intelligence tests has produced precise specification of mental retardation by level of intellectual performance, research in organic components of retardation has resulted in the elaboration of a complex medical nomenclature. The expanded AAMD medical classification system consists of 8 major classifications, 39 subclassifications, 35 sub-subclassifications, and 16 supplementary terms (Heber, 1961).

Professionalization of the Diagnostic Function

The clinical perspective leads to the professionalization of the diagnostic function. The more formal the norms and the more elaborate the measuring devices, the stronger the tendency to professionalize the diagnostic function and to adopt a clinical perspective. This is very evident in the highly formalized and professionalized processes that operate in the labeling of the mental retardate. Only those who have received special training are regarded as having the requisite skills for administering intelligence tests and/or making medical diagnoses. Persons with these skills now form a corps of professional diagnosticians who have official sanction to label deviants by using appropriate diagnostic instruments. In the capacity of legitimate labelers, they control who may enter many programs and statuses in American society. Low performance on carefully normed intelligence measures, administered by duly trained and licensed professionals, is the recognized criterion in some states for placing persons in special education classes, hospitals for the retarded, or in categorical aid programs for the totally disabled.

In the future, much greater use will undoubtedly be made of professional evaluations when courts are making judicial decisions in incompetency hearings. This has been strongly recommended in the *Report of the Task Force on Law* of the President's Panel on Mental Retardation (Bazelan and Boggs, 1963). This report also calls for more precise classification and identification of groups to whom particular laws may apply. The implications of this recommendation are far reaching. Forty states have laws regulating the involuntary hospitalization of the mentally deficient. While most states still rely mainly on judicial procedures in such commitments, some require that deficiency be manifested "in psychological signs." However, they do not specify the nature of the signs nor who is to certify that they are present (Lindman and McIntyre, 1961).

If a person is judged incompetent by reason of mental disability, this has significant repercussions for him as an individual. Twenty-seven states have sterilization laws applicable to the mentally retarded, 37 states prohibit marriage of persons designated variously as "idiots," "imbeciles," and "feebleminded," and 8 states permit the annulment of an adoption of the child is subsequently found to be "feebleminded." Although terms used in legislation are ambiguous and their referents are not always clear, it appears that in most states a mentally retarded person cannot be issued a driver's license nor can he vote, hold public office, or perform jury duty (Lindman and McIntyre, 1961).

Presumption of Correctness of Official Definitions of Retardation

The clinical perspective leads to the assumption that the official definition of behavior is the "right" definition. If persons in subgroups of the community do not concur with official findings and refuse to define a member of their group as "retarded," the clinical perspective assumes that persons in the subgroups are wrong. It follows that those who do not concur with official labels must be educated so that they understand the "real" nature of the problem. If they refuse to be converted to the official definition of the situation and resist "enlightenment," then the clinical perspective is prone to interpret their recalcitrance as psychological denial and to act accordingly (Mercer, 1965).

Disagreement with official definitions of deviance are most likely to occur under two circumstances: when members of the subculture have not been socialized to the core-culture norms represented by the diagnostic instruments used by the clinician, and when the amount of deviance is minimal. If the person labeled deviant is visibly disabled or deformed physically or if his behavior shows gross incompetence in motor or perceptual skills or the ability to speak and to understand language, he will probably be regarded as deviant by any human social system in which he participates (Kanner, 1957).

If his incompetence is primarily in skills valued and cultivated by certain segments of society but not valued or cultivated by other segments of society, then he will not be viewed as subnormal by the latter. Nevertheless, there is a strong tendency in the clinical perspective to elevate verbal and mathematical competence, so valued and cultivated by the dominant culture, into a universal standard by which all persons in all subsystems are judged. Failure may mean being labeled pathologically subnormal—a mental retardate. The essential ethnocentricity of this position is frequently overlooked in the concern for the size of the standard error of the mean and fitting the best theoretical mathematical curve to the empirical data obtained from statistical measures.

Research done from a clinical frame of reference accepts the diagnostic procedures, nomenclature, and systems of labeling that have been developed by professional diagnosticians. It may, on occasion, become concerned with improving diagnostic procedures, with refining classification systems so that they are more precise, or with developing more adequate social structures for screening and labeling persons as retarded. However, this type of endeavor does not violate the assumptions of the clinical conceptual system. On the contrary, it is focused on sharpening the tools of that system.

Research done within a clinical framework accepts as the focus for study those individuals who, by processes recognized as legitimate in the society, have been labeled as deviant. Having accepted the societal definitions as valid, the investigator proceeds to study individuals so identified. In so doing, he has adopted the values of the social system that defined the person as deviant and has assumed that its judgments are the valid measure of deviance.

Impact of the Clinical Perspective— the Terminology of Mental Retardation

The impact of the medical model is striking when we analyze the terminology used by clinicians in communicating about mental retardation. Their vocabulary reveals how they are conceptualizing the issues involved. Consequently, the similarity between the terminology used in discussing diseases and that used in discussing mental retardation is significant.

A review of mental retardation terminology based on a content analysis of the literature on retardation clearly demonstrates the influence of medical conceptualizations on the field (Davitz, Davitz, and Lorge 1964). We can infer from the widespread use of such concepts as etiology, symptom, syndrome, diagnosis, prognosis, and prevalence that persons using these terms are perceiving mental retardation as an individual disorder somewhat akin to the disease processes to which these terms are usually applied. Analysis of the meaning of each of these concepts reveals the perspective being adopted by persons using these terms.

Etiology is the examination of a supposed causal link. *Syndrome, symptom,* and *diagnosis* are all closely related medical terms, which also imply specific, identifiable dysfunctions in the individual. The word *symptom* refers to signs indicating the presence of a disease, while a *syndrome* is a group of symptoms which occur together and characterize a disease. When these terms are used to describe mental retardation, there is the clear assumption that mental retardation involves perceptible changes in the functioning of the individual that will be manifested through a series of indicators, i.e., symptoms. When these symptoms are organized into patterns, they can be recognized as specific syndromes indicating the presence of a particular subvariety of retardation. Diagnosis is the determination of the existence or nonexistence of mental retardation and involves the task of recognizing the presence or absence of symptoms characteristic of various varieties of mental retardation. The act of searching for symptoms in order to make a diagnosis implies the belief that mental retardation exists in the individual as a verifiable condition that can be assessed.

The term *prognosis* is also borrowed from the medical vocabulary, where it is commonly used to designate a forecast made about the probable course which a disease will take. The notion of making a prognosis for mental retardation implies that it is a pathological process, a condition that may be "curable" or "incurable," "remedial" or "irremedial."

Considerable debate has centered around the issue of whether mental retardation that is "curable" is "really" mental retardation. Doll took the view that the "criteria of incurability is essential to the definition of the term" (Doll, 1941). Tredgold argues that it seems unwise to "accept the permanence of a mental defect as a necessary criterion in its diagnosis. It would surely be illogical to jettison a diagnosis made on clinical grounds for the sole reason that a cure has been found" (Tredgold, 1956). The history of this debate will be reviewed in a later section. At this point, resolution of the issue of whether mental retardation is curable or incurable is irrelevant to our discussion. What is significant are the terms in which the argument is couched. Both sides assume that mental retardation is a condition about which a prognosis can be made in the same sense that one can make a prognosis about the probable course of a disease. Doll is simply saying that, if a condition carries a prognosis of curability, it should not be called mental retardation in the first place.

The term *pseudofeebleminded,* widely used in the field of mental retardation, also reveals the contours of the clinical perspective. Synonyms frequently used for this concept are "pseudosymptomatic retar-dation," "apparent feeblemindedness," and "impermanent mental defective." The prefix "pseudo" denotes a false or counterfeit relationship that feigns or bears a deceptive resemblance to the "real" object. If there can be "pseudofeeblemindedness," then the clear implication is that the opposite must exist, "real feeblemindedness." Just as a clinician may misdiagnose a case of rheumatic fever or polio, so a clinician may misdiagnose a case of mental retardation. There is extensive literature on the manner in which inadequate examiners, a poorly selected test battery, language barriers, emotional disturbance, physical handicaps, educational and social neglect, and other variables may complicate the diagnostic process and produce a misdiagnosis.

We must conclude from the terminology commonly used by practitioners in the field of mental retardation that their frame of reference has been greatly influenced by disease orientations and medical concepts. Etiological, diagnostic, and prognostic concepts are applied to all levels and all forms of mental retardation.

In our study of mental retardation in Riverside, the field survey was conceptualized and conducted from the clinical perspective and is a clinical epidemiology in the traditional sense.

Chapter 2

THE SOCIAL SYSTEM PERSPECTIVE

An estimated three per cent of the population (or 5.4 million children and adults in the United States) are afflicted with mental retardation, some severely, most only mildly. Assuming this rate of prevalence, an estimated 126,000 babies born each year will be regarded as mentally retarded at some time in their lives.

Mental retardation ranks as a major national health, social, and economic problem:

It afflicts twice as many individuals as blindness, polio, cerebral palsy, and rheumatic heart disease, combined. . . .

About 400,000 of the persons affected are so retarded that they require constant care or supervision, or are severely limited in their ability to care for themselves and to engage in productive work; the remaining five million are individuals with mild disabilities.

Report of the President's Panel on Mental Retardation, 1962

Who are the mentally retarded—the estimated 5.5 million persons who collectively rank as a "major national health, social, and economic problem"? What is the nature of their "affliction"? Why are they "regarded as mentally retarded"?

According to the medical, clinical perspective described in chapter 1, the answers to these questions can be found by conducting a clinical epidemiology. The investigator designs a study in the standard tradition of medical epidemiologies, and defines the symptoms of the disorder and how they will be diagnosed. He then sets about to "study the distribution of the disease in space and time within a population and the factors that influence this distribution" (Lilienfeld, 1957).

It became apparent very early in our research enterprise that the medical model for conceptualizing mental retardation in the community was inadequate. Although a medical-pathological model might suffice for research conducted primarily in a hospital setting and focused mainly on biologically damaged persons, the complexity and variety of the situation in the larger society could not be comprehended within the narrow assumptions of this perspective. Consequently, the conceptual map for the study was redrawn in broader terms in which the clinical perspective is included as the single most socially significant framework for thinking about mental retardation. However, that perspective is placed within a broader social system context. Delineating this broader perspective became the major conceptual task of the research project.

The social system perspective on mental retardation stems mainly from the sociological tradition and the study of deviant behavior. To understand this perspective, it is essential that the reader be familiar with certain basic sociological concepts: status, role, role expectations or norms, sanctions, and socialization.

Social Statuses and Social Roles

The sociologist visualizes the social structure as a network of interlocking social systems. Each of these social systems is composed of social statuses, social roles, and social norms.

Social statuses are the positions in a social system. In structured, formal systems, the positions have names or titles, and occupants are known by the title of the position they hold in that system. For example, in a school system there are the positions of principal, school secretary, teacher, kindergarten student, student in a special education class, custodian, and so forth. In a family, the primary positions are those of mother, father, son, and daughter. Each status exists as an entity regardless of its occupant at any given time. Statuses in less formal social systems may not have titles, but they can still be identified and studied. A social role is the behavior of status occupants, the part each plays in a group. For example, the teacher's role is to direct instruction, make assignments, read and grade papers, and so forth.

Finally, statuses and roles are usually classified into those which are "ascribed" and those which are "achieved." Ascribed statuses are those which an individual holds by virtue of attributes that are not acquired and cannot be modified. Among the major ascribed statuses are those based on sex, age, and ethnic group. Achieved statuses are those to which a person is assigned because of his own behavior and the manner in which his performance is evaluated by the group. Achieved statuses are acquired by virtue of individual competence or incompetence as judged by others in the system. Frequently, it is difficult to determine, for any particular status, whether it is primarily ascribed or achieved. However, the differentiation is still analytically useful.

Who Is "Normal"?

Persons participating in a social system share common expectations as to how the occupants of various statuses in the system ought to play their roles. The teacher has certain expectations about how a student ought to play his role, and the student, in turn, has certain expectations about the way in which a teacher ought to behave. The role expectations for each status involve certain obligations and privileges which the occupant of the status has in relation to other persons in the system. These shared expectations are the norms of the social system.

The term *normal* from a social system framework does not refer to an individual's statistical position in relation to his peers nor to the absence of pathological signs. Normal behavior is role performance that conforms to the norms and expectations of the social system being studied. Deviant behavior is behavior that varies sufficiently from the expectations of the group to trigger group strategies aimed at coping with the deviance. Thus, the extent of deviation is determined not only by the behavior of the individual, but also by the norms used by the definer in making his judgments.

From a social system perspective, the term *normal* is strictly descriptive and nonevaluative. It carries no implication that a particular behavior is either "good" or "bad" in any universal sense. What is "normal" depends on the norms of the particular social system in which the person is functioning at any given time.

An equally important aspect of the normative structure of a social system consists of the sanctions that are used to enforce the norms and to assure that persons perform their roles in an acceptable fashion. Positive sanctions are the rewards which other members of the system give to those who perform their roles satisfactorily. These rewards may be tangible—such as money or prizes—or they may be symbolic, such as praise from other system members, prestige in the group, or an A on a report card. Among the most prized symbolic rewards are assignment to special achieved statuses that are valued by the group. For example, being chosen chairman of the committee, valedictorian of the class, or captain of the team are positive sanctions, which serve as motivations to exemplary role performance.

Social systems also use negative sanctions to punish those whose role performance is judged inadequate. Negative sanctions may take the form of physical punishment such as a spanking, imprisonment, or restriction of activity, or they, too, may be primarily symbolic. Ridicule, deprivation of privileges, and low marks on one's report card are some examples of symbolic negative sanctions. Just as social systems have valued statuses, which may be achieved by outstanding performers, they also have devalued statuses, which may be achieved by those who fail to meet role expectations. In school, the role failures may find themselves assigned to the slow reading group, the group of children who have failed a grade, the continuation school, or, in extreme cases, the class for the mentally retarded. The most drastic negative sanction that any social system has at its disposal is the removal of the offending person from his status in the system. Stripped of his status and deprived of his role, he has had the ultimate sanction of the social system used against him.

There are five aspects of the normative structures of different social systems that are relevant to the study of the labeling of the mentally retarded: the content of their norms; the focus of their norms; the level of their norms; the extent to which the norms have been formalized and codified; and the extent to which the system tolerates deviance from normative behavior.

Critical Aspects of Normative Structures

The Content of the Norms

Different social systems frequently value different types of behavior. What is "normal" behavior, i.e., behavior that fulfills system norms, in one social system may be regarded as abnormal in another. Different social systems, because of their different functions in society, may be concerned with different types of behavior. We can indirectly assess the content of the norms of a social system by studying the kinds of information that are collected by that organization about persons labeled as mentally retarded. Behavior that one system regards as significant when labeling a person as mentally retarded may be completely disregarded in another. For example, persons operating from the medical-pathological model of normal may see no necessity for an IQ test in diagnosing cases with clear evidence of biological anomalies. The statistical norm is, for them, irrelevant in such cases. Conversely, persons operating from the statistical model of normal may see no need for the medical-pathological model in reaching a diagnosis of mental retardation if the statistical norm is failed. Other systems may use both models.

The Focus of the Norms

Even systems that have similar normative content may focus on different aspects of behavior in evaluating role performance. For example, probation officers focus on behavior that violates the legal code and have only a secondary interest in intellectual achievement. On the other hand, the schools focus on the intellectual dimension and may have only a peripheral interest in the legal norms. Medical persons focus mainly on biological manifestations, and we would expect that persons identified as retardates by the County Health Department or pediatricians will show a higher rate of physical disability than those diagnosed by nonmedical agencies. Families, friendship groups, and neighborhood social systems have normative expectations that de-emphasize academic performance and are more likely to focus on interpersonal skills. When we examine the norms of social systems distant from the official agencies of society, we would expect to find sizable differences from the values of middle-class institutions.

Level of Expectation

Just as social system norms may vary in content and focus, they may also vary in the quality or level of performance expected of system members. Although the same type of behavior may be valued and rewarded in both systems, it may take a higher level of performance to be rewarded in one system than in another. For example, the norms of the public schools in Riverside permitted a child with an intelligence test score of 79 or below to be placed in a special education class for the mentally retarded. However, persons are not eligible for placement in a California Department of Mental Hygiene Hospital for the retarded unless they have an intelligence test score of 69 or below. Although both systems focus on the intellectual dimension, they have different levels of expectation. The public school norms were more stringent.

Even within a school system there are differentials. A child attending an elementary school in an upper-middle-class neighborhood must perform at a higher level academically to meet the system expectations of his school than a child attending a school located in a neighborhood of lower socioeconomic status. For example, there were 35 children with IQs below 85 in five Catholic parochial schools serving middle-class populations, and 83% of them were nominated as slow learners by their teachers. On the other hand, there were 18 children with IQs below 85 in the Catholic school serving the segregated, minority community, but only 44% were nominated by their teachers as slow learners (McCartin et al., 1966).

Formalization of the Norms

The norms of various systems also differ in the extent to which they are formalized and codified. Some social systems have a very rudimentary and informal patterning of positions and roles. Role expectations are not clearly defined nor sanctions for deviance clearly delineated. The pattern of interrelationships is highly flexible, and mutual expectations are implicit and amorphous rather than explicit and definitive. Examples of such social systems are neighborhoods, friendship groups, and families. Conversely, other social systems have positions that are clearly defined and titled; have role expectations that are formally stated and may even be written into rules or bylaws; have mutual obligations and responsibilities precisely outlined; have specified norms for evaluating successful role performance; and clearly detail the positive and negative sanctions that will be forthcoming for various levels of performance. Large bureaucracies, such as the public school system, illustrate this type of formalized and codified social system.

Tolerance of Deviation from the Norms

Finally, social systems vary in the extent to which they tolerate deviation from their norms. Although all systems permit status occupants some latitude in role performance, some systems are much more rigid than others. Each system has "ideal" norms, which specify the optimum role performance for various statuses. Few systems actually demand optimal performance from their members. Instead, there is a tolerance limit, a shadow area around the norm, within which behavior is regarded as less than ideal but still tolerable.

We can visualize each norm as having a series of boundaries that define the extent to which a particular behavior deviates from the ideal. These boundaries, which we will call the normative penumbra, range from ideal through permissible, to tolerable and intolerable. An analysis of deviance in a particular social system involves discovering the types of role behavior that are defined as optimal, permissible, tolerable, and intolerable in that system for various statuses. Direct inquiries of system members are likely to reveal the ideal norms. Observation of the types of behavior that precipitate positive and negative sanctions of varying degrees of severity is more likely to reveal the normative system as it actually operates.

Strategies in Coping with Deviance

When a participant's behavior pushes the limits of the normative penumbra, his deviant behavior threatens the integrity of the system and tends to undermine its normative structure. There are at least three strategies which a social system may use in coping with such a deviant member.

(1) Other members of the system may attempt to "normalize" the deviant's behavior by applying positive or negative sanctions or by intensifying the socialization process through education, psychotherapy, or rehabilitation.

(2) If normalization fails, as it frequently does in working with biologically damaged individuals, the other persons in the system may assign the deviant member to a devalued status within the system, a status reserved for those who cannot or will not conform to system norms. If no such status exists, as in the case of the family with a mental retardate, the social system may develop a new status especially for the deviant member. This special status has role expectations tailored to the deviant member and norms that apply only to him and others like him in the system. This strategy of creating a new status for the deviant requires changing both the normative structure and the status structure of the system in order to provide a role in which the deviant member can function.

(3) Finally, the system may use the strategy of "estrangement" and deprive the deviant of his status in the system. This strategy defines the deviant as a "stranger," an outsider who is beyond the norms of the group. This is what happens when the school expels a student or a family places a child in a foster home or institution.

A social system accomplishes two objectives when it employs one of these strategies in coping with the deviant behavior of one of its members. These responses reinforce the normative structure by demonstrating to other participants in the system the negative consequences of deviation. In addition, such action sets the limits of the normative penumbra, i.e., the boundaries between optimal, permissible, tolerable, and intolerable behavior. Other participants in the system, noting the kind and amount of deviation tolerated before sanctions are invoked, learn the location of the normative boundaries. Thus, coping strategies both reinforce the norms of the system and define its normative boundaries.

We turn now to a discussion of how these basic sociological concepts will be used to understand and interpret mental retardation in an American community.

A Social System Definition of Mental Retardation

From a social system perspective, "mental retardate" is an achieved social status and mental retardation is the role associated with that status.[1] A mental retardate is one who occupies the status of mental retardate and plays the role of the mental retardate in one or more of the social systems in which he participates. To clarify this point, let us consider the public school system. In addition to such statuses as teacher, principal, and custodian, the school system also has statuses for children: the status of student in a regular class; the status of accelerated student; the status of retained student; the status of educable mental retardate; the status of trainable mental retardate; and so forth. Children achieve these statuses just as adults achieve the status of teacher, principal, or custodian. We can analyze the process by which a child achieves the status of mental retardate just as surely as we can analyze the process by which a person achieves the status of teacher or principal.

From a social system perspective, the term mental retardate does not

[1] Some of the early writers recognized that normative expectations vary from one group to another, and that some of the behavior diagnosed as evidence of mental retardation may be culturally determined. As early as 1933, E. O. Lewis (1933) differentiated between "pathological" and "subcultural" types of retardation, stating that pathological retardation results from organic defect while subcultural retardation represents the lower end of the normal distribution. He noted that "as civilization becomes more complex, more persons will be deficient. . . . We see that the subcultural variety of mental defect is an inevitable concomitant of progress." Here, clearly, is the recognition that as the norms of society become more intellectually demanding, society, in a sense, creates retardates because there will be more persons who cannot meet the more exacting standards.

In 1947, T. L. McCulloch came closer than any of the earlier thinkers to the perspective presented in this volume. He noted that different communities have different tolerance thresholds for social deviance, hence the validity of objective measures fluctuates as these thresholds vary from one locus and time to another. In his opinion, social incompetence is frequently correctable and, hence, mental deficiency may be curable (McCulloch, 1947). He contended that mental deficiency is essentially an "administrative" concept relating to the need to sort and assign persons to various programs. "The tolerance line for incompetence may be extremely variable, so that it may not be practicable to establish rigid lines of demarcation for defectives as a group. The concept is accordingly essentially administrative in nature, and, as such, is exceedingly useful for purposes of sorting a certain group of individuals, and of providing most wisely for their welfare. Recognition of the administrative nature of the concept is not an innovation. Burt advanced essentially the same notion in his analysis of deficiency in the public schools of London some decades ago" (p. 134).

Ann M. Clarke hints at a relativistic view of mental retardation when she discusses theoretical issues in the classification of mental deficiency. "To the extent that mental retardation is a social concept, with fluctuating thresholds of community tolerance,

describe individual pathology but rather refers to the label applied to a person because he occupies the position of mental retardate in some social system. In this volume we have used the term "labeled retardate" to designate persons who are retarded from a social system perspective. This differentiates them from "clinical retardates," persons who are retarded from the clinical perspective because they fail particular clinical measures. Labeled retardation can then be described as a process —the process of playing the role of mental retardate and meeting the role expectations which others in the system have for those who occupy the status of mental retardate. In this context, it is possible to describe the status of mental retardate and the role behavior expected of a person occupying that status without reference to the particular individuals who are playing that role. If a person does not occupy the status of mental retardate, is not playing the role of mental retardate in any social system, and is not regarded as mentally retarded by any of the significant others in his social world, then he is not mentally retarded, irrespective of the level of his IQ, the adequacy of his adaptive behavior,

---

classification is bound to be somewhat arbitrary and no system is likely to be either comprehensive or permanent" (Clarke and Clarke, 1958, p. 64). However, this notion is not developed any further and a clinical frame of reference is used throughout the rest of her discourse.

Among the clinicians, it is Kanner who has most clearly recognized the relativity of deviance to the role expectations of the social system in which the person is functioning. "The one type [of mental retardation] consists of individuals so markedly deficient in their cognitive, emotional, and constructively conative potentialities that they would stand out as defectives in any existing culture. . . . They would be equally helpless and ill-adapted in a society of savants and in a society of savages. They are not only deficient intellectually but deficient in every sphere of mentation.

"The other type is made up of individuals whose limitations are definitely related to the standards of the particular culture which surrounds them. In less complex, less intellectually centered societies, they would have no trouble in attaining and retaining equality of realizable ambitions. Some might even be capable of gaining superiority by virtue of assets other than those measured by the intelligence tests. . . . They would make successful peasants, hunters, fishermen, tribal dancers. They can, in our own society, achieve success as farm hands, factory workers, miners, waitresses, charwomen. But in our midst their shortcomings, which would remain unrecognized and therefore nonexistent in the awareness of a more primitive cultural body, appear as soon as scholastic curricula demand competition in spelling, history, geography, long division, and other preparations deemed essential for the tasks of feeding chickens, collecting garbage, and wrapping bundles in a department store. . . . It is preferable to speak of such people as intellectually inadequate rather than mentally deficient (Kanner, 1957, p. 71).

Sarason and Gladwin assume a somewhat culturally relativist position when they suggest the importance of differentiating between "mental deficiency" and "mental retardation." They would limit the latter term to persons who have no central nervous system pathology for, as they comment, "The frequent practice of labeling

or the extent of his organic impairment. From a social system perspective, a low score on an intelligence test is not a symptom of pathology but rather a behavioral characteristic, which is likely to increase the probability that a person will be assigned to the status of mental retardate in some American social systems.

If mental retardation describes an individual's role in a particular social system, then it is useful to study the personal characteristics of those who play the role of mental retardate in various social systems. Such a study will reveal the norms of each system and the process by which the system assigns persons having differing characteristics to the various statuses available in that system. The primary focus in a social system epidemiology is on the process by which a person achieves the status of mental retardate, the characteristics of persons who occupy the status of mental retardate in various social systems as compared with persons who do not hold that status, and the nature of the norms that define the person as retarded.

Within this framework, mental retardation is social system specific

---

these individuals 'subcultural' reflects that fact that their functioning reflects cultural rather than constitutional variables" (Masland, Sarason, and Gladwin, 1958, p. 152).

However, it is the writing and thinking of Lewis A. Dexter and Stewart E. Perry that most closely approximates the social system perspective as presented here. Dexter contends that "stupidity, in fact, is one of the commonest social valuations," and that fear of appearing stupid is, next to fear of sexual impotence, the most widespread anxiety in American society. He characterizes American society as "intelligence mad," using worry over intellectual failure as the chief goad to achievement. In the past, persons need not be embarrassed if they could not read, write, and cipher. But today, the insistence upon compulsory public education of a highly intellectual and abstract nature for everyone in American society has resulted in such an emphasis on academic brightness that individuals have no "cultural alternative," in Linton's sense, to acquiring skills in reading, writing, and arithmetic or being held in contempt by their peers. He holds that, just as the social institution of the clan "structured, targeted, and re-enforced" the blood feud, the social institution of public education has been the social mechanism for structuring contemptuous attitudes toward stupidity (Dexter, 1964, p. 13).

In an analysis of research problems in mental subnormality, Dexter suggests the basic premise of the social system perspective, "Mental retardation may, in large measure, *be* a social role, acquired as a result of experience, by high-grade retardates, who have been assigned certain statuses as a result of manifest psychobiological characteristics. And the major characteristics of the role may have as little necessary relationship to the psychobiological base as, for example, the Victorian conception of 'Woman' had to the actual differences between the male and the female of *Homo Sapiens*" (Dexter, 1960, p. 838).

Stewart E. Perry also makes a break with the traditional view of mental retardation and predicts that "mental deficiency will be viewed as a situational complex of many processes, of which the intellectual ones are only a very small part—and sometimes a

and can only be comprehended within the boundaries of a particular social system. Mental retardation cannot be conceptualized as an abstract category transcending social systems, for it is tied to a specific status and role in a specific social system. In this context, prevalence rates, in the traditional, epidemiological sense, are meaningless.

The role of retardate in a particular social system may be either active or latent. An active status is one that is currently filled by an incumbent or is structurally defined in the system, although not currently occupied. Vacant statuses in social systems, such as unfilled places in mental retardation classes in the public schools, tend to be filled relatively quickly by new recruits. The formal existence of an empty status seems to generate activity to recruit and assign someone to the vacancy.

A latent social status is one that is not structurally specified in the organization of the system but exists as a social category that can be activated and developed into a status if the need arises. For example, mental retardate is not a social status that is part of the usual complement of statuses in the American family. However, if an individual appears in the family social system who is unable to meet the role expectations of the regular statuses in the system, the family may develop a mental retardate status for him. It is a social category that exists in

---

rather unimportant part. Instead of primarily organic etiologies as the focus of interest, workers in this field will try to abstract many other different kinds of processes from the mental defective complex as being important etiologically" (Perry, 1965, p. 113).

He proposes that interpersonal processes may be a fruitful area of study for etiological factors in the so-called cultural-familial type of mental retardation and that viewing mental retardation as a defense mechanism might also provide a viable hypothesis. "Subnormal intellectual functioning can grow out of the experiences and attitudes with which a child is met in his very early life. . . . It is possible to develop a hypothesis of mental deficiency that would characterize it as something like a defense mechanism—an adaptive response—of an interpersonal nature. . . . Children can be brought up to be mentally retarded, just as they can be brought up to be schizophrenic or manic-depressive. . . . Yet, caught early enough, this sort of induced, trained mental incapacity can be reversed, as Skeels demonstrated experimentally. Deprivation leading to mental dullness is, then, not only understandable as an interpersonal phenomenon, but also as a matter of the social and cultural conditions of life for whole groups of people" (Perry, 1965, p. 115–116).

The most explicit statement of the perspective taken in this volume, however, was developed in the field of mental illness rather than mental retardation. Thomas J. Scheff (1966) develops the theoretical position that mental illness is essentially a learned social role and elucidates a social system model for mental illness. His work is a logical, theoretical extension of the social systems models of deviance evolved in the writings of Becker (1963; 1964), Kitsuse (1964), Erikson (1964), and Cicourel (1964). The works of all of these men are intellectual antecedents to the social system perspective presented in this volume.

American society and can be activated by the family as a role, if necessary.[2]

Thus, achieving the status of mental retardate, e.g., becoming a labeled retardate, is a social process. Although an individual's biological characteristics may increase the probability that he will be assigned the status of mental retardate, the two are not perfectly correlated. There are many alternative statuses to which persons with comparable biological equipment may be assigned. Differential diagnosis is the process of social decision-making which determines whether a particular person is assigned the status of educationally handicapped, cerebral palsied, autistic, mentally retarded, or some other social category. Mental retardation is not a characteristic of the individual, nor a meaning inherent in his behavior, but a socially determined status, which he may occupy in some social systems and not in others, depending on their norms. It follows that a person may be mentally retarded in one system and not mentally retarded in another. He may change his role by changing his social group.

The life space of the individual is a vast network of interlocking social systems through which the person moves during the course of his lifetime. Those systems which exist close to one another in the social structure, because of overlapping memberships and frequent communi-

[2] There are social systems, however, that do not have either active or latent mental retardate statuses. In such systems, it is not possible for anyone to hold the status or play the role of mental retardate, because mental retardation as a viable social category does not exist. It is important that we not be misunderstood at this point. A society with a population of any size will probably contain some persons whose behavior and/or appearance would make them eligible for the status of mental retardate if they participated in the social systems of modern America. However, if the status of mental retardate does not exist in the social systems in which they participate, they cannot be assigned to that status nor can they play the role of retardate.

The relativity of the existence of mental retardation as a social status is best seen in cross-cultural comparisons. Other societies have developed other kinds of social statuses for persons who, in American social systems, might play the role of retardate. In some societies, such persons are treated with awe, fear, and respect, and may play roles that involve control of magical and supernatural powers. Their seizures, lapses from consciousness, unusual physical appearance, or incomprehensible behavior may fulfill the role expectations which other members of the system have for persons holding a magical status.

Other social systems may place such persons in the status of buffoon, one who is ridiculed and regarded as ludicrous. Such a person is expected to violate the rules of decorum and is permitted certain types of behavior forbidden to other members of the system, because his behavior is not viewed as involving evil intent. Consequently, he is regarded with amusement rather than punished (Klapp, 1949). Still other social systems have no status of any kind for persons who would be classified as mental retardates in American society. Some such systems practice infanticide.

cation, evolve similar standards for what is "normal" role performance. Most individuals are born and live out their lives in a relatively limited segment of this social network and tend to contact social systems that share a common normative consensus. When an individual's contacts are thus restricted to a circumscribed segment of the structure, this gives stability to the evaluations that are made of his behavior and the roles that he plays in various systems.

However, when the person's life career takes him into segments of the social structure that are located at a distance from his point of origin, as when a minority child enters the public school, he may be judged by new and different norms. Behavior that was acceptable in his primary social systems may now be judged as evidence of "mental retardation."

An individual's participation in various social systems in the community also changes in the course of his lifetime. Persons age in and out of various social systems. In so doing, they may age in and out of deviant statuses. For example, many persons are labeled as mentally retarded only by the public schools. Many are not regarded as mentally retarded until they age into the school system and many are no longer regarded as retarded when they leave the purview of the schools.

System Factors in Prevalence

Even if a social system has a status designated mental retardate, we would hypothesize that the characteristics and numbers of persons assigned to the status of mental retardate will vary with the five characteristics of the normative structure discussed earlier in this chapter: content, focus, level, formalization, and tolerance for deviance. The kinds of behavior which the social system regards as indicative of mental retardation will influence the kinds of persons who occupy the status. The focus of the norms will specify which kinds of deviance will receive the most attention. The level of the norms will determine the percentage of persons likely to occupy the status of retardate in the system. The formalization of the norms will influence the thoroughness with which persons are scrutinized and hence the rate of identification for mental retardation. Finally, the less tolerance for deviance, the more persons who are likely to be placed in deviant statuses.

Levels of Retardation from a Social System Perspective

In American society, an individual constantly plays roles in various social systems—his family, his school, his work group, his neighborhood, his church, his friendship groups, and so forth. His performance is constantly being evaluated by members of those social systems. If he plays the role of mental retardate in every social system in which he participates, he is "totally" retarded. He always holds the status of mental retardate and is always playing the role of a retardate. If he never plays the role of mental retardate in any system, then he is not retarded, i.e., he is "normal." If he plays the role of a retardate in some of the social systems in which he participates and not in others, then he is retarded part of the time and normal part of the time, depending on the social system in which he is participating. In other words, he is "situationally retarded." Thus, individuals can be ranged along a continuum from the "normals," who never play the role of a mental retardate, through the "situationally" retarded, who play the role intermittently depending on the social system in which they are participating, to the "totally" retarded, who play the role of retardate in all the social systems in which they participate.

Socialization to the Role of Retardate

Just as he learns the expected role behaviors for other statuses, an individual is socialized to play the role of mental retardate once he has been placed in that status by the social system. As his fellows reward and reinforce role behaviors that conform to expectations and punish role behaviors that deviate from expectation, he internalizes the role that he plays. If he is socialized to meet the role expectations for the status of mental retardate, he will internalize the requisite pattern of behaviors. He will come to perceive himself as a retardate and incorporate the status of mental retardate as part of his concept of self.

Klapp (1949) has described the process by which social systems assign persons the status of the fool and then socialize them to perform the appropriate role. He has called this the "fool-making" process. There are many similarities between the process he describes and socialization to the role of a mental retardate.

When a person has been assigned the status of retardate by a professional diagnostician and has been systematically socialized to the role, it is difficult for him to escape the status even in thinking about himself. The struggle of ex-patients from an institution for the mentally retarded to escape the status of the mental subnormal is movingly described by Edgerton (1967).

The Legitimate Labelers

Who assigns persons to the status of mental retardate? Informal social groups have no procedure for identifying mental retardates, and the definition is likely to emerge gradually as members of the group become aware that one of their number is unable to meet role expectations. In large, structured organizations, the evaluation process is formalized. The social system does not rely entirely on emergent definitions.

In American society, a corps of professional diagnosticians has developed who are charged, officially, with the task of identifying persons who are violating societal norms. The professional diagnosticians, i.e., the legitimate labelers, base their evaluation procedures on the assumptions of the clinical perspective. As their clinical definitions have been codified into law and have been operationalized through intelligence testing, there has been an increasing professionalization of the diagnostic function. With his diagnostic instruments, the professional diagnostician determines who is deviant and the nature and the amount of that deviance. He determines which persons will be assigned to deviant statuses and the status to which each will be assigned. Consequently, the legitimate labeler plays a central role in defending the integrity of the normative structure of formal organizations by allocating symbolic rewards and punishments in the form of special statuses.

In addition to labeling deviants, professional diagnosticians frequently have the task of deciding upon the strategy which a system will use in coping with deviance. The strategy may be to prevent deviance before it occurs by restricting membership in the group to those who are able and willing to conform to its norms. In this role, professional diagnosticians act as screening agents who are responsible for preventing potential mental retardates from gaining entreé to certain educational, occupational, and other statuses.

Once a person becomes a member of a formal organization, the professional diagnostician is likely to be involved in determining the strategy to be used if his behavior deviates beyond the tolerance limits of the norms. He helps to decide whether the strategy should be normalization, placement in a deviant status, or elimination from the system. Refinement of diagnostic instruments and elaboration of the diagnostic nomenclature now provide a more precise basis for assigning persons who are labeled as "mental retardates" to the many different substatuses available. The legitimate labeler figures significantly in deciding which of these many substatuses the person will occupy. He may assign the "retardate" to the status of EMR (educable mental retardate) or TMR (trainable mental retardate). He may qualify the person to occupy the status of mental retardate in the community or in an institution. Within the institution, the professional diagnostician is important in deciding who may have campus privileges, who may attend the school, who participates in the activities at the rehabilitation center, who is treated as a custodial patient, and so forth.

Professional diagnosticians are organized into a social system that operates from the clinical perspective and has its own configuration of statuses, roles, and norms. Participants are primarily persons trained in medicine or psychology. Because professional diagnosticians are drawn from two disciplines which provide distinctly different types of training and orientation, each group brings its own set of norms and procedures and its own system of classification to their common task. Persons playing medical roles think in terms of the pathological model for "normal," use medical diagnostic instruments, and assign persons to medical classifications, i.e., Down's syndrome, Klinefelter's syndrome, Huntington's Chorea, and so forth. Persons playing psychological roles apply the statistical model for "normal," use psychological diagnostic instruments, and assign cases to psychological classifications, i.e., profoundly retarded, severely retarded, moderately retarded, and so forth.

Entrance to the clinical social system has become highly formalized. Legal restrictions assure that only persons who have been socialized to the clinical perspective and have internalized the norms of the clinical system become legitimate labelers because they are the only ones who understand the diagnostic tools, the intricacies of the nomenclature, and the norms of the system. It is the legally recognized, professional diagnostician who is the culture bearer for the clinical perspective. Because this group has the legal authority to place persons in the status of mental retardate, it is the single most important social system in the sociological study of mental retardation. Clinical norms pervade most of the literature and research on mental retardation and have diffused to other social systems. Other social systems borrow the labels applied by professional diagnosticians. Persons in other systems hesitate to define an individual as retarded until their judgment has been confirmed by the professional diagnostician. Only then are they assured that the individual is "really" retarded. In turn, professional diagnosticians accept responsibility for educating nonclinicians to view the world from the clinical perspective.

Summary

The essential differences between the clinical and social system perspectives are summarized in the following list:

Social System Perspective	*Clinical Perspective*
(1) Mental retardation is an achieved status in a social system and the role played by persons holding that status.	(1) Mental retardation is individual pathology that can be diagnosed by using the medical-pathological and/or statistical models of "normal."
(2) Mental retardation is specific to the social system. A person may be retarded at one time during the day or at one period during his lifetime and not be retarded at another time, depending on whether he is labeled by the system in which he is participating.	(2) Mental retardation is an individual characteristic that transcends cultures and sociocultural groupings. A person either "is" or "is not" mentally retarded. However, there are varying types and degrees of retardation, and, admittedly, borderline cases are hard to identify.
(3) A person is "normal" if he meets the expectations of the norms of the social system in which he is operating. Prevalence rates, in the traditional epidemiological sense, are meaningless. Sociocultural factors are intimately involved in the labeling process, i.e., the clinical diagnosis.	(3) Mental retardation is a condition in the individual that exists regardless of whether it is diagnosed. If a person has the symptoms of mental retardation, he is mentally retarded. Prevalence and incidence rates can be calculated by determining the number of persons with symptoms. Sociocultural factors need not be taken into account in making a clinical diagnosis.
(4) The prevalence rate for mental retardation will be relative to the content, focus, level, formalization, and tolerance limits of the norms of a particular social system, and the extent to which the status of "mental retardate" is differentiated within the structure.	(4) The "real" prevalence rate for mental retardation in any social system can be determined without regard for the norms of a particular social system, given adequate research design and instruments. Characteristics of the social structure may facilitate or impede the research process but will not affect in any way "true" prevalence or incidence.
(5) Each social system has a normative structure that functions to define the reciprocal privileges and obligations of persons occupying various	(5) Two models for normal are used interchangeably. Medical persons prefer the pathological model and search for biological symptoms. Psy-

roles in that system. Behavior that conforms to these norms is "normal," regardless of how it may be viewed by outsiders from other social systems with different norms.

chologists and educators prefer the statistical model and define "normal" as the average performance of a population. Intellectual subnormality can be discovered by the trained diagnostician. Because he has more sensitive instruments at his disposal, he may detect abnormalities not apparent to lay persons. Thus, it is his task to educate those who do not recognize the symptoms of mental retardation so they will comprehend the "real" situation.

(6) Intelligence tests and clinical instruments are codifications of the middle-class behavioral norms of the American core culture. Except for physical, motor, and perceptual disabilities so gross as to be labeled abnormal in any human society, it is not possible to conceptualize intelligence as existing apart from the sociocultural matrix which creates that intelligence. Problems with present attempts to measure innate ability are conceptual rather than technical.

(6) Present intelligence tests and clinical measures have certain well-documented deficiencies that need to be overcome. With further technical refinements, it should be possible to eventually develop valid, reliable instruments that are not influenced by cultural factors. In the meantime, we use the best instruments we have and try to take their shortcomings into account. Problems with present attempts to measure intelligence are essentially technical rather than conceptual.

Chapter 3

THE RESEARCH SETTING: RIVERSIDE, CALIFORNIA

The purpose of the research effort was to comprehend the nature and extent of mental retardation in an American community. Riverside, located fifty miles east of Los Angeles, was selected as the site for the study for several reasons. With a population of about 85,000 at the time of the fieldwork, it was large enough to yield a sufficient number of cases for statistical analysis and yet small enough to facilitate fieldwork (*U. S. Census of Population and Housing, 1960*). It is a city with its own history and identity and not merely a suburb of Los Angeles. Approximately 93% of the employed adults work either in the city or in Riverside County, and only 3% commute to Los Angeles. It is a community with a relatively long history during which a social structure containing a full range of social levels has evolved. At the top of the structure are families descended from early settlers. Their wealth stems mainly from citrus orchards and land investments. At the bottom are farm laborers and their families, who work in the citrus groves and packing houses. Its English-speaking Caucasian population includes all socioeconomic levels but is primarily middle-class. In southern California, English-speaking Caucasians are frequently called "Anglo-Americans," a designation we shall use to differentiate them from the Caucasian population of Mexican heritage. At the time of the study, 8.5% of the total population was of Mexican heritage and 4.7% of Afro-American heritage.[1]

Riverside's location, twenty-five miles from the research headquarters located at the Pacific State Hospital, was also advantageous. A community located closer to this hospital for the mentally retarded might contain an overrepresentation of families with retarded members. On the other hand, a community located at a greater distance from the hospital would have made it difficult for staff members to commute between the field office and research headquarters. Finally, the willingness of significant persons in the community to assist and cooperate

[1] The accepted nomenclature for the various ethnic groups varies from one region to another and from time to time as historic events make some designations more acceptable than others. We have decided to use the terms Anglo, Black, and Mexican-American rather than the more recently popular identification, Chicano. The traditional term is more universally understood, is less regional, and less time specific.

with the research project was important in the final decision to study Riverside.

Historical Roots of the Riverside Social Structure (1774-1885)

In 1774, Juan Bautista de Anza led an exploratory expedition into the dry, warm valley, bisected by the Santa Ana River and ringed by low mountains, which is now occupied by the city of Riverside. After Mexican independence, Don Juan Bandini, a respected member of Spanish colonial society, was granted seven leagues of land (31,080 acres) and induced several native Mexican families to settle on the border of his rancho to serve as a military buffer against stock-raiding Indians. Other grandees established ranchos by using Indian labor to raise cattle. Settlers from the United States began arriving but did not become the dominant influence until after the disastrous flood of 1862 and the drought of the following year. This catastrophic flood inundated the grape vineyards and orchards of the ranchos with sand and silt, and the drought decimated their herds, forcing them to sell their lands in parcels to the new American settlers. The flood also changed the character of the bottomland, so that, henceforth, it had to be irrigated.

The topography of the land, the historical land-grant patterns, and access to water were critical factors in establishing the ecological patterns that persist in present-day Riverside. The Santa Ana River, which now forms the northwestern boundary of the city, had a heavy spring flow from mountain snows and, together with Spring Brook, provided water for irrigation. The valley floor slopes gently upward from the river toward the mountains. It is bisected by a deep arroyo, which acted as a natural boundary between the northern and the southern portions of the valley. Within this topography, there were three types of land holdings, each of which attracted a different type of settler.

The Colony Association

After the flood, Bandini's land grant was broken up, and 6,000 acres of the section east of the Santa Ana River and north of the arroyo were sold to the Colony Association. This company was composed of thirteen stockholders led by a midwestern judge, who was respectable, financially solvent, an abolitionist, and one of the founders of the University of Minnesota. The Association surveyed a mile-square area into 2½-acre plots, which were subdivided into home sites to sell for $25 to $250 each. Land adjoining the "mile square" sold for $10 to $20 per acre with water rights. They also began building irrigation canals and advertising throughout the East and Midwest for "100 good families who can invest $1,000 each in the purchase of land." However, persons of lesser means who were "of good character," and "have not the money in hand to defray traveling expenses and pay the full price for the land at once," were also encouraged to make arrangements to pay a part of the money down and the rest in yearly installments (Brown and Boyd, 1922).

The promoters anticipated that the money from the sale of the land would pay not only for the original purchase price of the land but for surveying the lots and building the irrigation canals. The sale of water was envisioned as a profit-making venture, which would continue after all land plots had been sold.

The first settlers attracted to Riverside were from the Midwest, mainly Iowa and Illinois, and from Ontario, Canada. They formed an ethnically, economically, and culturally homogeneous, English-speaking, middle-class, Protestant community.

Almost immediate plans were made to construct a large irrigation system, to test the feasibility of various crops, to establish a school, to erect a church, to found a library, and to build midwestern-style homes. By 1878, the business center of town had all the components of a typical American village: mercantile stores, livery stable, blacksmith shop, saloons, drugstores, hotels, bakery, butcher shop, post office, and a newspaper. After the discovery of the excellent adaptation of the navel orange to the soil and climate, agricultural emphasis shifted from growing raisin grapes to planting citrus orchards.

The Proprietary Lands

Four years after the Colony Association purchased its land, a large 8,000-acre section of land south of the arroyo was purchased by two entrepreneurs, who subdivided it into ten-acre plots, each designed to face on a street. They, too, planned to use money from the sale of land to pay for the original purchase and to finance the building of a canal system. They also planned to sell water as a private profit-making venture. When the proprietors were unsuccessful in negotiating for the right to connect their canals to those of the Colony Association, they proceeded to buy a controlling interest in the Association and to unite the two settlements by bringing the entire valley into one water system.

Wealthy Easterners bought the large plots south of the arroyo, planted citrus orchards, and proceeded to build spacious homes along two of the earliest fully landscaped boulevards in the state. Although ethnically and religiously similar to the Colony settlers north of the arroyo, they were wealthier and proceeded to develop an elite society centered around a Country Club, Tennis Club, Polo Club, and an elegant theater.

The Dry Farmers

The third group of settlers in the early social structure of Riverside consisted of those Easterners who homesteaded on the government land surrounding the Colony Association and proprietory holdings. They were not as wealthy as their neighbors, and were without water rights, hence the name "dry farmers." Their battle for water rights was an early political issue, which clearly divided the more affluent from the less affluent groups in the community. An early settler described the dry farmers as follows. "The dry government lands came to be settled by a different class of men, men with families who had faith that these fine lands with a climate unsurpassed would not be always dry and barren and wind swept and treeless. Men who had little but their labor to sell brought their families and put down wells, put up windmills and the plains began to be dotted with homes" (Brown and Boyd, 1922, p. 374).

In 1885, the population of Riverside consisted almost entirely of English-speaking Protestants from the East and Midwest who were clearly divided into three socioeconomic status levels: the wealthy landowners south of the arroyo; the middle-class merchants and farmers north of the arroyo; and the dry farmers homesteading on government land surrounding the two other settlements. A few persons of Mexican descent lived in Spanish Town, but most traces of the hacienda society had disappeared. The Indians provided a sporadic labor supply for the dominant population and gradually disappeared. There were few, if any, wage laborers, for, in the words of an early settler: "There was but little call for labor when every man did his own work on the outside and his wife did hers on the inside" (Brown and Boyd, 1922).

The Citrus Era (1885-1945)

After the railroad completed its lines through Riverside and the orange growers organized cooperatives to pack, brand, and market their fruit in the East, orange production expanded from 6,000 to 40,000 railroad carloads per year. Wage laborers were needed to pick the fruit, build the packing boxes, and pack the oranges. Mexican families were encouraged to migrate to Riverside and to settle near the packing houses, which surrounded the three railroad stations—Arlington, Casa Blanca, and Mile Square. Consequently, Mexican settlements, which still persist, developed around each railroad station. At the time of the study, the Mexican community near the Mile Square station contained approximately 2,600 persons, or 39% of the Mexican population; the Casa Blanca community had about 2,200 persons, or 33% of the Mexican population; and the Arlington community had about 400, or 7% of the Mexican population. The remaining 21% were scattered throughout the community.[2]

The Mexican-Americans who originally settled near the Mile Square area were neighbors to the Anglo settlers who were homesteading on government land, were close to the business center of the community, and thus were less isolated from the Anglo community. On the other hand, Mexican-American families who settled near the Casa Blanca and Arlington stations were isolated from the business center of town and lived a rural, pastoral type of life with a greater social distance between themselves and the wealthy Anglo fruit growers who owned the large orchards. This situation created "barrio" communities insulated from many of the ideas and activities of the Anglo world.

In the period preceding World War II, Riverside grew by an average of 6,000 new inhabitants every ten years, but the social and ecological patterns of the city remained relatively stable.

The Post-World War II Era

Even before World War II, the Anglo-Saxon, Protestant character of Riverside was slightly modified by the arrival of persons from Southern and Eastern Europe, most of whom were Catholic. However, World War II produced the largest discontinuity with the past. During the war, the Riverside population increased by 12,000–29%. During the 1950s, it added an additional 38,000 persons to its population—an 80% increase. Although most of the migrants were Caucasians, about 3,000 Blacks, primarily from southeastern states, moved into the city—an increase of over 300% between 1940 and 1960. Black migrants found that public accommodations, such as restaurants and hotels, were closed to them, and they were restricted to housing in the areas of the city already occupied by Mexican-American families. Most Black families settled on the eastside, near the Mile Square area, but a few families found homes on the fringes of the Casa Blanca Mexican community. At the time of the study, there were approximately 4,000 Blacks living in Riverside. About 3,000, or 75% of the Black population, lived on the eastside, and about 750, or 19%, lived in the Casa Blanca area.

2 Special Census Data by Enumeration District from the 1960 U.S. Census.

Blacks were more highly segregated than Mexican-Americans, for only 6% of the former, compared with 21% of the latter, were living in predominantly Anglo areas.

The economic base of Riverside diversified significantly after the war. At the time of the study, a major air force base near the city employed over 6,000 servicemen and almost 1,000 civilians, many of whom lived in the city. A naval ordnance laboratory a few miles away employed approximately 1,100 full-time workers, over half of whom were professional personnel, scientists, engineers, and administrators. An air force supply depot and missile development center in a nearby town also employed some Riverside people. These military installations contributed sizable numbers of highly educated persons to the population as well as persons from diverse religious and ethnic backgrounds.

Following the war, manufacturing became more important than agriculture in the economy. The number of persons employed in manufacturing tripled in less than a decade, and the manufacturing payroll increased by 460% (*The Growth and Economic Structure of San Bernardino and Riverside Counties,* 1960). The rate of employment in manufacturing, 27.7 per 1,000 population at the close of World War II, had risen to over 47.0 per 1,000 by the time of the study. Aircraft industries and parts accounted for 40% of those employed in manufacturing. Food canning ranked second although it employed only one-third as many persons as aircraft, while stone, clay, and glass products ranked third, followed by primary metal industries, electrical equipment, and machinery manufacture.

About seven years before the study, a general campus of the University of California was established in Riverside, bringing 3,000 students and over 1,000 University employees and faculty members to the city. All of these changes brought more diversity to the community but did not significantly alter the basic middle-class, Anglo-Saxon, Protestant character of the general population.

Riverside at the Time of the Study

At the time of the study, we found the boundaries of the original land grants and settlement areas still clearly etched in the street pattern of the city. The "Mile Square" was predominantly commercial. Many of the large homes of a former generation had been subdivided into small apartments or converted to commercial use in a deteriorating area around the central core of the city. Many of the grand mansions of the once elite society south of the arroyo had been torn down or converted to commercial or civic functions. The building that once housed the fashionable Tennis Club had been remodeled and leased to a small fundamentalist church. The wealthy and influential now lived in large ranch-style or split-level homes on the high land in the eastern foothills or on the bluffs overlooking the Santa Ana River. Former government land below the arroyo was filled with tract homes,

Table 1: Modal Sociocultural Configurations for Characteristics of Households in Which Persons under 50 Years of Age Were Living

Sociocultural Characteristics	Modal Configurations			
	Riverside (N = 6,998) %	Anglos (N = 5,744) %	Mexican-Americans (N = 667) %	Blacks (N = 490) %
Occupational Structure				
% SES Index of Head 30+	69.5	78.7	20.4*	30.5*
% SES Index of Spouse 30+	72.7	81.5	21.5*	25.9*
Head Has White-collar Job	55.5	64.2	40.1*	18.9*
Spouse Has White-collar Job	71.3	80.2	21.0*	22.6*
Education				
Head Graduated from High School	74.9	82.3	20.4*	60.3*
Spouse Graduated from High School	72.7	81.4	17.6*	48.4*
Religion				
Religious Preference—Protestant	66.4	71.6	8.3*	87.3*
Geographic Origins				
Head Reared in U.S.A.	95.6	97.6	78.6*	100.0
Spouse Reared in U.S.A.	93.4	95.5	76.6*	99.0
Head Reared outside Southeast	86.4	88.8	91.2	50.4*
Spouse Reared outside Southeast	86.5	88.9	95.8	44.1*
Head Reared in Town Over 10,000	63.6	64.3	61.2	56.5
Spouse Reared in Town Over 10,000	65.9	67.0	63.4	54.9*
Housing				
Housing Value on Block $10,711 or higher	77.2	85.4	31.1*	42.6*
Own or Buying House	70.1	72.6	63.7	60.2
Housing Condition Sound	89.7	92.3	72.9*	81.0
Family Structure				
Family Consists Couple and Children	81.4	81.5	85.5	74.7
Five or Fewer Members in Family	72.4	77.5	42.4*	56.3*
Male Head of Household	91.5	91.9	92.7	84.1
Head Married, Living with Spouse	89.9	90.4	90.9	81.8
Language				
Speak English All the Time at Home	88.9	96.8	17.1*	96.5

* Group varies more than 10% from the modal configuration.

which housed the middle-class population of the city. The eastside Mexican-Black and the Casa Blanca communities were the most poverty stricken in the city.

From information collected in the household survey that we conducted as part of the clinical epidemiology we developed a profile of the modal sociocultural characteristics of the population of Riverside at the time of our fieldwork. Table 1 presents the most salient characteristics of this modal configuration for persons under fifty years of age, the age group with whom we were concerned in the epidemiological study.

The first column presents the modal configuration based on all persons in the sample of 6,998 in the field survey. The other three columns present the configuration for each of the three main ethnic groups in the population.

The Modal Configuration for the Community

Most persons lived in families in which the head of the household had a white-collar job (55.5%) and a job that was rated 30 or above on the Duncan Socioeconomic Index (69.5%) (Reiss, 1961).[3] An even higher

[3] The purpose of Duncan's socioeconomic rating was to obtain an index for each occupation in the detailed classification of the 1950 census of population. The aim was for ratings to have face validity and sufficient predictive efficiency with respect to the NORC scale to serve as an acceptable substitute for them. Median education and median income of the experienced civilian labor force in 1950 in each of the 45 occupations on the NORC scale that were comparable with the census categories were correlated with the NORC score. Correlations of .83 and .85 respectively were found. It was decided to use education and income as the measures of the socioeconomic status of each occupation. The variable to be predicted is the NORC score. These scores were calculated by a different method from the original scale used, but produced essentially the same ranking. NORC occupations were ranked according to the proportion of "excellent" and "good" ratings given the occupation.

Definitions and summary statistics for education and income: "Education" is the percentage in each occupation who are high school graduates or beyond. "Income" is the percentage in each occupation reporting incomes of $3,500 or more in 1949. An adjustment was made for the age composition of various occupations on the assumption that youthful earnings are less, and even if other things are equal, two occupations differing in their age compositions would be expected to have different average incomes. The age adjustment is slight in magnitude for all but a few occupations with highly unusual age distributions, such as newsboy. Combining the two predictors produces a multiple correlation of $R = .91$. The values of the age-adjusted education and income indicators for each occupation are substituted into the multiple regression equation, and this produces the "socioeconomic index" for that occupation. ($X_1 = .59X$ [Age-adjusted income] $+ .55X$ [Age-adjusted education] $- 6.0$). In this fashion, the index score for any occupation for which education and income data are given in the census reports can be calculated. The authors present evidence that these index weights, derived from only 45 occupations for which prestige ratings were available, have only a slightly higher error than that for the

percentage of the spouses of the heads of these households had been employed or were employed at the time of the study in white-collar jobs. Most heads of households had graduated from high school (74.9%), as had their spouses (72.7%). The middle-class Protestant (66.4%) character of the community was still identifiable at the time of the study.

The geographic origins of the population had also not changed noticeably from early years. Most of the persons in the sample were living in households in which the head had been reared in the Unitel States (95.6%), and this was also true for their wives (93.4%). Specifically, most heads of households (86.4%) and their wives (86.5%) had been reared outside the southeast and southcentral states, and over 60% had been reared in places having a population over 10,000 persons. Thus, the modal configuration was for persons in Riverside to live in households in which the head and his spouse had been reared in an urban area in the western, midwestern, or northeastern region of the United States.

Most persons in Riverside (77.2%) lived in neighborhoods in which the median value of housing was $10,711 or higher, according to the United States Census data. Most (70.1%) lived in dwellings which the family owned or was buying and which were rated in sound condition by the interviewer (89.7%). The typical family configuration of Riversiders under fifty years of age consisted of a married couple and their children (81.4%). The family had less than six family members (72.4%) and a male head of household (91.5%), who was married and living with his spouse (89.9%). Finally, most persons in Riverside lived in families that spoke English all the time (88.9%).

The Anglo Modal Configuration

With numbers as large as those in table 1, small differences can achieve statistical significance, although they may have relatively little social significance. Rather than using statistical significance as the criterion, we have used a 10% difference as one likely to be large enough to affect enough persons in an ethnic group to be of some social significance. In table 1, an asterisk was placed beside the percentage for each ethnic group that varied more than 10% from the modal configuration of the community. Anglos, who comprised 82% of the population of the city, of course, had the greatest influence on the modal configura-

original 45. Some limitations: (1) Occupational categories are broad, and specific jobs classified in the same category may vary widely in tasks, duties, education required, and income. (2) The index only indicates the prestige standing of the occupations and will not give optimal prediction of individual standing in a local community.

tion. The modal configuration and the Anglo configuration of sociocultural characteristics in Riverside did not vary more than 10% on any characteristic.

The Mexican-American Modal Configuration

The configuration of the sociocultural characteristics of the household in which the Mexican-Americans in Riverside were living differed in many respects from the modal configuration for the community. Occupational differences were striking. Approximately 80% of the occupations of the heads of households in which Mexican-Americans were living rated between 0 and 29 on the Duncan Socioeconomic Index Score, and only about 20% rated in the modal category for the community. Twenty-one percent of the Mexican-American population lived in households in which the spouse had a white-collar occupation, and only 40.1% of the heads of households had a white-collar job.

Over 80% of the heads of households and their spouses had less than a high school education. Over 90% of the Mexican-Americans were Catholic, 8.3% Protestant. The modal configuration for the Mexican-American population on these characteristics was in direct contrast to that for the community as a whole. Mexican-Americans were primarily Catholics from lower socioeconomic and educational levels in a predominantly middle-class, Anglo-Saxon, Protestant community.

Their geographic origins also differed from the modal configurations for the community. Almost 25% of the heads of households and their spouses were reared outside the United States. Housing values were distinctly nonmodal. Only 31.1% of the Mexican-American dwellings were on blocks with a median housing value of $10,711 or higher, compared with 77.2% for the community. Only 72.9% of these units were rated as sound, compared with almost 90% for the community as a whole.

The modal Mexican-American family had more than five members. Only 17.1% of the Mexican-Americans in the sample lived in households in which English was spoken all the time, compared with 88.9% for the community as a whole. Thus, the percentage of Mexican-American persons living in families with socioculturally modal characteristics deviated more than 10% from the community-wide percentage for thirteen of the twenty characteristics studied. In many cases, the differences were much larger than 10%.

The Black Modal Configuration

Black families were similar to the Mexican-American families occupationally. Only one-fifth of the heads of households and their spouses had white-collar jobs. More Blacks than Mexican-Americans lived in families in which the head of household had graduated from high school, but the percentage was still less than the mode for the community, 60.3%, compared with 74.9%. Differences were greater when the spouses of the heads of households were compared, 48.4%, compared with 72.7% for the community. More Blacks were Protestant than the community-wide percentage.

Only 50.4% of the Blacks lived in households in which the head was born outside the South, compared with 86% for the community. In addition, slightly more Black heads of households and their spouses were from a rural background than other groups in the community. Thus, adult Blacks in Riverside were more likely to have been reared in the rural South than adults from the other two ethnic groups.

Blacks came from larger families than the modal configuration for the community, 56.3% had five or fewer members, compared with 72.4% for the community. However, other differences in family structure varied less than 10% from the modal configuration. The Black modal configuration varied more than 10% from the modal configuration of the community on twelve of the twenty comparisons.

It is apparent from this analysis that both Mexican-Americans and Blacks in the city of Riverside at the time of our study were living in households that differed in many significant ways from the modal configuration for the community. These sociocultural differences and their impact on labeled mental retardation will subsequently be analyzed.

How Typical Is Riverside?

The ecological and social structures of Riverside are a unique product of its geographic location and history. For this reason, it will not be possible to generalize findings from the Riverside epidemiology directly to other communities. However, it is still useful to compare four of the ethnic and socioeconomic characteristics of Riverside with those of 58 other cities in the 1960 census with populations 70,000 to 90,000. To facilitate comparisons, the 58 cities were grouped by three geographic areas: Pacific and Mountain States; the Midwest and Northeast; and the South Atlantic and Central States.[4]

[4] The Pacific and Mountain States are California (excluding Riverside), Washington, Oregon, Alaska, Hawaii, Montana, Idaho, Wyoming, Colorado, New Mexico, Arizona, Utah, Nevada. The South Atlantic and South Central States are Arkansas, Louisiana, Oklahoma, Texas, Kentucky, Tennessee, Alabama, Mississippi, Delaware, Maryland, Virginia, West Virginia, North Carolina, South Carolina, Georgia, and Florida. The

The percentage of Mexican-Americans (Spanish surname) in Riverside's population (8.5%) was similar to the percentage in other communities in the Pacific and Mountain States but greatly exceeded the percentage in other regions of the country. The proportion of Blacks (nonwhites) in Riverside (4.7%) was comparable to the proportion found in other cities in the West, Midwest, and Northeast (6.5%), but southern cities had almost four times as many Blacks as Riverside (19.1%).

In Riverside, both the total population and the Black population had a higher median number of years of education than elsewhere, but the differential was most striking for Blacks. The median number of years of education for adult Blacks in Riverside was 11.5 years, compared with 9.0 years in other western, midwestern, and northeast communities of comparable size, and 7.5 years in South Central and South Atlantic States. On the other hand, the median years of education for Mexican-Americans was lower in Riverside than in other Pacific and Mountain States (7.6, compared with 9.2 years) but was higher than that for Mexican-Americans in southern states, mainly Texas, where the median education was only 4.7 years.

At the time of the census, the percentages of unemployed males in the labor force over fourteen years of age for all ethnic groups was lower in Riverside then elsewhere. Unemployment rates for Blacks were slightly higher in other Pacific and Mountain States and in the South but were twice as high in the Midwest and Northeastern States as in Riverside. Unemployment for Mexican-Americans was more than twice as high in other Pacific and Mountain States and in the South as in Riverside. Median family incomes for all ethnic groups were lower in Riverside than elsewhere in the West but were higher than in the Midwest, Northeast, and South.

When comparisons were made by ranking all 58 cities on these four characteristics, Riverside was near the median for percentage of "white" and percentage of "nonwhite" in the population; ranked third in median education for the total adult population; ranked fourth for median education of the nonwhite population; ranked twentieth for median income for the total population; and ranked tenth on median income for the nonwhite population. It also ranked seventh in the percentage of the total population employed in professional and tech-

---

Midwestern and Northeastern States are Minnesota, Iowa, Missouri, North Dakota, South Dakota, Nebraska, Kansas, Ohio, Indiana, Illinois, Michigan, Wisconsin, New York, New Jersey, Pennsylvania, Maine, New Hampshire, Vermont, Massachusetts, Rhode Island, and Connecticut.

nical jobs. We found that the occupational and educational level of the Riverside population placed it near the top for cities of its size on the West Coast and in the Mountain States and made it relatively comparable to cities in the Midwest and Northeast. The greatest dissimilarities existed between the population of Riverside and that of southern cities.

These few comparisons indicated that Riverside did differ from other cities of its approximate size in the United States at the time of the epidemiology, and that findings from a study of Riverside cannot be projected directly to other cities. This would have been true regardless of the city selected for study. Such differences need to be kept in mind in interpreting findings. For this reason, the analysis of population subgroups is more useful as a basis for generalization than the description of the total population.

The remaining chapters are divided into three parts. Part 2, The Social System Epidemiology, reports findings from the study of the characteristics of persons in the city of Riverside who were holding the status of mental retardate. The epidemiology was conducted according to the assumptions of the social system perspective. Part 3, The Clinical Epidemiology, reports the general procedures and findings from the field survey, which was conducted within the clinical perspective according to the assumptions of the medical-statistical model of "normal." Part 4, Current Issues in the Clinical Perspective, contrasts the findings from the two approaches, discusses the implications of the clinical perspective for American society, and suggests some modifications in clinical procedures and definitions that would bring the clinical model closer to social system definitions.

Part II

THE SOCIAL SYSTEM EPIDEMIOLOGY

Chapter 4

WHO LABELS WHOM?

A social system epidemiology proceeds from the social system definition of mental retardation. In that definition, "mental retardate" is an achieved status and mental retardation is the role associated with the status. A mental retardate is one who occupies the status of mental retardate and plays the role of mental retardate in one or more of the social systems in which he participates. A social system epidemiology of the community discovers which persons are holding the status of mental retardate in the various social systems of the community and studies their characteristics. It studies how the normative structures of various subsystems vary and thus influence the number, characteristics, and distribution of mental retardates in the community. Finally, the social system epidemiologist studies how persons achieve the status of mental retardate in specific subsystems.

Procedures in a Social System Epidemiology

Two hundred and forty-one formal organizations, both private and public, covering every facet of community life were contacted. Each organization was asked to nominate for the study all mentally retarded persons known to that organization and to share whatever demographic and clinical information the organization knew about each nominee. After being assured that all information would be held in strictest confidence, all of the organizations that were approached agreed to participate.

For the social system epidemiology, the term *mental retardate* was deliberately left undefined. When the staff of an organization requested a definition, as they frequently did, they were asked to use whatever definition was customarily used by their staff. It was explained that the research project was interested in studying differences between organizations and did not wish to impose a standard definition. Assured that their judgments were acceptable to the study, each organization produced a comprehensive list of mental retardates together with the clinical and demographic information about each nominee available in organization records. Some organizations had their own staff members fill out the information protocols on nominees while others preferred to have our research staff do the necessary clerical work.

Approximately 1,500 nominations were received from formal organizations. Any nominee with a home address outside the city limits of Riverside was eliminated so that the geographic boundaries of the social system epidemiology would be coterminous with those for the clinical epidemiology. Duplicate nominations were identified and the case register consolidated so that each individual appeared only once. All information from various organizations about a particular individual was collected into one record. Every nominee was traced to determine if he was still living at his Riverside address during the census month. When consolidated, the central case register contained 812 nominees who had been nominated 1,493 times by the formal organizations of Riverside. These were the individuals who were holding the status of mental retardate in one or more of the formal organizations in the community, mental retardates by social system definition.

In order to simplify the social system analysis, the 241 formal organizations were grouped into eight categories: the Public Schools; Law Enforcement; Private Service Organizations; Private Organizations for the Mentally Retarded; the California State Department of Mental Hygiene; Medical Facilities; Public Welfare and Vocational Rehabilitation; and Religious Organizations.[1]

Table 2 gives the total number of persons nominated by each type of organization, the number of persons nominated only by that type of organization, the number of persons also nominated by one or more

[1] The following organizations were included in each category. Public Schools: the Riverside Unified School District; Law Enforcement: Riverside County Probation Department, California Youth Authority, Riverside Police Department; Private Service Organizations: Crippled Children's Society, Family Service Association, the Community Settlement House, the Home of Neighborly Service, Arlington Children Center, Boy and Girl Scouts, Christian Day School, YWCA, Nursery Schools, the Epilepsy Society, Elks Major Project, YWCA, the Junior Indoor Sports Club, Gheel House, and adult service clubs; Private Organizations for the Mentally Retarded: Retarded Children's Association and the Cresthaven School for the Retarded, private homes, nurseries, and recreational groups for the retarded; California State Department of Mental Hygiene and related facilities: Pacific State Hospital admitted and preadmission registers, the Bureau of Social Work of the Department of Mental Hygiene, Riverside Mental Hygiene Clinic, Patton State Hospital, preadmission files at the Riverside Probation Department; and Medical Facilities: the Riverside County Department of Public Health, Crippled Children's Services, pediatricians, psychiatrists and psychologists in private practice, the Visiting Nurse Association, Riverside Community Hospital; Public Welfare-Vocational Rehabilitation: Riverside County Welfare Department, State of California Department of Vocational Rehabilitation; Religious Organizations: ministers and priests in all Protestant, Catholic, and Jewish churches located in Riverside, all nurseries associated with churches, the Salvation Army, the Jewish Welfare Association, the Holy Innocents Guild, and the Catholic Welfare Bureau.

Table 2: Numbers of Persons Nominated as Mental Retardates by Eight Types of Formal Organizations

Type of Organization	Nominated Only by That Type of Organization	Nominated by One or More Other Types	% Overlap	Total Nominations by That Type of Organization
Public Schools	340	89	21	429
Medical Facilities	97	69	41	166
Law Enforcement	28	20	42	48
Department of Mental Hygiene	55	64	54	119
Public Welfare–Vocational Rehabilitation	28	40	59	68
Religious Organizations	33	52	61	85
Private Organizations for the MR	16	56	78	72
Private Service Organization	12	37	54	68

NOTE: There were 812 persons nominated by one or more formal organizations in the community.

other types of organizations, and the percentage of overlapping cases. The Public Schools contributed 429 persons to the central case register, 340 of whom were not nominated by any other organization. The next largest contributors were Medical Facilities with 166 nominees, 97 of whom were not nominated by other organizations, followed by the Department of Mental Hygiene with 119 nominees, 55 of whom were not duplicated. All other types of organizations contributed less than 100 cases to the central case register, and two of them—Private Organizations for the Mentally Retarded, and Private Service Organizations—made less than 20 unduplicated nominations. Persons served by these types of organizations are more likely to be labeled as mentally retarded by other organizations in town than those labeled by the Public Schools or Law Enforcement.

Who Are Labeled by Formal Organizations?

The labeled retardates, those holding the status of mental retardate in one or more of the social systems of Riverside, were not a random selection from the population of the city. The 812 persons holding the status of mental retardate in the various formal organizations of the city were compared by age, sex, ethnic group, and socioeconomic status with the general population of the community.

Age

The age profile for persons under 50 years of age in the general population of the community shows that 13% were 4 years of age or younger; 39% were between 5 and 19 years of age; and 48% were 20 through 49 years of age. The age profile of all 812 individuals nominated by formal organizations shows an underrepresentation of persons under 5 years of age holding the status of mental retardate (7%), an overrepresentation of persons 5 through 19 years of age (72%), and an underrepresentation of persons 20 and older (21%). This pattern was especially marked for the Public Schools (0% preschool, 79% school-age, 21% adult) and Law Enforcement Organizations (4%, 83%, 13%), and also persisted for the Department of Mental Hygiene (2%, 67%, 31%). Public Welfare–Vocational Rehabilitation was the only category nominating a majority of persons over 20 years of age (0% preschool, 41% school-age, 59% adult). At the other extreme, Medical Facilities nominated almost exclusively persons under 20 years of age (27%, 67%, 6%). It was the only group to nominate a higher percentage of preschool children than are found in the general population. Labeled retardates in Riverside are primarily school-age children. Every type of organization in the city contributed to this disproportion except Public Welfare–Vocational Rehabilitation.

Sex

Although the general population of Riverside had a slight surplus of females, 50.5% female to 49.5% male, every type of organization except Private Service Organizations reported more males holding the status of mental retardate than females. The surplus of males was greatest for Law Enforcement (65% to 35%) and the Department of Mental Hygiene (63% to 37%), but was sizable for Medical Facilities (61% to 39%), Public Welfare–Vocational Rehabilitation (57% to 43%), and the Public Schools (55% to 45%). Only Private Organizations for the Mentally Retarded (51% to 49%), Private Welfare (50% to 50%), and Religious Organizations (52% to 48%) had nearly equal percentages by sex. Males are more vulnerable to being labeled as mentally retarded than females, especially by public agencies.

Social Status

A home address was the only piece of information available in every file. Therefore, value of housing on the census block was the only measure of socioeconomic status available for most cases in the central case register. The distribution of the general population by housing-value decile was 40% in deciles 1–5 and 60% in deciles 6–10. Disproportionately more of the 812 labeled retardates were from the five lower deciles: 59%, compared with 41% in the higher deciles. Unlike age and sex differentials, socioeconomic differentials did not characterize all formal organizations. Those organizations which had the greatest overrepresentation of low-status persons and underrepresentation of high-status persons were Law Enforcement (92% low vs 8% high), Public Schools (72% low vs 28% high), Public Welfare–Vocational Rehabilitation (66% low vs 34% high), and to a lesser extent, Private Service Organizations (53% low vs 47% high). On the other hand, those labeled as mental retardates by the Department of Mental Hygiene facilities, Private Organizations for the Mentally Retarded, and Medical Facilities conform closely to the socioeconomic distribution of the community. Religious organizations are the only group that nominated a higher proportion of high-status persons than exists in the population of the community and proportionately fewer persons from deciles 1 through 5.

Ethnic Group

Anglos, who constitute 82%of the population under 50 years of age make up only 54% of the 812 labeled retardates. Mexican-Americans, who compose 9.5% of the under 50 group, contribute 32% to the labeled retardates—more than 300% more than would be expected from their proportion in the population. Blacks, who constitute 7% of the population under 50, contribute 11% to the register of labeled retardates. Ethnic disproportions are very marked in the Public Schools (37% Anglo, 45% Mexican-American, and 16% Black). Disproportions also exist in Law Enforcement (21%, 58%, 19%), Public Welfare–Vocational Rehabilitation (59%, 29%, 12%), and, to some extent, in Private Service Organizations (71%, 23%, 4%). These are the same organizations that nominated a disproportionately large number of persons from low socioeconomic status. The Department of Mental Hygiene facilities (80%, 15%, 2%) and Medical Facilities (78%, 13%, 6%) show only a slight underrepresentation of Anglos and overrepresentation of Mexican- Americans. Both the Private Organizations for the Mentally Retarded (90%, 4%, 6%) and Religious Organizations (91%, 7%, 2%) had an overrepresentation of Anglos and an underrepresentation of members of minority groups.

Who are the labeled? In general, most formal organizations of Riverside have proportionately more males and more school-age persons occupying the status of mental retardate. However, organizations vary in their selection for socioeconomic status and ethnic group. Those organizations that nominate disproportionately more persons from lower socioeconomic levels—such as the Public Schools, Law Enforcement, and Public Welfare–Vocational Rehabilitation—tend to be nonmedical, publicly supported agencies. They also are likely to nominate disproportionately more persons from minority groups, especially Mexican-Americans. Those organizations that nominate from a cross section of all socioeconomic levels do not show large ethnic disproportions. They are more likely to be privately supported or to be publicly supported, medically oriented agencies. Examination of the normative structures of these different agencies provides a clue to some of the reasons why the demographic and social characteristics of persons holding the status of mental retardate vary greatly from one type of formal organization to another.

Comparative Normative Structures

In chapter 2, we described five aspects of the normative structure of social systems that will influence the types of persons defined as deviant: the content of the norms; the focus of the norms; the level of the norms; the extent to which the norms have been codified and formalized; and the extent to which the system tolerates deviance. The nature of the information in the central case register available for persons nominated by each kind of formal organization provides indirect evidence on the first three of these aspects of the normative structure.

The Content of the Norms

Most of the formal organizations contacted in the social system epidemiology were staffed by professional persons who had either been trained as professional diagnosticians or had had a college education in which they had been introduced to the clinical perspective. Therefore, we expected to find most organizations operating from a clinical perspective and did not expect to find wide differences in the content of their organizational norms. However, as noted in chapter 1, the clinical perspective has evolved from two traditions: the medical tradition, which has used a medical-pathological model for "normal," and the psychological tradition, which has historically used a statistical model for "normal." The medical-pathological model defines abnormality in terms of symptoms that are diagnosed and classified by medical syndromes, while the statistical model defines abnormality in terms of deviation from the mean of the population. We expected that organizations oriented toward the statistical model would be more prone to evaluate and describe persons in terms of an IQ.

We can assess whether an organization emphasizes medical or statistical norms by analyzing the nature of the data available in the files for persons labeled as mentally retarded by that organization. If an organization has a medical diagnosis for a large percentage of its nominees, then it is using medical norms. If it has an IQ for most nominees, it is using statistical norms. Private Welfare and Religious Organizations were omitted from this analysis because they tended to borrow labels from other agencies and had very little diagnostic information on individuals whom they nominated.

The statistical model of normal is the most widely used norm in formal organizations. Over 80% of all the records of all labeled retardates on the case register had a recorded IQ. The medical model is much less widely used. Only 29% of the labeled mental retardates had a medical diagnosis in their files. There were significant differences by types of organizations in the use of the two normative models. These differences tended to correspond with the extent to which persons from lower socioeconomic status and ethnic minorities were overrepresented among those labeled as mentally retarded by that type of organization.

Table 3 presents the rank order of organizations by the extent to which persons from lower socioeconomic statuses and ethnic minorities were overrepresented among those labeled as mentally retarded. Law Enforcement and the Public Schools were the two organizations with the greatest overrepresentation of minorities and persons from lower socioeconomic status, and they were also among the highest ranking organizations in using the statistical norm (90% and 99%) and the lowest ranking in using a medical-pathological norm (19% and 13%). The Department of Mental Hygiene used both the medical and statistical models of normal simultaneously and almost universally. It ranked highest in the use of a medical norm, with 92% of its case records containing a description of the mental retardate couched in medical, diagnostic language, and also ranked second highest on the percentage of cases with an IQ (95%).

Other types of organizations tended to range between the two extremes. Over half of the cases from Public Welfare–Vocational Rehabilitation (63%), Private Organizations for the Mentally Retarded (57%), and Medical Facilities (52%) in the community contained a medical diagnosis. An even larger percentage of case records from these agencies reported an IQ: 78%, 78%, and 65%, respectively.

Table 3: Characteristics of Persons (in percent) Labeled by Various Formal Organizations

			Content of Norms		Focus of the Norms			Level of Norms	
	Lowest 5 Housing Deciles	Black and Mexican-American	Medical Diagnosis	IQ Test Score	Learning Problems	Health Problems	Acting-out Behavior	IQ above 70	No Reported Disabilities
Law Enforcement	92	77	19	90	56	21	67	54	71
Public Schools	72	61	13	99	90	27	30	46	62
Public Welfare–Vocational Rehabilitation	66	41	63	78	78	51	27	34	38
Private MR Organizations	43	10	57	78	77	57	38	14	25
Department of Mental Hygiene	40	17	92	95	70	70	51	11	11
Medical Facilities	38	19	52	65	50	70	26	[a]	16

[a] Insufficient data.

In short, both the Law Enforcement agencies and the Public Schools depend almost exclusively on the statistical model for their normative frame. They are also the two organizations with the largest overrepresentation of persons from lower socioeconomic status and ethnic minorities. Department of Mental Hygiene facilities consistently use both medical and statistical models of "normal" and do not show ethnic and socioeconomic disproportions in the populations nominated. Other types of formal organizations use the medical-pathological model in about half of their cases. They do not have very marked socioeconomic or ethnic disproportions. We concluded that the medical-pathological model is less likely to produce socioeconomic and ethnic disproportions in the labeling and that heavy reliance on the statistical model without concomitant use of the medical model is associated with such disproportions.

Focus of the Norms

When staff members of formal organizations referred labeled mental retardates to the study, they were asked to describe the person's "problems." File readers were instructed to record, verbatim, any "problems" mentioned in the file. The term *problem,* like the term *mental retardate,* was left undefined so that each agency described "problem behavior" from its own frame of reference. Verbatim descriptions were coded into three major categories for analysis, learning problems, acting-out behaviors, and problems associated with health and physical disabilities.[2] Categories are not mutually exclusive. A nominee could be reported to have all of these problems, none of these problems, or any combination of problems. For this reason, the percentages reported will total more than 100% in any given agency.

The "problem profiles" of persons labeled as mentally retarded by various organizations in Riverside were quite varied. These differences undoubtedly reflect differences in the characteristics of participants in various social systems, but they also reflect the varied foci of the norms of different types of organizations as staff members select the terms in which they describe the nature of each individual's deviance.

Table 3 presents the percentage of cases in which "learning" was

2 The following types of verbatim responses were coded into each of the analytic categories. Learning problems: academic deficiency, low achievement test scores, language difficulty, reading problems, poor work habits, slow learner, etc.; acting-out behaviors: deviant, disobedient, hostile, aggressive, hyperactive, short attention span, impulsive, outbursts of temper, poor social adjustment, lying, runaway, stealing, vandalism, and so forth; problems associated with health and physical disability: mention of specific physical handicaps, illnesses, or diseases, epilepsy, maturational difficulties, neurological problems, and so forth.

listed as a "problem" behavior. The Public Schools ranked first with 90% of its case records containing some mention of learning problems. They were followed by Public Welfare–Vocational Rehabilitation (78%), Private Organizations for the Mentally Retarded (77%), Department of Mental Hygiene (70%), Law Enforcement (56%), and Medical Facilities (50%). Organizations were ranked in almost exactly the same order when classified by the percentage of cases in which health and physical disabilities were *not* mentioned as problems. Only 21% of the Law Enforcement records and 27% of the Public School cases mentioned health or physical disability problems. At the other extreme, approximately 70% of the persons nominated by the State Department of Mental Hygiene and Medical Organizations had health or physical disability problems reported. The other two types of organizations ranged between the two extremes. The rank ordering for agencies by the percentage focusing on learning problems and not focusing on health and physical disability problems is almost identical to the rank ordering for organizations that have an overrepresentation of low socioeconomic status persons and ethnic minorities.

Law Enforcement ranked first in reporting acting-out problems, 67% of the cases, followed by the Department of Mental Hygiene (51%). Other agencies reported acting-out problems in one-fourth to one-third of their cases. It is significant that the two types of agencies in which mental retardates are institutionalized, Law Enforcement and the Department of Mental Hygiene, which administers the hospitals for the mentally retarded, report significantly more acting-out problems among their nominees than those agencies that serve persons still living in the community. This is the chief characteristic that apparently differentiates persons who are removed from a community setting.

Level of Expectation

Formal organizations also vary in the level of performance used as a criterion for subnormality. Persons nominated by some organizations were significantly more deviant physically and intellectually than persons nominated by other agencies. The lower the mean IQ and the larger the mean number of physical disabilities of persons holding the status of mental retardate, the less stringent the demands of a system.

Fifty-four percent of the persons nominated by Law Enforcement had an IQ of 70 or above, as had 46% of the persons holding the status of mental retardate in the Public Schools and 34% of those nominated by Public Welfare–Vocational Rehabilitation. The average IQ of the mental retardate nominated by these three organizations was 70.3, 67.4, and 60.2, respectively. These three types of organizations label more persons who are less deviant intellectually than any of the other groups, and also rank highest in the percentage of persons from low socioeconomic status and ethnic minorities who are nominated as mentally retarded. Only 14% of those nominated by Private Organizations for the Mentally Retarded, and 11% of those holding the status of mental retardate in a Department of Mental Hygiene facility had an IQ of 70 or above. The average IQ of the mentally retarded in these organizations was 50.4 and 42.5, respectively. These averages are significantly lower than the averages for the three highest ranking organizations.

It was possible to secure some direct or indirect information on six major physical disabilities for most of the cases on the register: speech, ambulation, arm and hand use in self-care, vision, and hearing. The ratings were made using four-point scales ranging from no difficulty to extreme difficulty and give some indication of the extent to which labeled retardates have serious physical disabilities of the type that are likely to be noted in organizational files. If a person was reported as having "no difficulty," he received the score of 0; "some difficulty," a score of 1; "much difficulty," a score of 2; and "extreme difficulty," a score of 3. An individual received 0 if there was no mention of an illness, accident, or operation involving the central nervous system; and a score of 1 for each involvement mentioned. Finally, if no seizures were mentioned, he received a 0 on that item. If seizures had occurred in the past but were no longer present or the frequency was not given, he received a score of 1. If he currently had seizures less than once a year, or few times a year, he received a score of 2. If he currently had seizures once a month or more, he received a score of 3. An individual's physical disability index score was the sum of his ratings on these items. Theoretically, scores could range from 0 through 21; however, actual scores range between 0 and 13.

The rank order of organizations by the percentage of individuals with no reported physical disabilities was approximately the same as it was for IQ above 70. Again, Law Enforcement and the Public Schools are the two types of agencies with the most stringent norms. Seventy-one percent and 62.0% of the persons they labeled as mentally retarded had no reported physical disabilities. Their average scores were less than 1 on the physical disability index. The Department of Mental Hygiene, again, had the least stringent norms. Only 11% of the mental retardates in that system were without physical disabilities, and the average physical disability score was 3.9. Those nominated by Medical Facilities were almost as disabled as those from the Department of Mental Hygiene. Only 16% of them were without physical disability, and their average score was 2.9. Private Organizations for the Mentally Retarded and Public Welfare–Vocational Rehabilitation fell between the two extremes reporting no physical disabilities for 25% and 38%

of their labeled retardates and mean disability scores of 2.5 and 2.2. The three formal organizations ranking highest in nominating persons from low socioeconomic status and ethnic minorities are the three organizations nominating persons with the fewest physical disabilities as mentally retarded. Mental retardates nominated by the Department of Mental Hygiene were the most deviant intellectually and physically, with other formal organizations falling between the two extremes.

There was insufficient evidence in the central case register to assess the extent to which formalization of the norms and tolerance for deviance may influence rates of labeled retardation in various social systems. These two aspects of social structure will be examined in detail for the one agency we studied in depth, the Public Schools.

Interlocking Social Systems

Thus far, we have studied each organization separately by noting the demographic and clinical characteristics of persons who hold the status of mental retardate in each type of organization. A study of the interlocking pattern of nominations made by various types of social systems revealed the anatomy of the larger social system formed by agencies which label mental retardates.

Each person in the central case register was scored according to the total number of times he was nominated by formal organizations. Totals ranged between 1 and 15. When we compared the mean number of times persons were nominated by various types of organizations as mentally retarded, we found large differences. The average number of nominations for persons holding the status of mental retardate in the Public Schools was only 1.7, and for Law Enforcement it was 2.0. The mean number of nominations was much higher in other organizations: 2.5 for Medical Facilities; 2.9 for Public Welfare–Vocational Rehabilitation; 3.3 for Private Service Organizations; 3.4 for Department of Mental Hygiene; 3.9 for Religious Organizations; and 4.8 for Private Organizations for the Mentally Retarded. A comparison of the percentage of shared nominations for each type of organization reveals the same pattern (see table 2). For example, over 78.0% of the persons holding the status of mental retardate in Private Organizations for the Mentally Retarded and Private Service Organizations were nominated by other organizations, as were 61% of those holding the status of retardate in Religious Organizations. At the other extreme, only 21% of those nominated by the Public Schools were mentioned by any other organizations. Clearly, persons holding the status of mental retardate in some types of formal organization are significantly more likely to hold that status in other formal organizations. What is the nature of this interlocking network of roles and statuses?

Figure 1 presents a diagram of the constellation of interlocking social systems based on the number of persons nominated jointly by various types of organizations. In order to simplify the diagram and highlight the major patterns, joint nominations of 12 or fewer were not recorded.

Figure 1: Constellation of Organizational Networks for Labeled Mental Retardates[a]

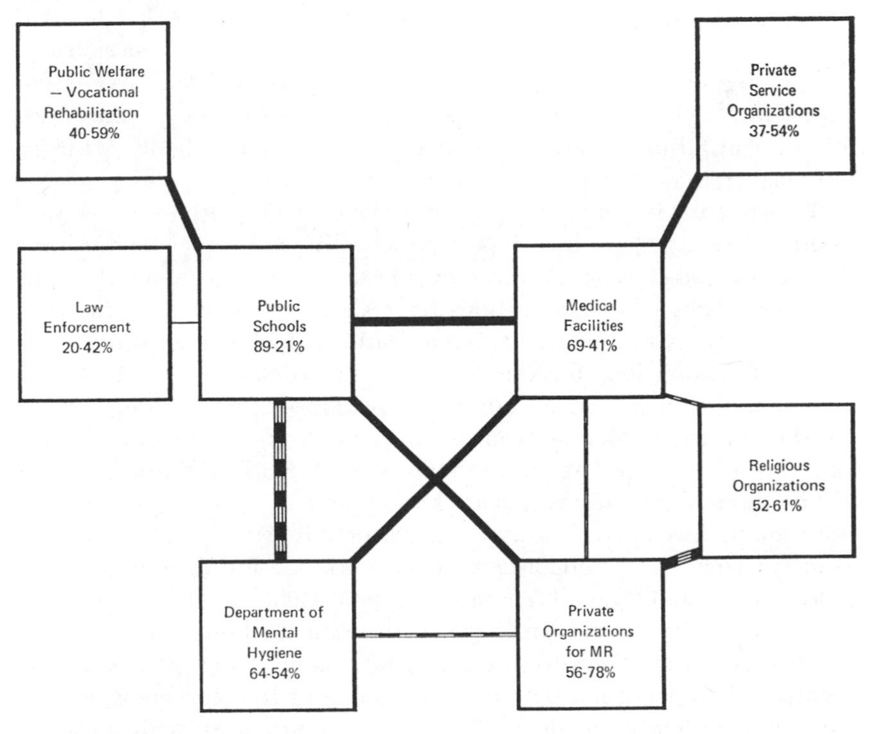

[a] Figures in boxes are the number and percentage of cases nominated that overlap with one or more other organizations.

The Public Schools clearly hold a commanding position in the community constellation. They have significant overlap with six other types of agencies including two, Public Welfare–Vocational Rehabilitation and Law Enforcement, which are not connected in a significant way with any other type of formal organization. The only overlap that dropped below 12 cases was with Private Service Organizations and Religious Organizations. The central case register contained 429 nominees from the Public Schools, of whom 89, or 21%, were shared with other organizations. Thus the Public Schools had the largest total overlap with other organizations, but also had the smallest overall percentage of overlap. There are 340 cases nominated by the Public Schools who are not holding the status of mental retardate in any other type of formal organization in the community.

Medical Facilities are the second most central organization in the community constellation having a sizable overlap with five other types of organizations. They are the only type of organization that has an important overlap with Private Service Organizations. However, they have no significant contact with Law Enforcement or Public Welfare–Vocational Rehabilitation. The percentage of cases they share with other organizations is larger than that for the Public Schools (41.0%) but smaller than that for other central organizations.

Department of Mental Hygiene and Private Organizations for the Mentally Retarded are each linked closely with four other types of organizations and thus hold a third-level position in the community constellation. Religious Organizations have significant overlap with only two other types of community organizations, Medical Facilities and Private Organizations for the Mentally Retarded. Over half of the cases from these three organizations are overlapping nominations: 54% for Department of Mental Hygiene, 61% for Religious Organizations, and 78% for Private Organizations for the Mentally Retarded.

The three organizations that ranked highest in nominating persons from low socioeconomic statuses and ethnic minorities are linked in a distinct triangle in the organizational network: the Public Schools, Law Enforcement, and Public Welfare–Vocational Rehabilitation. They are also the organizations nominating persons with the highest IQ and the fewest disabilities. They are the organizations most likely to be using a statistical model of normal (IQ test) and least likely to be using the medical-pathological model. The three organizations with proportionately fewer persons from lower socioeconomic statuses and ethnic minorities are also clearly linked in a triangle within the community network: Department of Mental Hygiene, Private Organizations for the Mentally Retarded, and Medical Facilities. They are most likely to use the medical-pathological model for normal and to label persons with significantly lower average IQs and more physical disabilities than the other group. The normative structure of community organizations is linked to the social characteristics of persons whom they are likely to label as mentally retarded. The content, form, and level of the norms of community organizations is a critical factor determining who will hold the status of mental retardate in the community.

Chapter 5

WHO ARE LABELED BY CLINICIANS?

Decisions made by many clinically trained professionals in selecting, evaluating, and labeling their clients in many different social organizations of the community combine to create the clinical case register. It is not possible to know, ex post facto, what factors were weighed in each case. However, we can gain some insight into the overall labeling process and the impact of the clinical perspective by a careful study of the end results of these interlocking, multiple decisions. By comparing the characteristics of persons labeled by professional labelers with the characteristics of persons labeled by nonprofessionals and with persons in the general population of the community, we can discover which groups in the population are most likely to be labeled retarded by clinical nominators and to be playing the role of retardate in the community.

Characteristics of Those Labeled by Professional Labelers Compared with Those Labeled by Nonprofessionals

The case register of persons nominated by formal organizations was divided into two parts: persons nominated by organizations that are not staffed by persons professionally qualified to make a clinical diagnosis of mental retardation, and persons nominated by clinically trained professionals or organizations that systematically make use of clinically trained persons in arriving at a diagnosis of mental retardation.

Persons nominated by the Public Schools, the Department of Mental Hygiene, the Department of Vocational Rehabilitation, the Retarded Children's Association, the Department of Public Health, the Aid to the Totally Disabled program of the County Welfare Department, the School for the Deaf, and psychiatrists, medical doctors, and psychologists in private practice were grouped in the clinical case register. Persons nominated by churches, service clubs, youth groups, private service organizations, and so forth were classified in the nonclinical case register. These classifications are not mutually exclusive. Some persons were nominated by both clinical and nonclinical organizations and appear in both categories.

When we compared persons nominated by clinical organizations with those nominated by nonclinical organizations, we found only minor differences in their social and clinical characteristics. About 9% of the persons on both registers were living in institutions, and approximately 45% of both groups had no reported physical disabilities. The mean IQs for both groups were essentially the same, 63.3, compared with 62.6. The nonclinical register contained 13% more Anglos, 8% more persons in housing deciles 6 through 10, and 10% more preschool children than the clinical register, making those nominated slightly more like the community as a whole than persons nominated by clinical organizations.

We concluded from these comparisons that staff members in most formal organizations, regardless of whether they are professionally trained diagnosticians, are placing persons in the status of mental retardate who have approximately the same clinical and social characteristics. The clinical perspective is the perspective of most formal organizations in Riverside, regardless of whether they have medically or psychologically trained diagnosticians on the staff.

Intellectual Performance of Individuals on the Clinical Register

Of the 687 persons on the clinical case register, there were 619 for whom an intelligence test score was available in the dossier, 91% of the total. Persons having no IQ in the dossier tended to be significantly younger ($p<.05$); were more likely to be Anglo ($p<.01$); were more likely to come from higher socioeconomic backgrounds ($p<.05$); were less likely to have been referred by the public schools $p<.001$); and were more likely to have been referred by the Public Health Department or the Retarded Children's Association ($p<.01$). The mean disability scores were 1.5 for those with available IQs and 2.7 for those without a recorded IQ ($p<.01$). There were no differences by sex or differences in the total number of organizations nominating the person to the clinical register. Many of the persons without an intelligence test score were diagnosed by a medical doctor as mentally retarded. The nominees' high social status and numerous physical disabilities may have made their deficiencies sufficiently obvious to the clinician that he felt an intelligence test unnecessary and used a medical model for diagnosis. In the case of the very young, the inadequacies of IQ measures may have influenced the clinician to make a diagnosis using a pathological model without a psychometric, statistical evaluation.

Most of the dossiers that had intelligence scores in them contained scores based on individually administered intelligence tests, mainly the Wechsler Intelligence Scale for Children, the Wechsler Adult Intelligence Scale, the Stanford-Binet, or the Kuhlmann-Binet. Frequently, a file contained more than one intelligence test score. If the person had an intelligence test score based on one of the individually administered intelligence tests, that score was given preference over scores based on group tests. If he had more than one individually administered test in his record, the most recently administered test was given preference. If his file contained only group intelligence test scores, the most recent score was given preference.

There were 30 cases for whom an intelligence test score was recorded, but the dossier contained no information about the test used nor the date of the test. Of the 589 cases with information available about the date and type of IQ test, 97% were evaluated using an individually administered test. Fifty-two percent were measured with some form of the Stanford-Binet, and 42% with some form of the Wechsler. Thus, 94% of the cases for whom information was available were evaluated by one of the two standard psychometric tools.

While almost half (45.5%) of the tests had been administered within the two years prior to the study, there were 133 cases (22.6%) with tests administered three to four years prior to the study and 188 cases (31.9%) whose most recent test score was recorded five or more years prior to the study. Periodic retesting is not a common practice in most clinical agencies.

There is a clustering of IQ test scores in the range between 55 and 85, indicating a high concentration of cases in the categories clinically defined as the mildly retarded and the borderline. On the basis of the AAMD classificatory system, 34.6% of all labeled retardates for which IQs were available would be termed borderline, 34.1% mildly retarded, 13.6% moderately retarded, 5.5% severely retarded, 5.4% profoundly retarded, and 6.8% would be considered normal. This latter group consisted of 42 persons with intelligence test scores of 85 and above. They were significantly more likely to be young, male Anglos with physical disabilities nominated by medically trained clinicians.

If we treat cases with an IQ of 85 and above as misdiagnosed and eliminate them from consideration, the following percentage distribution results: 73.7% of the clinical register would be cases of borderline or mild retardation, 20.5% would be moderately or severely retarded, and 5.7% profoundly retarded. This distribution parallels that found in other studies. For example, in his 1929 study of England and Wales, Lewis found that the ratio of "idiots," "imbeciles," and "feebleminded" to each other was 5:20:75 (Primrose, 1962). Tizard studied the "ascertained prevalence" of mental retardation in London, that is, the mental retardates known to governmental agencies and listed in the central governmental registers. He produced a sample of 11,172 labeled retardates by selecting one case in 12 from the governmental register. Of this number, 2,736 were diagnosed as "imbeciles or idiots," with IQs under 50. There were 8,436 diagnosed as "feebleminded," with IQs 50 through 70. These individuals were those excluded from the educational system as "unsuitable for education in school." The ratio of "imbeciles or idiots" to "feebleminded" was thus approximately 25:75 (Tizard, 1964). This ratio is similar both to that found by Lewis and to the findings in Riverside.

The fact that the distribution of IQs on the clinical register in Riverside is very similar to that found in other studies gives some assurance that the 10% of the Riverside cases for which no IQ was available were not significantly different in intellectual ability from those for whom we had IQs.

Physical Disabilities of Persons on the Clinical Register

As noted in chapter 4, it was possible to secure some direct or indirect information on six major physical disabilities for approximately 90% of the cases on the clinical register. On the register, 9.1% of the cases were unratable on arm-hand use, 7.9% on ambulation, 13.6% on speech, 9.2% on hearing, and 10.4% on vision.

The most frequently reported difficulty was with speech. Fully 30.2% of the persons on the clinical case register had some or much difficulty with speech, and 4.3% could not speak at all. Over 15% had some or much difficulty with ambulation, and 3.4% could not walk at all. Arm-hand use ranked third. Approximately 15.0% of the persons on the clinical register had some or much difficulty with arm-hand use, and 1.0% had no arm-hand use whatsoever. Twelve percent of those on the register had difficulty with vision, which could not be completely corrected with glasses. No one was reported to be totally blind. Over 9% of the labeled retardates had some or much difficulty with hearing. The California State School for the Deaf contributed 1.8% of the cases on the register, cases which were probably over and above those that would be expected in a community with no such school. When these 11 cases are subtracted, 7.7% of the clinical register had some reported hearing difficulty.

Central nervous system involvement as a result of serious illness was mentioned more frequently than involvement resulting from either accidents or operations. Thirteen percent of the dossiers reported that the person had had a serious illness involving the central nervous system, 4.1% reported an accident involving the central nervous system, and 2.5% reported an operation involving the central nervous system. Seizures in the past or present were reported in 13.1% of the cases.

Using the physical disability index described in chapter 4, 46.5% of those on the clinical case register had no reported physical disabilities: 18% had a score of 1, 13.5% a score of 2, 6.4% a score of 3, 3.4% a score of 4, 3.4% a score of 5, and 8.8% had scores of 6 or more.

The relationship between IQ test score and physical disabilities was curvilinear. Those with the highest and lowest IQs had the most physical disabilities ($p<.001$). The profoundly retarded (IQ 0–19) and severely retarded (IQ 29–39) had very high average disability scores, 6.6 and 3.5 respectively. The mean disability score for trainable retardates (IQ 40–59) dropped to 1.7, and that for educable mental retardates (IQ 60–79) was a negligible .7. Persons labeled with an IQ of 80 or above had as many physical disabilities as trainable mental retardates, 1.7. Those nominated without an IQ test had almost as many physical disabilities (2.7) as the severely mentally retarded (3.5). The presence of physical disabilities appears to influence the clinicians' perceptions of the person so that he may diagnose a physically disabled person with relatively high intellectual ability as a mental retardate. The presence of physical disabilities also increases the likelihood that a diagnosis will be made without an intelligence test. Most persons in both these categories were diagnosed and nominated by medically trained diagnosticians who, presumably, were using a medical-pathological model as their diagnostic frame of reference.

This finding graphically illustrates the divergence between pathological and statistical models of "normal" in actual diagnostic decision-making and documents the uneasy marriage of the pathological and statistical models in current diagnostic practice. The medical professional, trained in the pathological model, which focuses on biological signs, reaches a diagnosis of mental retardate on the basis of biological symptoms. This diagnosis may diverge from the diagnosis that would be reached based on a statistical model and using an intelligence test. Because the two models are used simultaneously in the field of mental retardation, the statistical model by psychologists and the pathological model by medical professionals, many discrepancies are bound to appear. That these discrepancies are due primarily to differences between the statistical and pathological models of normal is shown by the fact that both groups who deviate from the statistical model, i.e., those with high IQs and those without IQ data, have more physical disabilities and were nominated, primarily, by medically trained people.

Sex of Persons on the Clinical Register

There were significantly more males than females on the clinical case register than in the population of the community. The clinical case register contained 392 males (57%) and 295 females (43%), although 49.5% of the general population were males and 50.5% were females ($p<.001$). The average IQ of females on the clinical case register, 61.2, was significantly lower than that for males, 64.9 ($p<.02$). The lower female mean is due in part to the large number of males (49) compared with females (16) who were labeled as mentally retarded with IQs of 80 or above. Stated in another way, 55% of the persons with an IQ of 79 or below were male, and 75% of those with an IQ of 80 or above were male ($p<.01$).

This tendency does not entirely account for the overrepresentation of males on the clinical register. There are still significantly more males among labeled retardates who meet the educational definition of mental retardation—an IQ of 79 or below. The usual interpretation for similar findings in other studies is that there simply are more males than females who are clinically retarded, and this discrepancy is a real difference between the sexes. However, we did not find a significant surplus of males in the field screening, which is reported in part 3 of this volume. Why should there be proportionately more males than females nominated for the clinical register? Why do labeled males have lower IQs than labeled females? Why are more males with IQs over 80 nominated than females? Could it be that society is able to tolerate a greater amount of intellectual subnormality in a woman than in a man? If only the most visibly subnormal females are referred and labeled, this factor could account for our finding that labeled females have lower IQ test scores than labeled males.

The average disability scores for the two sexes were identical, 1.7. When physical disability was held constant, males and females were equally likely to come to the attention of the clinician and to be labeled mentally retarded. A female with physical disabilities and a low IQ was just as likely to be labeled as a mental retardate as a male with similar disabilities and a similar IQ. The normal-bodied female with a lower IQ, however, was less likely to be labeled a mental retardate than a normal-bodied male with a comparable IQ. The typical configuration of female social roles, especially for adults, makes fewer demands for achievement than the typical male configuration. Women may marry, have children, and keep house. They are not expected to compete in the occupational world and may drop out of educational competition with fewer social consequences. Simpler social roles and lower societal expectations may serve as a refuge allowing women with marginal IQs to perform acceptably, while males with comparable IQs are referred to clinicians and labeled as incompetent.

Age Characteristics of Persons on the Clinical Register

Figure 2 presents a bar chart which compares the age distribution of persons on the clinical case register with the age distribution of the population of the community for persons under 50 years of age. The sexes have been combined because there were no significant sex differences in age distribution. The age profile of the community is shown by the shaded area, and the age profile of the clinical register by the heavy double line.

Figure 2: Age and Socioeconomic Distribution of the Clinical Case Register Compared with the General Population of the Community Under 50 Years of Age

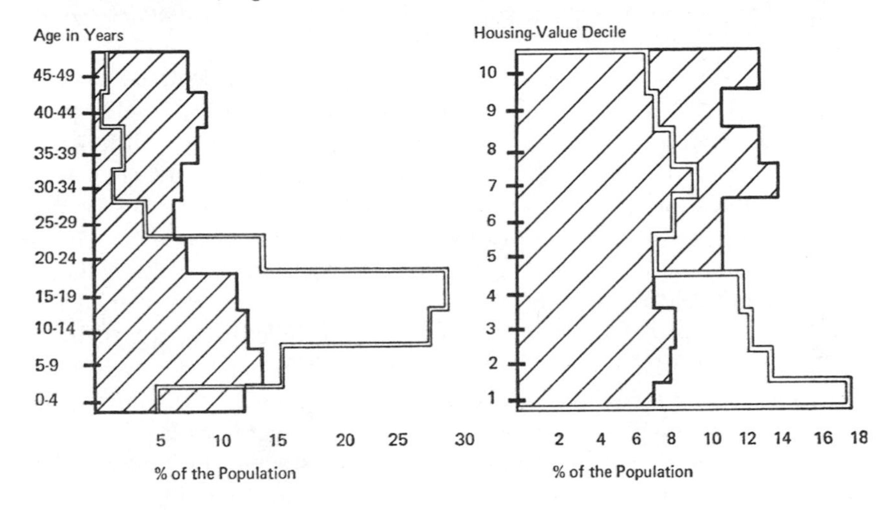

Note: Shaded area is the community population and the double line outlines the distribution of the clinical register. When age distributions were compared $X^2 = 487.9$, 10df, $p < .0005$. Mean housing-value decile for the clinical register was 4.7, for the survey sample, 6.1. $t = 12.4$, $p < .0005$.

The differences between clinical case register and community are both visually apparent and statistically significant ($p < .001$). There are only one-third as many persons on the clinical case register under 5 years of age as would be expected from their percentage in the general population. On the other hand, there are 10% more persons on the register between the ages of 5 and 9 than would be expected, more than twice as many persons between 10 and 19 as would be expected, and 64% more than would be expected between 20 and 24.

Persons of 25 years of age and over are noticeably underrepresented. The age group 25–29 has only 59% as many persons as would be expected; the age group 30–34 has 21% as many; and 35–39 has 30% of the number expected. The age groups 40–44 and 45–49 are even more drastically underrepresented. They have only 3% and 9% as many persons as would be expected from their proportion in the general population. Similar age differentials have been reported in other studies that used informants to develop a case register (Gruenberg, 1955).

Why are preschool children and adults underrepresented on the clinical case register, and school-age children overrepresented? Are school-age children "over-labeled"? There were 42 persons nominated as mentally retarded who had a reported IQ of over 85, and 36 of them were school-age children. Most clinicians would consider these cases misdiagnosed. Yet, even if we subtract these 36 cases from the school-age population, school-age children are still significantly overrepresented on the clinical register.

Perhaps the overrepresentation, as in the case of females, occurs because only the most mentally abnormal and physically disabled preschool children and adults are known to agencies, while children in school with relatively fewer disabilities are screened and labeled.

Most preschool children were nominated by medical professionals, and in only one-third of the cases was an IQ test score reported. However, preschool children on the case register definitely did have more reported physical disabilities than school-age children, an average of 3.4, compared with 1.5 ($p<.05$). The adults on the clinical case register (26 through 49 years) had a mean IQ of 51.0, significantly lower than the mean of 61.3 for school-age persons ($p<.001$). Only two adults with IQs of 80 or above were nominated as mentally retarded, while 58 school-age persons and four preschool children were nominated with IQs in this range. At the other end of the distribution, 43.5% of the adults had an IQ below 50, while only 16.3% of the school-age persons were this intellectually subnormal. Adults also had significantly more physical disabilities than school-age children ($p<.001$). Only the most intellectually and physically abnormal adults are known to agencies.

We can only speculate why the community enforces more stringent norms on school-age children. However, community reaction is probably related to societal expectations and the social roles played by persons of different ages in American society. Role expectations are very amorphous and lenient for the preschool child. His cognitive skills are not systematically cultivated and evaluated. If a preschool child has no obvious physical disabilities and his behavior is not visibly unusual, his family and relatives are not likely to be critical of minor variations. Many persons under five who later are labeled as clinically retarded may not be labeled earlier because they are able to meet the demands of the family environment and are not perceived as subnormal by anyone in their social group. In addition, diagnostic instruments developed for use with young children are neither as reliable nor as valid as those for older persons. Thus, only the most mentally subnormal and physically disabled are labeled until the child begins to play the role of student in the public school. School role expectations requiring cognitive skills, verbal facility, and intellectual achievement present arduous demands never before encountered. *In the competitive context of the school, each child is continuously evaluated by standarized tests and teacher's tests that use the statistical model of "normal." This model assures that somebody will fail. Every "normal" distribution has, by definition, a negative tail and generates its own subnormals.*

What about adults? They differed even more from school-age children than did preschool nominees. Here, again, the nature of societal demands appears to be a key factor. There is no single social institution comparable to the public school in which all adults must participate. The social groups in which they do participate are not constantly sorting and labeling persons, using the statistical definition of "normal," nor are they mainly concerned with cognitive and verbal abilities. Women may meet societal expectations as wives, mothers, and housekeepers even if their reading skills are rudimentary and their mathematical computations erratic. Men may find work in occupations that require relatively little intellectual acumen. They disappear into the general population. As adults, only the most physically and mentally deviant are still labeled by community organizations as mental retardates and continue to play that role. What social purpose is served by labeling a person as retarded during the school years if he is able to play productive roles in the community as an adult and is no longer labeled as a retardate?

Socioeconomic Characteristics of Persons on the Clinical Register

The average housing decile for the population of the community was 6.1; for the clinical register, it was 4.7 ($p < .001$).[1] Figure 2 compares the

[1] We would expect that the average housing decile for the community would be about 5.0 instead of 6.1 ($t = 12.4$, $p < .0005$). The reason that the average housing decile is higher than 5.0 is that new homes constructed in the community between

distribution of housing values on the blocks where persons on the clinical case register lived with the distribution for the general population of the community. The shaded areas represent the community distributions, and the area enclosed by double lines represents the clinical register. The differences are very striking. Above the fourth decile, there are fewer mental retardates on the clinical register than would be expected from the proportion in the population of the community. In the fourth decile and below, there are more persons on the clinical register than would be expected. The gap between expected and actual cases is particularly large in decile 1, with more than twice as many labeled retardates as would be expected by the proportion of persons in decile 1 in the population.

There were more males than females nominated at every socioeconomic level. The average IQ of persons on the clinical register did not vary in any systematic way with socioeconomic status. The mean IQ for persons in deciles 1 through 4 was 63.6. The mean IQ for persons in deciles 5 through 10 was 63.0.

However, age and physical disabilities did differentiate high-status persons on the clinical register from low-status persons. The average age of mental retardates in deciles 1 through 4 was 17.0 years, and that for persons in deciles 5 through 10 was 14.9 years ($p<.001$). High-status nominees also had significantly more physical disabilities. The average physical disability score for deciles 1 through 4 was 1.18, and that for deciles 5 through 10 was 2.05 ($p<.001$). Thus, clinically labeled mental retardates from higher socioeconomic levels were younger and more physically disabled, while those from lower levels were older and had few physical disabilities.

In another study, two distinct groups of mental retardates were identified through latent class analysis in the hospital population of the state hospital for the mentally retarded which serves Riverside (Miller, Eymen, and Dingman, 1961). One group consisted of young, physically disabled mental retardates from higher socioeconomic backgrounds, and the second group consisted of older, normal-bodied mental retardates from lower socioeconomic levels. Thus, the same basic clusters of persons by socioeconomic level, age and physical disabilities found in Riverside were also found in the hospitalized population of retardates.

Why should high-status nominess be younger and more physically

the 1960 census, on which the decile categories were established, and 1963, when the fieldwork was done, were almost entirely tract homes that ranged in value from $15,000 upward. This new building added to the number of dwellings in the upper deciles and reduced, proportionately, those in the lower deciles.

disabled than low-status nominees? Could this reflect a systematic pattern in the clinical labeling process? A child reared in a high-status family participates in a social milieu that provides him the opportunity to acquire the knowledge and skills needed to do well on Anglo "intelligence" tests because the adults in his social world have the necessary skills and knowledge. In this situation, the children who do not acquire the minimal skills needed to pass an Anglo "intelligence" test are mainly those who have some kind of biological dysfunction that interferes with their ability to learn from their social environments. Being physically disabled, they are likely to be labeled as deviant by their families at an early age and referred to a clinician. They would qualify as clinically retarded by both the pathological and the statistical definitions of abnormal.

On the other hand, a child reared in a low-status environment or in a minority subculture has less opportunity to acquire the knowledge and learn the skills needed to do well on an Anglo "intelligence" test, because the adults who are socializing him do not have such skills and knowledge. In this situation, not only children with biological dysfunctions but those with no physical disabilities may fail to acquire the knowledge and skills necessary to pass such tests. Since many who are not learning these skills are not physically disabled and do not deviate noticeably from the expectations and performance of adults in their social worlds, they are not labeled as deviant by their families. When they are older, probably in school, they are labeled as retarded by teachers and psychometrists, who evaluate mainly verbal and cognitive skills and use a statistical definition of subnormal that compares their performance with that of children from more advantaged environments and children from the dominant Anglo culture.

The high-status and low-status children with organic anomalies and the physically normal low-status child all appear together on the clinical register, but their routes to the register have been very different. In general, labeled high-status children, who were more likely to have physical disabilities, were defined as abnormal by their parents at an early age and labeled as retarded by a medical doctor using a pathological model. On the other hand, labeled low-status children, most of whom had no physical anomalies, were not perceived as abnormal by their parents nor anyone in their social milieu until they were older and had reached school. At that time, they were referred by a teacher and labeled mentally retarded by a school psychometrist using a statistical model for evaluating "normal" performance. If this process operates, then high-status labeled retardates would be mainly persons with biological dysfunctions who were not able to learn from their social environment, and low-status retardates would consist not only of the physically disabled who were not able to learn but also of the physically normal who did not have an opportunity to learn. All three groups would perform poorly on clinical measures, such as an IQ test, and would be indistinguishable clinically.

Ethnic Characteristics of the Clinical Register

We compared the ethnic distribution of the entire community under 50 years of age with the ethnic distribution of the entire clinical case register. Eighty-two percent of the community population was Anglo, 9.5% Mexican-American, and 7% Black. If Mexican-Americans were represented in proper proportion, we would expect about 10% of those on the clinical register to be of Mexican heritage. Instead, 32% were Mexican-Americans, three times the expected proportion. We would expect 7% of those on the clinical register to be Black; instead, 12% are Black. We would expect 82% to be Anglos but find 53% instead. Because ethnic group and socioeconomic status are interrelated, Mexican-American and Black rates could be higher mainly because most of them are from a lower socioeconomic background. We must hold socioeconomic status constant in order to assess the extent to which ethnic group operates as a factor in being labeled as a mental retardate independent from social status.

Socioeconomic Distributions within Ethnic Group

We classified persons on the clinical case register into three socioeconomic levels by housing-value decile. We found that there were fewer Anglos on the clinical register from each of the three social status levels than would be expected from their proportion in the community population. The differential decreased as status increased. In deciles 1 through 3, we would expect 53% Anglos and found only 19%; in deciles 4 through 7, we would expect 87% but found 69%; in deciles 8 through 10, we would expect 98% and found 89%.

The reverse was true for the Mexican-American population. While we would expect about 29% of the labeled retardates in deciles 1 through 3 to be of Mexican heritage, we found 61%. Instead of the expected 6% in deciles 4 through 7, we found 16%. Instead of 1% in deciles 8 through 10, we found 7%. There were significantly more persons of Mexican heritage labeled as mental retardates than would be expected from their percentage in the population, and this was true of all social status levels.

Differentials for the Black population disappeared when socioeconomic level was held constant. In deciles 1 through 3, we would expect 18% to be black and found 17%; in deciles 4 through 7, we would expect 7% and found 12%; in deciles 8 through 10, we would expect 1% and found 2%. Thus, control for socioeconomic status tends to eliminate the overrepresentation of Blacks on the clinical register, but it does not account for the overrepresentation of persons from a Mexican heritage. This same phenomenon occurred in the household survey screening, which is described in part 3 of this volume. When social status differences were controlled, higher rates of intellectual subnormality based on a statistical model disappeared for Blacks, but differentials still remained for Mexican-Americans. Socioeconomic differences were a major factor in Anglo-Black differences, but controlling socioeconomic factors did not eliminate Anglo-Mexican differences. We will return to this issue in a later chapter.

Age Distributions within Ethnic Group

Sex differentials in labeled retardation hold for all ethnic groups. Each ethnic group at each status level had more labeled male retardates than females and in approximately the same proportions. However, there were significant differences when the three groups were compared by age. Anglo retardates were both younger and older than retardates of Mexican or Black heritage. There were disproportionately more preschool labeled retardates and retardates 30 years of age and over in the Anglo group than in the two minority groups ($p<.001$). Differences are greatest when only low-status persons in deciles 1 through 3 are compared ($p<.001$), although the same pattern persists for middle-status persons, deciles 4 through 7 ($p<.05$). No comparisons were made for high-status persons because only 10 Mexican-American and 3 Black labeled retardates were from homes in deciles 8 through 10.

We reported earlier that high-status labeled retardates on the clinical register were significantly younger than retardates from low-status homes. This age differential persists for Anglos, and the trend remains for Mexican-Americans but not for Blacks. The mean age of low-status Anglos was 19.3, middle-status, 16.0, and high-status, 14.7 ($p<.01$). For Mexican-Americans, the average age of low-status persons was 16.9 and that of middle-status persons was 14.1, but these differences did not quite achieve statistical significance. The average age for Black retardates was 14.4 for deciles 1 through 3 and 14.7 for deciles 4 through 7.

Table 4 shows that labeled mental retardation is a more age specific condition for Mexican-Americans and Blacks than it is for the Anglo population. All the preschool retardates and most of the adult re-

Table 4: Comparison of Age, IQ, and Physical Disability Scores by Ethnic Group

Variable	Anglo (N = 361) %	Mexican-American (N = 221) %	Black (N = 79) %	Significance Level[a] %
Age				
0–4	8.0	0	0	
5–19	67.6	76.5	86.1	<.001
20–29	16.6	21.3	12.6	
30–49	8.0	2.3	1.3	
IQ				
0–19	6.5	2.8	1.3	
20–39	9.4	2.8	6.6	
40–59	22.1	22.2	32.9	<.001
60–79	47.4	67.6	55.3	
80+	14.6	4.6	3.9	
Physical Disability Scale				
0	32.1	61.5	71.3	
1	19.4	17.2	10.0	
2	16.9	10.8	7.5	
3	9.3	2.3	5.0	<.001
4	5.1	1.4	2.5	
5+	17.2	6.9	2.5	

[a] A chi-square test was used because of the nature of the distributions for Age and IQ. The mean scores on Physical Disability were Anglo 2.18, Mexican-American .99, and Black .81. Using one-way analysis of variance $p < .001$.

tardates over 30 labeled by clinical organizations are Anglos. Labeled mental retardation is even more "school specific" for Blacks than for Mexican-Americans. Of the Black retardates on the register, 86% were between 5 and 19 years of age, compared with 76% of the Mexican-Americans and 68% of the Anglo retardates of the same age. This finding supports our earlier argument that the families and relatives of persons from lower socioeconomic levels, a high percentage of whom are persons from minority groups, are not likely to perceive their children as mentally retarded during the preschool years and do not refer them to a clinician. Anglo parents are more likely to make this initial referral. Once in school, teachers begin to make referrals, and minority children are labeled for the first time. When they leave school, minority persons are no longer under the close purview of clinical organizations and are either able to find a place for themselves in adult society or are labeled as something other than mentally retarded by the organizations which serve them. Fewer Anglos are able to make this transition. Could it be that Anglos have lower IQs and more physical disabilities before they are placed in the status of a mental retardate and, hence, are less likely to make the transition to the status of "normal" adult?

Distribution of IQ within Ethnic Group

Table 4 groups the labeled retardates from each ethnic group into five levels by IQ. With IQ as with age, Anglos have a higher percentage of persons with very low and very high IQs. The percentage distributions show that 15.9% of Anglos of all status levels have IQs below 40, while only 5.6% of all Mexican-American retardates and 7.9% of all Black retardates have IQs that low. At the other end of the distribution, 14.6% of all Anglos on the clinical register had IQs above 79, while only 4.6% of the Mexican-Americans and 3.9% of the Blacks had IQs that high ($p<.001$). This persists even when social status is held constant ($p<.001$). Once again, the peculiar characteristic of the labeled Anglo population is that it has a higher percentage of persons at both extremes, while Blacks and Mexican-Americans are highly concentrated in the middle ranges, IQs between 40 and 79.

Physical Disabilities within Ethnic Group

Table 4 reveals ethnic differences in physical disability that are large and consistent. Anglos have an average disability score of 2.18, while that for Mexican-Americans is .99 and for Blacks .81 ($p<.001$). Only 32% of the labeled Anglos had no disabilities, while 61% of the labeled Mexican-Americans, and 71% of the labeled Blacks were without reported physical disabilities.

When only low-status persons (housing deciles 1 through 3) are compared, the differences persist, although they are slightly reduced ($p<.01$). The average Anglo disability score drops to 1.6, and the percentage of persons with no disabilities increases to 41%. Mexican-American and Black scores remain about the same as for the total group. Among middle-status retardates, the average disability score of Mexican-Americans increases to 1.7, becoming more like the Anglo pattern. The Black mean remains significantly lower ($p<.01$). However, there are still a sizable percentage of labeled Mexican-Americans (51%) and Blacks (70%) who have no reported physical disabilities, compared with Anglos (30%).

Physical disabilities appear to be the intervening variable explaining ethnic differences in age and IQ among labeled retardates. More Anglos have physical disabilities. Physically disabled persons are more visibly deviant and, hence, are more likely to be identified early by their families and more likely to be taken to a medical doctor for evaluation. The medical doctor, using a medical diagnostic model, may diagnose some referrals as mentally retarded when, in fact, they have IQs which are "normal" by statistical norms. This produces a disproportionate number of Anglos with high IQs. On the other hand, physical disability is correlated with IQ. In general, those who are organically damaged have significantly lower IQs, producing a disproportionate number of Anglos in the lowest IQ categories. Organically damaged persons are less likely to be able to move out of the status of retardate than normal-bodied persons; hence, there are more Anglo adult retardates.

Most Mexican-American and Black retardates are labeled by the schools, which use a strictly statistical model of normal. Therefore, they are labeled later in life, and there are very few who are labeled with an IQ over 79. Labeled Mexican-Americans are very homogeneous in age, IQ, and physical disabilities. Ninety-eight percent of the labeled Mexican-Americans are between 5 and 29 years of age, 90% have an IQ between 40 and 80, and 62% do not have any physical disabilities. Labeled Black retardates are an even more homogeneous population than Mexican-American retardates. Ninety-nine percent of them are between 5 and 29 years of age; 88% have IQs between 40 and 80; and 71% have no physical disabilities. Labeled Anglos are significantly more intellectually subnormal and physically disabled than persons labeled as mentally retarded from minority groups. Because most labeled minority retardates are normal-bodied, they are able to escape the status of retardate once they are out of school. Consequently, there are only a few minority adults, usually the physically disabled, who remain identified as subnormals. For persons from minority groups, labeled retardation is more age specific and more closely tied to the statistical model of normal and performance on an intelligence test than for Anglos.

The low-status, school-age Mexican-American male is the most vulnerable to the dynamics of the labeling process. He is the most intellectually and physically normal of all persons on the clinical case register. At the other extreme, preschool and adult Mexican-Americans and Blacks are essentially immune to the labeling process. There were no preschool minority children nominated by clinicians for the register, and only a few adults over 30 years of age.

Chapter 6

THE SITUATIONALLY RETARDED

Having investigated the formal organizations of the community from a social system perspective with special emphasis on social systems operating from the clinical perspective, we will now examine the characteristics of persons perceived as subnormal by two informal social systems, the neighborhood and the family.

Methods Used to Secure Neighbor and Family Nominees

Nominations from neighbors and from each family were secured during the field survey interview. Interviews were conducted on 500 of the approximately 1,000 census blocks in Riverside, and all geographic areas and socioeconomic levels in the community were represented in their proper proportion.

Neighbor Nominees

Near the end of each field survey interview, after all of the screening questions for adaptive behavior had been completed, each respondent in the household survey was asked three open-ended questions about mental retardation. These were the only questions in the interview in which the word "retarded" was used. The first two questions described a moderately retarded and a severely retarded person, respectively, and then asked the respondent what he thought the parents of such a person should do with him and whether he believed the Public Schools should provide special classes for him.[1] Following these two opinion questions, respondents were asked the following question, "Often families with

[1] The two questions preceding the request for nominations were as follows: (1) "In this study, we are especially interested in people who are slow learners, who are retarded. Some retarded people will never be able to read better than about the fourth-grade level. They will always be like a nine-year-old child and will always need someone to look after them. If parents have such a child what do you think they should do with him? Do you think that the Public Schools should provide special classes for such a child?' (2) "There are some people who are extremely retarded. When they grow up they will never be able to dress themselves or even to feed themselves. They will always need someone to look after their needs and to care for them. If parents have such a child, what do you think they should do with them? Do you think the Public Schools should have a special program for such a child?"

retarded persons have special problems, and we are interested in knowing about any retarded persons who live in Riverside. Do you know of anyone in Riverside who is retarded? Is this a child or adult? What is his/her sex? Where does he/she live? Do you know his/her name"? The interviewer was instructed to continue to probe in order to secure as much information about the nominee as possible, especially his name, address, sex, and approximate age.

The question asking for nominees was placed at the end of the series of three questions about retardation because we believed that respondents would be reluctant to nominate persons for the case register if they were asked to name mental retardates without any preparatory inquires. However, the two questions describing a moderately and a severely retarded person did set the context within which respondents made their nominations. To this extent, the interview itself provided a framework for the response and this factor should be borne in mind when interpreting the findings. Thirty percent of the respondents nominated one or more persons as a retardate. Altogether, there were 243 persons nominated for whom the respondent provided sufficient information so that it was possible to verify whether their address at the time of the study was within the geographic boundaries set for the study. We have called these persons the "neighbor nominees."

Family Nominees

We did not feel that we should ask respondents directly whether they believed any member of their own family to be retarded, nor did we feel it would be acceptable to ask the respondent to rate the behavior of other adult members of the family. Therefore, we did not ask respondents to make evaluative ratings of adults in the family nor did we ask explicitly for mental retardates. Instead, each respondent, usually the mother, was asked to rate all persons in the family under 16 years of age by placing a mark on a 13-centimeter line drawn between five pairs of adjectives. The first adjective pair, sickly–healthy, was used as a sample rating to be certain that the respondent understood what was expected. The four remaining adjustive pairs were active–inactive; lazy–ambitious; obedient–disobedient; and bright–slow. We interpreted the ratings given a child on the bright–slow dimension as a rating of perceived intelligence.

The 2,760 children rated by respondents were assigned a score by measuring the distance, in centimeters, between the "slow" end of the continuum and the mark made by the respondent. Hence, the "brighter" the mother's perception of the child, the higher the score.

Ratings were negatively skewed. The 444 children who had scores of 7.2 centimeters or less were the 16% who received the lowest ratings and have been designated as family nominees.

Professional Labelers vs Neighbors and Family

Differences between the social characteristics of persons nominated as subnormal by clinicians and those nominated by neighbors and family are very significant. Sex is the only variable that did not differentiate nominees from these groups. All groups nominated more males as subnormal than females (clinicians 57.1%, neighbors 55.1%, and family 55.6%).

Significantly more of the persons nominated by neighbors were under 16 years of age than were persons nominated by clinical organizations ($p<.001$). Apparently, neighbors are more likely to perceive and to report children as subnormal than adults. Age comparisons were not possible for family nominees because only persons under 16 were rated by respondents.

The ethnic disproportions so characteristic of those labeled by clinical organizations did not occur for either neighbor or family nominees ($p<.001$). The proportion of Mexican-Americans and Blacks nominated by neighbors (10.1% and 3.4%) and families (15.3% and 8.8%) approximates the proportion in the community as a whole.

The same is true for socioeconomic status. In fact, neighbor nominees consist of slightly more Anglos (86.5%) and more high-status persons (36.6% in deciles 8–10) than are found in the community. Family nominees mirrored the community distribution with 28.4% from deciles 1–3, 41.2% from deciles 4–7, and 30.4% from deciles 8–10. This finding indicates that the labeling of large numbers of persons from low socioeconomic levels and minority ethnic groups as subnormal is a characteristic of the clinical perspective that is not shared by lay persons in the community. Neighbors of low socioeconomic persons and of ethnic minorities do not perceive and nominate them as subnormal more often than neighbors of high-status persons. Families of low-status persons and ethnic minorities do not rate a disproportionate number of their children as "slow." Such evaluations result from the application of clinical norms.

In chapter 4, we reported that the social characteristics of persons nominated by different types of formal organizations varied significantly from one organization to another. The sociocultural characteristics of neighbor nominees and persons rated as subnormal by their families not only conform more closely to the sociocultural characteristics of the community but are more similar to the characteristics of persons nominated by the Department of Mental Hygiene, Private Organizations for the Mentally Retarded, Medical Facilities, and Religious Organizations of the community than to public agencies such as the Schools, Law Enforcement, and Public Welfare–Vocational Rehabilitation. The latter agencies nominated disproportionately more persons from low socioeconomic statuses and from ethnic minorities than did other formal organizations in the community.

Content of Neighbor and Family Norms

When neighbors and families nominate a person as a mental retardate or rate a child as "slow," are they assessing the same kinds of behaviors that clinicians assess when they nominate a person as a mental retardate?

The Content of Neighbor Norms was studied by using the total number of neighbor nominations received by each person on the central case register as the dependent variable in a stepwise multiple correlation analysis in which IQ and physical disabilities were used as independent variables. It was assumed that those persons nominated most frequently by their acquaintances and neighbors would exemplify the characteristics most likely to influence their visibility as subnormals to persons in the community. There were 697 persons on the comprehensive case register for whom there was complete information on all the variables being studied. IQ was the most significant single variable when correlated with number of neighbor nominations ($r = -.31$, $p<.001$). The lower the individual's IQ, the more persons in the community who were likely to nominate him as retarded. The correlation with physical disabilities was almost as high ($r = .24$). Persons with more physical disabilities were more likely to be nominated by neighbors as retarded. The multiple correlation coefficient for the two characteristics taken together was .35, accounting for 12.3% of the variance in the number of neighbor nominations. Correlations with social characteristics such as housing value ($r = .19$), ethnic group ($r = -.11$), segregation of neighborhood ($r = .19$), and marital status of parents ($r = -.11$) indicated that sociocultural characteristics were less salient than either IQ or physical disabilities in neighbor norms and were correlated in the *opposite* direction to that found for clinical organizations in the community. Anglos from higher socioeconomic status, from families living in segregated majority neighborhoods, who had parents who were married and living together were significantly more likely to receive multiple nominations from their neighbors ($p<.001$). Persons who were in an institution were also more likely to receive multiple nominations by neighbors and acquaintances ($p<.05$).

Level of Neighborhood Norms

It is clear from the preceding analysis that neighbors and acquaintances are applying a normative system that is similar in content to that embodied in clinical measures. IQ level and physical disabilities are significantly correlated with the number of neighbor nominations. If that is the case, why should there be such discrepancies between the sociocultural characteristics of persons nominated by neighbors and acquaintances and the characteristics of persons nominated by clinical organizations? Could it be that lay nominators are using a comparable normative framework for making evaluations but have different levels of expectations than those applied by clinicians?

The mean IQ for neighbor nominees was 55.0, while the mean IQ for retardates labeled by clinical organizations was 63.1 ($p<.001$). The mean IQ of neighbor nominations was significantly lower than that of persons nominated by Law Enforcement Agencies (70.3), by the Public Schools (67.4), and by Public Welfare–Vocational Rehabilitation (60.2). Only retardates nominated by Private Organizations for Mental Retardates and the State Department of Mental Hygiene had lower mean IQs than neighbor nominees, 50.4 and 42.5, respectively.

Persons nominated by neighbors and acquaintances also had more physical disabilities than persons nominated by either the Public Schools or Law Enforcement. There were 51.7% of the neighbor nominees who had one or more physical disabilities, while only 38% of the Public School nominees and 29.2% of the nominees from Law Enforcement had reported disabilities. Other clinical organizations, however, nominated more disabled persons than did neighbors. In general, the level of expectations of neighbors and acquaintances was similar to that of those organizations in the community which nominated persons whose ethnic and sociocultural characteristics were similar to the community as a whole and showed little or no surplus of ethnic minorities or low socioeconomic status persons: Private Organizations for the Mentally Retarded, Medical Facilities, and the Department of Mental Hygiene.

The level of expectations of lay nominators was undoubtedly influenced by the context in which the question was asked in the household survey, and we cannot draw any firm conclusions about what the level of expectations would have been if the question had been asked in another setting. However, the context of the question did not deter 15 respondents from nominating persons with IQs over 85. In general, however, it appears that the lay nominator requires more deviant behavior before he perceives and nominates a person as mentally retarded than is required by many professional labelers.

Content of Family Norms

To what extent do family norms correspond with the norms of the clinical perspective? Do persons rated as "slow" by their families have significantly lower IQs, more physical disabilities, and more adaptive behavior failures than those who are rated as "bright"? Is there any difference in family norms by ethnic group or socioeconomic status?

The ratings given children seven months through fifteen years of age on the "slow–bright" rating scale were correlated with IQ test score, adaptive behavior score, and physical disability as measured in the field epidemiology (see part 3 for explanations of these measures). Correlations were calculated separately for each ethnic group and for each of three socioeconomic levels categorized by the Duncan Socioeconomic Index Score of the occupation of the head of the household. The ratings given children by the respondent, usually the mother, were significantly correlated ($p<.001$) with their IQ test scores. The correlations were .34 for Anglos, .28 for Mexican-Americans, and .47 for Blacks. They were .36 for high-status persons, .36 for middle-status persons, and .35 for low-status persons. Children rated near the "slow" end of the continuum were significantly more likely to have low IQ test scores regardless of ethnic group or socioeconomic level.

Correlations with adaptive behavior were also statistically significant ($p<.001$), –.37 for Anglos, –.45 for Mexican-Americans, –.51 for Blacks, –.34 for high-status persons, –.42 for middle-status persons, and –.41 for low-status persons. Persons with the most adaptive behavior failures were rated lowest on the "slow–bright" dimension. Correlations with physical disability scores were much lower, although most were still statistically significant: –.07 for Anglos, –.29 for Mexican-Americans, –.14 for Blacks, –.02 for high-status, –.11 for middle-status, and –.15 for low-status persons. Parental ratings of children, regardless of the ethnic group or socioeconomic level of the parent, involved perceptions that were highly correlated with the kinds of assessments made in intelligence tests and the Adaptive Behavior Scales.

Certain demographic and sociocultural characteristics also influence parental ratings. There is a significant tendency in all ethnic groups and socioeconomic levels to rate older children as brighter than younger children, and girls as brighter than boys. There is also a slight tendency for more-educated parents to rate their children as brighter than less-educated parents. However, high-status parents do not rate their children as brighter than do low-status parents nor do Anglo parents give their children higher ratings for "brightness" than do Mexican-American and Black parents.

No inferences can be drawn about the level of the expectation of the family, as was done for the level of expectation of neighbors and acquaintances, because we did not ask directly about mental retardation in a family member. However, we can say with a high level of assurance that family evaluative frameworks and clinical evaluative frameworks are relatively parallel but the socioeconomic and ethnic differentials that appear in labeling by formal organizations are not reflected in parental ratings.

The Situationally Retarded

"We now have what may be called a 6-hour retarded child—retarded from 9:00 to 3:00 five days week" (Conference on Problems of Education of Children in the Inner City, 1969).

Individuals play roles in various social systems: their families, the school, work groups, neighborhood, church, and friendship groups. Their performance is constantly being evaluated by members of these groups. When mental retardation is defined as a social role played by a person holding the status of a mental retardate in a particular social system, mental retardation is social system specific. A person may play the role of the retardate in one social system and not in another.

In chapter 2 we proposed that levels of retardation, from a social system perspective, could be defined in terms of the number of social systems in which a person plays the role of retardate. If a person holds the status of retardate in all the social systems in which he participates and plays the role of retardate twenty-four hours per day, he is comprehensively retarded. Persons who are living in an institution for the mentally retarded are examples of the comprehensively retarded because all of their roles every day are bounded by the definition that they are a "retardate."

If a person lives in the community, he may play the role of the retardate in all of his social groups and may also be classified as comprehensively retarded, or he may play the role of the retardate in some systems in which he participates and not in others. In the latter case, he is a "retardate" part of the time and a "normal" part of the time. We have called the latter group the situationally retarded because their retardation varies with the situation or the social system in which they are participating at a particular time. We know how many formal organizations nominated each person as a mental retardate, how many neighbors and acquaintances nominated each person as a mental retardate, and whether a person is a resident of an institution or a home for the retarded. Using this information, we constructed a five-level rating of situational retardation, retardation from a social system perspective.

The 103 persons on the comprehensive case register who were living in an institution or a home for the retarded were given a score of "5." They are the most comprehensively retarded from a social system perspective. The 47 persons who were nominated 5 to 15 times by formal organizations and/or household survey respondents but were still living in a noninstitutional setting were scored "4." They are probably total retardates living in the community. The 77 noninstitutionalized persons who received a total of 3 or 4 nominations were scored "3," and the 111 who were nominated twice were scored "2." They are partial situational retardates. The 540 nominated only once were scored "1." They are the most situationally retarded.

Clinical and Sociocultural Characteristics of the Situationally Retarded

Each person on the comprehensive case register was classified into the proper group by his situational retardation score, and the clinical and sociocultural characteristics of the persons in each of the five groups were compared. Table 5 presents the comparisons for the two clinical and the three sociocultural characteristics for which we had relatively complete information.

The 540 persons who were minimally situationally retarded, i.e., nominated only once, had a mean IQ of 70.4, and the 111 persons nominated twice had a mean IQ of 69.8 Thus, approximately half the persons in these two categories would be rated as "borderline" by the AAMD definition and would not even be labeled as mentally retarded, using a traditional 3% criterion. The mean IQ dropped sharply for each successive category on the scale. Those nominated 3 or 4 times had a mean IQ of 61.3. The comprehensively retarded living in the community, group 4, had a mean IQ of 50.9, and the comprehensively retarded living in institutions had a mean IQ of 40.9. The correlation between IQ and situational retardation score was $-.55$ ($p < .001$). As a person became more comprehensively retarded from a social system perspective his IQ decreased.

Physical Disabilities showed a similar linear relationship to situational retardation. Those who were most situationally retarded had a mean physical disability score of .7, which increased for each successive category, 1.5, 2.3, 2.4, and 3.4. The correlation between physical disability score and situational retardation score was .12 ($p<.001$). Persons with IQs of 60 and below and two or more physical disabilities were highly visible, and more individuals and agencies in the community defined them as mental retardates than persons with borderline IQs and few physical disabilities.

The sociocultural characteristics of persons in the five categories also differed significantly and in linear fashion. In general, the percentage of Anglos increased progressively from the situationally to the comprehensively retarded. The percentage of Mexican-Americans and Blacks decreased progressively ($p<.001$). There were proportionately more comprehensively retarded Anglos in the community than in institutions and fewer comprehensively retarded Mexican-Americans and Blacks in the community than in institutions. The most important finding, however, is that situational retardation, i.e., playing the role of the retardate in some social systems but not in others, characterizes significantly more Mexican-American and Black retardates than Anglo retardates. The ethnic characteristics of the comprehensively retarded group closely approximated the ethnic distribution of the community. The situationally retarded were disproportionately drawn from minority ethnic groups.

A similar linear pattern holds for the other two sociocultural variables studied. The situationally retarded were from significantly lower socioeconomic statuses than the comprehensively retarded and were significantly more likely to live in segregated minority or integrated residential areas. The mean housing-value decile for the situationally retarded was 4.5, while that for the comprehensively retarded living in the community was 6.6, and that for the comprehensively retarded in institutions was 5.6 ($p<.001$). Over half the situationally retarded lived in minority segregated or integrated neighborhoods, but only 29.8% of the comprehensively retarded living in the community lived in such neighborhoods, and only 35.6% of the totally retarded in institutions had families that live in such neighborhoods.

In order to determine which of these five variables accounted for the greatest amount of variance in level of retardation from a social system perspective, we did a stepwise multiple regression using the situational retardation score as the dependent variable and the two clinical and three sociocultural variables as independent variables. When all five variables were used simultaneously, the multiple correlation coefficient was .59, accounting for 34.8% of the variance in situational retardation. The most important single variable was IQ ($r = .55$), accounting for

Table 5: Characteristics of Persons at Various Levels of Situational Retardation from a Social System Perspective

Clinical Characteristics	Situational Retardation—— 1 (N = 540)	2 (N = 111)	—Comprehensive 3 (N = 77)	4 (N = 47)	Retardation 5 (N = 103)	Significance Level[a] r	p
Mean IQ	70.4	69.8	61.3	50.9	40.9	−.55	<.001
Mean Physical Disabilities	.7	1.5	2.3	2.4	3.4	.12	<.001
Sociocultural Characteristics[b]							
% Anglo	48.1	66.7	68.8	85.1	71.8		
% Mexican-American	36.5	21.6	19.5	10.6	18.4	−.24	<.001
% Black	11.9	10.8	7.8	4.3	5.8		
Mean Housing Decile	4.5	5.1	5.3	6.6	5.6	.07	<.001
% Living in Segregated Minority or Integrated Area	52.2	45.0	39.0	29.8	35.6	.08	<.01

[a] Linear correlations were calculated between situational retardation score and IQ; Physical Disability Score; Housing Value Decile; Ethnic Group dichotomized Anglo vs Mexican-American and Black; and Residential Areas dichotomized Segregated Minority and Integrated vs Segregated Majority.

[b] Ethnic percentages do not add up to 100% because 28 persons were classified as "other."

Table 6: Situational Retardation Scores of Persons Nominated by Various Social Systems

Social System	Situational Retardation— 1 %	2 %	—Comprehensive 3 %	Retardation 4 %	5 %	Significance Level[a] r	p
Public Schools (N=429)	67.4	11.9	8.7	4.6	7.3	−.14	<.001
Medical Organizations (N=166)	48.2	16.9	14.5	10.8	9.6	.08	<.01
Law Enforcement (N=48)	37.5	33.3	14.6	4.2	10.4	.04	NS
Private Service Organizations (N=68)	36.8	7.4	19.1	22.0	14.7	.16	<.001
Religious Organizations (N=85)	30.6	11.8	22.4	27.0	8.2	.18	<.001
Public Welfare–Vocational Rehabilitation (N=68)	27.9	25.0	27.9	17.6	1.5	.10	<.01
Neighbor Nominees (N=244)	27.0	18.4	20.5	18.4	15.6	.37	<.001
Private Facilities for MR (N=72)	12.5	8.3	27.8	37.5	13.9	.30	<.001
Department of Mental Hygiene (N=119)	9.2	9.2	14.3	10.1	57.1	.57	<.001

[a] Linear correlations were calculated between situational retardation score and whether the individual was nominated by a particular social system as a mental retardate. N=878

30.2% of the variance, but the next most significant variable was ethnic group (r = .21), which increased the multiple correlation coefficient to .58. Housing value ranked next (r = .15), and physical disabilities ranked fourth (r = .12).

Source of the Situational Retardate

Which types of community organizations are most likely to nominate the situational retardate? Who is responsible for their labeling?

Table 6 shows the percentage of persons nominated by each of the nine sources of labeled retardates who fall into each category of situational retardation. The sources have been rank ordered by the percentage of their nominees scoring "1" on the index.

The Public Schools are the heaviest contributors to situational retardation. Over 67% of the persons labeled by them are in category "1," and almost 80% of their nominees are in categories "1" and "2." Looked at in another way, over half of the 540 persons (53.3%) who are situationally retarded were labeled by the Public Schools.

Almost half of the 166 persons labeled by Medical Organizations were also situational retardates. This figure undoubtedly reflects the relatively large number of persons with IQs above 80 who were nominated by medical doctors. Many of these persons were diagnosed using a medical model exclusively, and were not labeled as retarded by other organizations, especially those who rely on the statistical model of normal in making diagnoses. Law Enforcement Organizations ranked next in the proportion of their nominees who were situational retardates (37.5%), with Private Service Organizations close behind (36.8%).

Only about one-fourth of the persons nominated by neighbors or by Public Welfare–Vocational Rehabilitation were situational retardates, and almost none of those nominated by Private Facilities for the Mentally Retarded and the Department of Mental Hygiene were in this category. Persons in institutions were given a score of 5. The high rate of comprehensive retardation in the group nominated by the Department of Mental Hygiene is understandable because over half of those nominated by this agency were institutionalized. However, the extent of social system retardation for persons nominated by Private Facilities for the Mentally Retarded is very similar to that for the Department of Mental Hygiene, and most of these nominees were noninstitutionalized. If we add categories "4" and "5" together, the comprehensively retarded in the community and in institutions, 67.2% of the Department of Mental Hygiene nominees and 51.4% of the nominees from Private Facilities for the Mentally Retarded were comprehensively retarded.

To determine which source of nominees was most highly correlated with situational retardation scores, we did a stepwise multiple regression with the situational retardation score as the dependent variable and nominating organizations as the independent variables.

Being nominated by the Department of Mental Hygiene was most highly correlated with comprehensive retardation ($r = .57$), followed by being nominated by a neighbor ($r = .37$). These two sources of nominees together accounted for 41% of the variance in situational retardation score ($R = .64$). The next most highly correlated formal organization was Private Facilities for the Mentally Retarded ($r = .30$), which, together with the preceding two sources, accounted for 45% of the variance in situational retardation ($R = .67$). Persons reported by any one of these three sources as mentally retarded had a high probability of being nominated by other sources and of playing the role of retardate in many of the social systems in which they participated.

The Public Schools were at the other end of the continuum. There was a correlation of $-.14$ ($p<.001$) between nomination by the Public Schools and being comprehensively retarded. That is, persons who were comprehensively retarded were significantly *less* likely to have been nominated by the Public Schools. *Public School nominees were significantly more likely to be situationally retarded. Situational retardation is primarily a product of the labeling process in the Public School. The Public Schools, more than any other social system in the community, produce the "six-hour retardate."*

Summary and Conclusions

Our analysis has shown that the sociocultural characteristics of neighbor nominees conform closely to those of the community and differ significantly from the characteristics of persons labeled as mentally retarded by clinical organizations. Our findings indicate that lay persons are using an evaluation system in defining mental retardation that is similar to the dimensions measured by the IQ test and physical disability score. The difference between the sociocultural characteristics of persons defined as mentally retarded by neighbors and by clinical organizations appears to lie in their level of expectation. Persons nominated by neighbors have a significantly lower mean IQ and more physical disabilities than persons on the clinical case register.

The same is true for children rated in the lowest 16% on a "slow–bright" rating scale by their families. Minority ethnic groups and low socioeconomic levels are *not* overrepresented among persons perceived as subnormal by their parents even though parent ratings are correlated with IQ test score, adaptive behavior score, and, to a lesser extent, physical disability.

When situational retardation was measured using an index classifying labeled retardates according to the number of nominations received and their living arrangements, the situationally retarded were found to have significantly higher IQs and fewer physical disabilities than the comprehensively retarded. They were also more likely to be from minority ethnic groups, living in segregated minority or integrated neighborhoods, and from lower socioeconomic status than the comprehensively retarded.

We concluded that lay definitions do not result in the same sociocultural biases as clinical definitions and that the situational retardate is primarily a product of the labeling process in formal organizations in the community, especially the Public Schools.

Chapter 7

THE LABELING PROCESS IN THE PUBLIC SCHOOLS

The public schools were the most significant formal organization in the social system epidemiology of mental retardation in the community. The schools not only labeled more persons as mentally retarded than did any other formal organization but also held the most central position in the network of formal organizations in the community dealing with mental retardation. Many other organizations used the results of the labeling process in the public schools as the basis for assigning persons to the status of mental retardate, that is, they borrowed school labels. Finally, the public schools nominated more situational retardates than any other social system. For these reasons, we will conclude the section on the social system epidemiology with a study of the process by which a child achieves the social status of mental retardate in the public schools. The labeling process in the public schools has a significance that transcends the school system and has a profound impact on the characteristics of persons bearing the label of mental retardate in the entire community. The analysis of the operation of the school system in sorting, labeling, and placing children in the status of mental retardate is the most critical aspect of any *sociological* analysis of mental retardation as a deviant status in the community (Cicourel and Kitsuse, 1963).

The Social Structure of the Public School System

At the time of the study, the Riverside Unified School District had approximately 25,300 students enrolled in 22 elementary schools, 6 junior high schools, and 3 senior high schools. In addition, there was a special school for physically handicapped children. Although the schools varied greatly in the size of their student bodies and the size of their administrative staffs, all schools depended on the staff of the Public Personnel Department, located in the central administrative offices of the district, for psychological evaluations of children. The two primary responsibilities of the department were to organize and evaluate the findings from the extensive group-testing program of the district and to administer the individual intelligence tests that are required by state law before a child may be placed in a program for the mentally retarded. This department, directed by a psychologist with the rank of Associate Superintendent, controlled the movement of children into the many special programs offered by the school district. Any child who moved from the status of "normal" student in a regular classroom to "mentally retarded" student in a special education classroom had to have his new status certified and legitimated by one of the three certified psychologists working for the Pupil Personnel Department. Thus, the staff of this department played the role of legitimate labelers in the public school system. They, and only they, could certify a child as mentally retarded and eligible for special education.

Four sources of information were used to secure data for the analysis of the labeling process in the public schools: a study of the characteristics of all 1,234 children referred for any reason to the Pupil Personnel Department during a single school year, the "referral study"; a study of the characteristics of all children who had ever been labeled as mentally retarded by the schools and were still living in the geographic area of the study, the "retardate roster"; a content analysis of teachers' written evaluations of children who were referred as possibly mentally retarded, compared with children in the regular classroom, the "normative analysis"; and information from the household survey.

From the referral study, there emerged a relatively clear picture of eight stages through which children typically passed in achieving the status of mental retardate in the public schools. Each stage is identified by a pivotal decision made about the child. Each decision either moves the child closer to becoming a mental retardate or permits him to remain in the status of "normal" student. A child may proceed in regular progression through these stages to the status of retardate or he may return to his "normal" student status by means of various escapes depicted as slides in Figure 3.

Stage 1: Enrollment in Public School

The first step in becoming retarded in the public schools is to enroll in the public school system rather than one of the private schools available in the city. At the time of our study, 85.7% of the children six through fifteen years of age in Riverside were enrolled in public schools and, hence, exposed to the risk of being assigned to the status of mental retardate in the public schools. Of those not in public schools, 9.3% were attending one of the eight Catholic schools serving the community, 3.4% were attending other private schools, and 1.6% were in special schools of various kinds, such as the School for the Deaf, the school at Juvenile Hall, the Indian School, and the private school

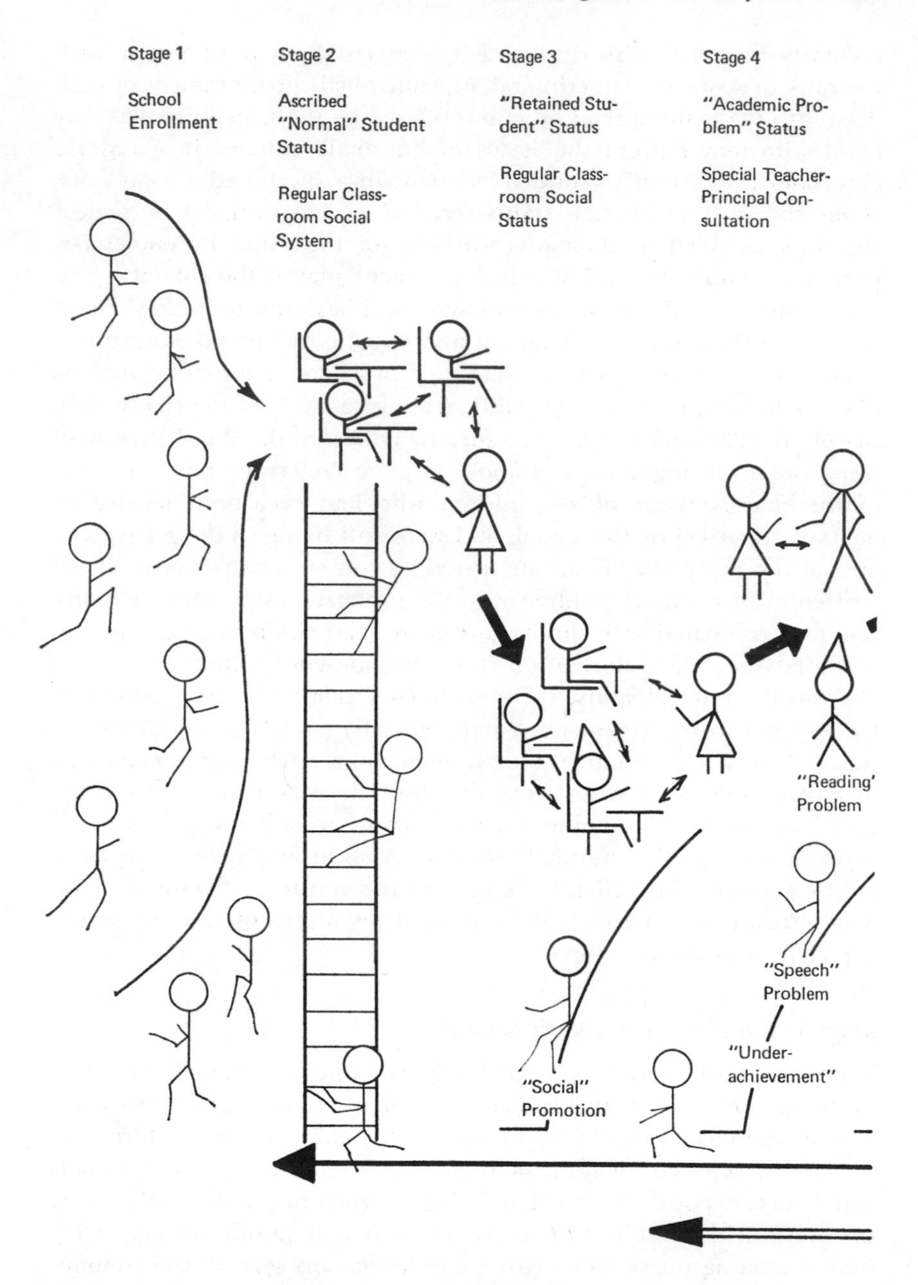

Figure 3: Achieving the Status of Mental Retardate in the Public Schools

Stage 5	Stage 6	Stage 7	Stage 8
"Case-to-be-evaluated" Status	"The Labeling"	Achieved "MR" Status	Vacating the "MR" Status
Psychological Testing and Evaluation	Status Assignment	Status Assumption in "MR" Class	Surrendering the Label

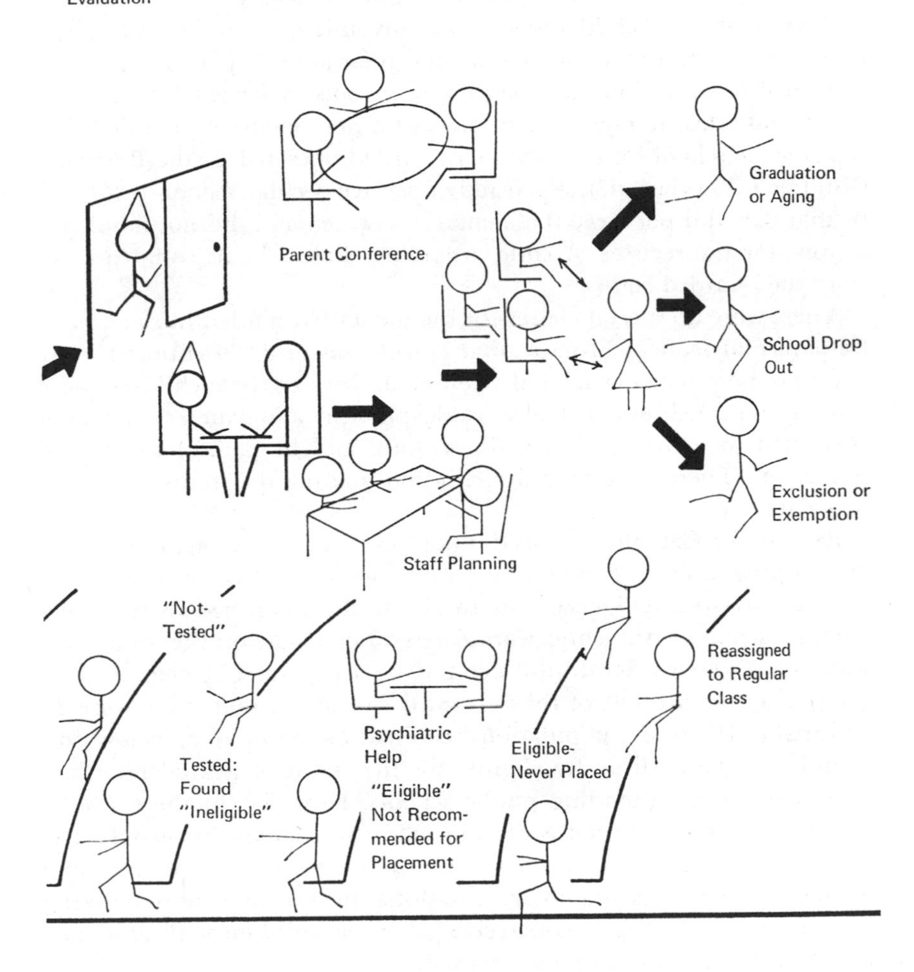

══ Return to "Normal" Student Status

for the mentally retarded operated by the Retarded Children's Association. Undoubtedly, some of the children not attending public schools at the time of our study had attended public schools in the past or might enroll in public schools in the future. However, at the time of our study, only about 86.0% of the school-age population could potentially be channeled through the Pupil Personnel Office and into the status of mental retardate in the public schools.

Does the school a child attends make any difference in the probability that he will achieve the status of mental retardate? As part of our study of formal organizations, all the private schools in Riverside were contacted and asked to nominate persons who were mentally retarded. Except for the school for the mentally retarded operated by the Retarded Children's Association, the privately operated secular schools informed us that they did not serve the mentally retarded and did not nominate anyone for the register. A child attending those schools could not occupy the retarded status.

There were no special classes for the mentally retarded in the Catholic parochial schools. From a total enrollment of 2,800 children, only two were nominated as mentally retarded. Both of these children were severely retarded and had observable physical anomalies. They were permitted to "attend" classes, do errands, and be part of the life of the school. There were no other children holding the status of mental retardate.

Because the Catholic schools did not have any achievement or ability testing program at the time of our study, we secured permission to administer group intelligence tests to all children enrolled in their elementary schools.[1] Any child who scored 90 or below on the group test was administered a Stanford-Binet LM by a psychologist employed by the project. As a result of this screening, we found that there were 27 children (1.1% of the population) who had an IQ of 79 or below and would have been clinically eligible for the status of mental retardate if they had been attending public schools. However, in the Catholic schools, they held the status of "normal" students and incurred little risk of being labeled as retarded, since there were no statuses available for mental retardates and no organizational mechanisms for diagnosing or labeling them. Teachers perceived them as children with academic problems but not as mentally retarded.

Who were the children who were not attending public schools and, hence, were not exposed to the risk of being labeled a mental retardate? How did their social characteristics differ from those of the children

[1] We thank the Educational Testing Services and the California Test Bureau for providing these intelligence tests for our use.

attending public schools? We compared the characteristics of the 1,565 children in the household survey between the ages of six and fifteen who attended Riverside schools with the 237 children in the survey not attending public schools and found them significantly different in age, sex, religion, socioeconomic status, education of parents, ethnic group, and school achievement. Significantly more of the children not in Riverside public schools were in the elementary grades (66.7% vs 50.1%) and were ten years of age or younger (56.5% vs 50.8%). Elementary school is the period during which a child is most likely to be referred for evaluation as a possible mental retardate. For example, of all the children on the retardate roster of persons who had ever held the status of mental retardate in the public schools, 85.0% were referred and placed during elementary school and only 15.0% were placed during secondary school. Since children attending private schools are more likely not to be enrolled in the public schools during the elementary school years, they are less exposed to the risk of labeling and placement.

Significantly more of the children in private than in public schools were males (55.3% vs 50.4%) and more of them were two or more years behind the grade normally expected for a child of their age (8.0% vs 4.0%). Because most of the private schools in Riverside are operated by the Catholic Church, it is not surprising to find that 74.2% of the children in private schools have at least one Catholic parent, and that this is true of only 27.2% of the children in the public schools. In spite of the fact that most Mexican-American families in Riverside are Catholic, the proportion of Mexican-American children in public schools is approximately the same as the proportion in private schools, indicating that most Mexican-American parents send their children to public schools regardless of their religious preference. On the other hand, about half of the Anglo families in Riverside with one or more Catholic parents were sending their children to parochial schools. Almost all Black children attended public schools. As a result, there were significantly more Anglo children in private schools and more Black children in public schools than would be expected by chance.

Public school children came significantly more often from lower-status homes and from homes in which the parents had had less education than the parents of children in private schools. For example, 36.1% of the public school children lived on blocks rated in the five lowest housing-value deciles, while only 27.8% of the children in private schools lived on such blocks. Of the mothers of public school children, 30.3% had less than a high school education, compared with 23.6% of the mothers of children in private schools.

To summarize, except for the children in the private school for the mentally retarded and the two children nominated by the Catholic schools, none of the children who were in private schools in Riverside held the status of mental retardate. However, there were at least twenty-seven children holding the status of "normals" in Catholic schools who would have been clinically eligible for placement in the status of mental retardate if they had been attending public schools. Children attending Catholic schools incurred relatively little risk of being labeled as mental retardates, unless they were visibly and severely deviant.

We found that there is a tendency for private schools to attract disproportionate numbers of children from the population which, in the public schools, has a higher risk of being suspected as mentally retarded: males, children below their age-grade norm, and children in the elementary grades. These children, who are thus removed from the risk of being labeled retarded, are also more likely to come from higher-status Anglo families.

These differentials cannot be accounted for on the basis of any systematic policy of exclusion on the part of the public schools. In the school year of the "referral study," only five children were permanently excluded from the public school. Two were 16-year-olds expelled for persistent truancies; a third was a 15-year-old involved with law enforcement agencies, who subsequently moved to another town; and only two had IQs low enough to qualify them for special education. One was a 17-year-old male with an IQ of 53; and the other, a 6-year-old male with an IQ of 55. Both had manifested bizarre behavior patterns in the classroom. Thirteen others were suspended because of psychiatric problems but were later readmitted. It is the parental decision to enroll a child in public rather than in a private school and not any action on the part of the public school itself which constitutes the first stage in the labeling.

Stage 2: "Normal Student" in the Regular Classroom

Almost all children begin their public school careers in the ascribed status of "normal" student in a regular classroom. They must achieve the many other statuses available in the school system, including that of mental retardate. The only exceptions to this rule are children with obvious physical disabilities who are either exempted from school or are immediately placed in the school for the physically handicapped. Some of these children are also labeled as mental retardates, but retardation tends to be a secondary diagnosis. Their school status is determined primarily by their physical rather than their intellectual limitations.

Within the boundaries of the regular classroom, children gradually differentiate into a variety of social categories as a result of interaction with their teachers and their peers. Although peer differentiation is important, it is primarily the expectations of the teacher that determines who will be identified and referred as a possible candidate for the status of retardate.

The teacher is expected to teach the children in her classroom the academic and intellectual skills prescribed for their grade level, to maintain the class as a functioning system, and to socialize children so that their interpersonal conduct is integrative rather than disruptive to the classroom. Her major leverage in this socialization is her control of the system of formal rewards and punishments of the school. Because a teacher is limited in the extent to which she may use physical coercion or material rewards and punishments, she mainly controls behavior with one type of sanction, symbolic rewards. Socializing children to be motivated by symbolic rewards is one of her primary tasks. The school's near total dependence upon symbolic sanctions has produced an elaborate evaluation system, which uses status assignments as important symbolic rewards and punishments. These educational statuses are differentiated on four levels. The first level is differentiation within the classroom.

The classroom teacher constantly grades each child on his academic performance and his interpersonal behavior. The significance of an A or an S is reinforced by assigning children to statuses within the classroom on the basis of their graded performance. They are sorted into "the fast reading group," the "average reading group," the "slow readers," the "first group in arithmetic," the "second group in arithmetic," and so forth. As children move into junior high school, they may be assigned to arithmetic or social studies sections according to academic proficiency. In high school, they are sorted into various curricula, some leading to college and some leading to a terminal high school diploma. All such assignments serve the latent function of reinforcing the norms of the school.They reward exemplary performers by assigning them to valued groups and curricula and punish those who fail by assigning them to devalued positions.

All of the above statuses are within the boundaries of the regular classroom system. However, there are children whose behavior deviates sufficiently from that of "normal" student so that they intermittently hold statuses beyond those in the classroom system. At this second level of differentiation, students who excel may achieve valued extra classroom statuses such as being appointed a street-crossing guard, a lunch-room arranger, or room representative to the student government. Those with special interests and talents may achieve valued statuses in instrumental music, in the school chorus, or as tutors of younger students. At the other end of the scale, students who fail to meet the expectations of the pupil role may achieve disesteemed positions in the system, such as being sent for speech therapy, for remedial reading, for special tutorial assistance, or for detention after school. Although such statuses are devalued, the burden of stigmatization is relieved by the fact that the child occupies these positions intermittently and his primary status is still that of a "normal" pupil in a regular classroom.

A third level of differentiation within the school system is that of "retained" student. Every child is expected to move each year to successively higher grades. This role expectancy is relatively easy to achieve because there is a general policy favoring "social" promotions in order to keep children with their age peers. We found that 95% of the children six through fifteen years of age in our survey sample met the age-grade norm, that is, were within two years of the grade appropriate for their chronological age. The teacher usually is the one who first proposes that a child who is not performing at "grade level" be retained. Although the child who "flunks" is removed from his status with his age peers and is relocated with a group of younger children, he still remains with the "normals."

Finally, there is a fourth level of differentiation, which removes the pupil completely from the "regular" classroom by assigning him a status in a "special education" class. This removal clearly sets him apart as one so abnormal that he cannot operate effectively within "normal" classroom expectancies. Deviation in either a positive or negative direction may precipitate removal from the regular classroom. In Riverside, there were special accelerated classes for the gifted, those with IQs of 130 and over, as well as special classes for the "retarded," those with IQs under 80.

Thus, in addition to her more commonly recognized functions, the classroom teacher allocates status rewards and punishments to children in her classroom. Her focal position in the labeling process can be readily documented. Of the 1,234 children referred for evaluation to the Pupil Personnel Department during the year of our referral study, *two-thirds* were first referred by a classroom teacher. Of the 71 children eventually recommended for placement in special education during that school year, *all but two* were initially referred by a classroom teacher. *None* was referred by a parent or relative. Of the 271 children actively occupying the status of educable mental retardate in the public schools during the year of our study, 90% had originally been referred by a teacher and only 2% had originally been referred by parents or relatives. Three percent were referred by the Probation Department and 3% were interdistrict transfers who had been placed in special education in some other school system before coming to Riverside. Clearly, the classroom teacher is the primary gatekeeper to the status of mental retardate. If she does not perceive a child as deviant and initiate formal evaluation proceedings, that child is unlikely to be labeled as retarded.

As noted earlier, not all classroom teachers in the school system are in equally pivotal positions. The elementary teacher, especially the teacher in the first four grades, is the chief identifier. Once a child has passed the critical years, the probability of his being labeled mentally retarded declines markedly. For example, in the referral study we found that 52 of the 71 placed in special education during that school year (73%) were below the fifth grade at the time of referral. These 52 children were selected from 12,300 children enrolled in elementary classes, an incidence rate of approximately 4 per 1,000. The 19 referred from higher grades produced an incidence rate only half as high, about 2 per 1,000. Most of the children actually placed in special education during the year of the referral study were referred because the teacher regarded them as mentally retarded. Fifty-three, or 75%, of those placed during that year were specifically referred as candidates for special education, 14, or 20%, were referred for academic difficulty, and only 5% were originally referred for reasons unrelated to mental retardation and were subsequently found to be eligible for the status of mental retardate.

Of the 271 children in special education classes during our study year, 196 (73%) had first been referred before the fifth grade and 83% had been referred during elementary school. The elementary teacher is the primary labeler. Her norms determine which children will be exposed to the risk of holding the status of retardate.

What are the standards which the elementary teacher applies when she decides that a child is sufficiently deviant to be referred for psychological evaluation? What teacher expectations does the child violate who eventually achieves the status of mental retardate?

The Normative System of the Elementary Classroom Teacher

To answer these questions, we decided to analyze the evaluations made by elementary classroom teachers of children whom they referred as suspected mental retardates with a matched sample of children not referred. The cumulative record files of 74 of the children referred by teachers and placed in special education classes during the two-year period of the study contained verbal evaluations made by the regular classroom teachers before referral. In a separate data file, we had copies of the cumulative record of over 1,700 elementary school children in the regular classes of the school district.[2] From this data pool, it was possible to match the 74 children referred for special education with children in the regular class by sex, ethnic group, school, and grade at the time of referral. The matched samples were 57% male; 23% Anglo; 55% Mexican-American; 22% Black; and 92% in elementary school.

While only 18% of the children in the matched sample selected from the the regular classroom had repeated one or more grades, 74% of the children who were referred for evaluation as possible mental retardates had failed at least one grade, and 12% had failed two or more grades.

We calculated the grade point average for each child in motor skills, social skills, music and art, and academic subjects based on grades he received from his regular classroom teacher. All the regular classroom teachers, who had graded each referred child prior to placement were included because, together, they develop a collective definition of the child as "mentally retarded." These grade point averages were compared to grades given by the regular classroom teachers to nonreferred children.

The children referred for special education had been graded significantly lower in all four areas by their regular classroom teachers, than the matched children who were not referred ($p<.001$). The grade point averages for children referred and placed in the retardate status were 2.0 in motor skills, 1.8 in social skills, 2.0 in music and art, and 1.3 in academic subjects. The corresponding averages for nonreferred children were 2.3, 2.3, 2.4, and 2.1.

Every spring, each classroom teacher is expected to write a brief, verbal description of each child in her class. These descriptions are permanently recorded in the child's cumulative record folder and become part of the collective definition of the child from the viewpoint of the school. These evaluations are confidential and are intended to help subsequent teachers understand the child. Although the school system provides each teacher with a general guide containing a list of areas which she may wish to cover in her comments, she is free to record any observations she believes are important and is in no way bound by the guidelines. Therefore, the verbal evaluations of children are

[2] The children in this data file were part of the study of school desegregation funded by the California State Department of Education, Bureau of Intergroup Relations, McAteer Grants Nos. M5-14, M6-14, M7-14, and M8-14.

relatively spontaneous expressions of a teacher's opinion of a child after teaching him for one year.

Each verbal description was first divided into meaning units and each unit was coded independently. Every time a new idea was introduced or a new behavior described, that adjective or phrase, as the case might be, was coded as a separate meaning unit. Fifty categories for classifying the meaning units were developed on the basis of teachers' comments contained in over 500 cumulative records from the Riverside School District. Categories were defined so as to describe not only the nature of the behavior but the positive or negative direction of the evaluation. For example, there are separate categories for comments about low mental ability and high mental ability; high perseverance and low perseverance; good adjustment and poor adjustment; and so forth.

Three coders read the files, divided each record into meaning units, and classified each unit. In the reliability check of the coding of 1,500 randomly selected meaning units, there was complete coder agreement on 84.2% of the classifications and agreement between two of the three coders on 14.3% of the cases. Therefore, we concluded that the coding was sufficiently reliable to warrant analysis.

Three types of spontaneous teacher comments significantly differentiated the children referred as mentally retarded from those not referred ($p<.001$). A significantly larger percentage of the referred children's records contained spontaneous comments about their low mental ability (79.6% vs 35.4%), and a significantly smaller percentage of the referred children's records contained spontaneous comments about their high mental ability (1.6% vs 44.3%) or their academic competence (6.8% vs 30.4%). There was a tendency for those referred for special education to be perceived as having poor adjustment, low perseverance, and low competence in English, but these differences did not reach statistical significance in this sample. A child's ability to play the student role and appear busy were significant in another study in which a group of labeled children was compared with a group of nonlabeled children with IQs under 80 matched for ethnic group (Mercer, 1970).

Stage 3: The Retained Student Status

For most children, the next step toward retardation after failing the role expectations of the elementary classroom teacher is to be retained for a grade. Only 28.0% of the children who were in special education classes at the time of our study had gone directly into special education without first repeating at least one grade, 62.5% of them had repeated one grade, and 9.5% of them had repeated two or more grades.

Who were the children in the Riverside school system who were most likely to be retained? In the household survey, a child who was two or more years behind the grade that would be expected for his age was classified as failing the "age-grade" norm. When we compared the characteristics of children in the Riverside schools who were behind the age-grade norm, i.e., holding a "retained student" status, with the characteristics of children who were holding a normal student status, we found that significantly more males were below the age-grade norm (66.7% vs 49.7%). The children holding the status of retained student tended to come from homes that differ from the modal sociocultural configuration of the community. One-third fewer Anglo students were in the retained category than would be expected from their proportion in the population, but four times more Mexican-American children were behind age-grade norm than would be expected. Children holding a retained student status were more likely to come from homes in which the occupation of the head was a blue-collar job (69.4% vs 43.5%) and was rated 0–29 on the socioeconomic index (60.3% vs 28.6%). More of their homes were valued in the lowest five deciles (71.4% vs 34.6%). The characteristics of their families were also significantly different from those of children holding a "normal" status. Significantly more retained children came from families in which the head of household was not reared in the United States (22.2% vs 4.3%) and from families that did not use English all the time at home (39.7% vs 11.2%). They were significantly less likely to live in a family with a male head of household (81.0% vs 91.5%) and were more likely to come from wholly or partially dependent families (15.9% vs 6.5%). They were also more likely to come from families in which the head of household had lived in the United States less than ten years. This interrelated set of characteristics closely parallels the modal sociocultural characteristics of the community described in chapter 3. Children from socioculturally modal backgrounds were less likely to be behind grade in school.

Because of the disproportionately large number of children of Mexican heritage who were behind their age-grade norm, we decided to compare the Mexican-American children in our sample who were behind in school with those who were not behind. There were no sex differences within the Mexican group, indicating that the overall sex differences in school failure are produced primarily by the non-Mexican boys, who are significantly more likely to hold the "retained" student status than non-Mexican girls. Mexican-American children who were behind the age-grade norm were more likely to come from the homes that spoke Spanish most frequently; from homes in which the head of household was separated, widowed, or divorced; from families depending on welfare; from families living in homes valued at less than $10,000; from families in which the head of household had lived in the United States less than ten years; from families in which the head of household and his wife had less than an eighth-grade education; and from families rated 0–29 on the socioeconomic index based on the occupation of the head of household. The same sociocultural characteristics that were related to being labeled as a mental retardate also differentiated the Mexican-American children who failed in school from those who succeeded.

It is not possible from our data to determine which children were receiving "social promotions" and, thus, maintaining their "normal" student status in spite of low academic performance. However, it is clear that holding a "retained student" status is the first step on the path to retardation in the public schools, and the children who are held back in school have distinctive social characteristics that are very similar to the characteristics of children who are eventually labeled retarded and placed in special classes.

Stage 4: Referral by the Principal

When a child is retained and continues to fail the teacher's expectations, he has reached a critical phase in the labeling process, Stage 4. Few children are retained for more than one grade, because educators feel that every child should be kept with his age peers. Should he be given a "social promotion" for the next year, recommended for some special remedial program, or referred for psychological evaluation? At this point, the teacher is likely to confer with the principal because all referrals for psychological evaluation must go through his office.

There are many alternatives open to the principal. The child may be labeled a "late bloomer" and given a social promotion. He may be labeled a reading problem or a speech problem and referred for special help in these areas while remaining in the regular classroom. Or he may be sent for evaluation and diagnosis by a certified psychologist in the Pupil Personnel Department.

We have little information on the kinds of considerations that impinge on this crucial decision because we have no information on the characteristics of all of the children whom teachers discussed with principals in the context of making a possible referral for psychological evaluation. However, we can make some inferences about the nature of the process by analyzing the characteristics of all children actually referred to the Pupil Personnel Department by teachers and principals during the year of the referral study. The Pupil Personnel Department has a form that is completed by every principal making a student referral. This form contains information about each child's age, grade, sex, elementary school, the reason for referral, and a verbal description of the child's problem as seen by the principal and teacher.

During the school year of the referral study, 1,243 children were handled by the Pupil Personnel Department, and 747 of these children were referred by a teacher-principal team. All children referred during that year faced the risk of being tested by a psychologist and found eligible for placement in the status of mental retardate. None of the nonreferred children in the district were exposed to this risk.

Thirty-one percent of the 747 children sent by teachers and principals were referred as candidates for classes for the gifted. Another 29.8% of the children referred were sent primarily because of behavior and disciplinary problems, 19.5% were referred because of academic difficulty with no mention of special education, and 8.3% were referred for evaluation specifically because the teacher-principal team believed they should be placed in special education classes for the mentally retarded.

There was a consistent decline in the rate of referral as grade level increased. The total rate for all referrals dropped from 69.7 per 1,000 in elementary school to 30.1 per 1,000 in junior high school and 20.6 in senior high school. Thus, an elementary school child was twice as likely to be referred to the central offices as a junior high child and was three times more likely to be referred than a high school child.

There were also large differences in rates of referral per 1,000 when elementary schools were compared with each other. Some schools had a rate of referral five times larger than others. We found that these differences in rates were not related to the affluence of the neighborhood nor to the percentage of minority groups served by the school, but were related to at least two other factors: differences among principals and differences by school size. Some principals were more willing to refer problem cases to the central offices, while others regarded referral as a last resort. Schools with large enrollments tended to have lower rates of referral than smaller schools. The inverse ratio between size and rate was related to a procedure that scheduled each school for an equal number of days of psychological services, regardless of size. Principals in the large schools had to make selections from among students referred by teachers so as to reduce the number to be serviced to a size that could be managed in the time allocated. This practice resulted in a lower rate per 1,000 pupils for large schools but allowed principals in smaller schools considerable latitude in the selection process. Consequently, the child in the larger school had a lower probability of being referred for evaluation and was exposed to less risk of attaining the status of mental retardate than the child attending the smaller school (Robbins, Mercer, and Myers, 1967).

Table 7 presents the characteristics of children who were exposed to the risk of being labeled as mentally retarded at various stages in the labeling process and compares them with the characteristics of the sample of public school children six through fifteen years of age who appeared in the household survey.

When we looked specifically at only those children referred by the teacher-principal team and compared the characteristics of these children with the characteristics of all public school children of the same age in the household survey, we found that teachers and principals were referring significantly more boys (65.2% of referrals vs 50.4% in the school population), significantly more children who were behind their age-grade norm (27.2% of the referrals vs 4.0% of the school population), and significantly more children from the lower grades. The mean grade of children referred by teachers and principals was 4.1, while the average grade for the public school population between five and fifteen year of age was 6.0 ($p<.001$). Children of all ethnic groups were referred in their approximate proportions. Eighty-one percent of the school population was Anglo, 11.0% Mexican-American, and 7.9% Black. About 83% of the children referred by teacher-principal teams for evaluation were Anglo, 6.9% Mexican-American, and 10.3% Black. Mexican-American children were slightly underrepresented in the population referred, and Anglo and Black children were overrepresented. In addition, there was no difference in the average housing-value decile for the two groups. Thus, in the total initial referrals made to the Pupil Personnel Department by teachers and principals for any reason—behavior, special education, or gifted—there was no socioeconomic bias and only a slight ethnic bias, which tended to underrepresent Mexican-American children.

Stage 5: Psychological Testing and Evaluation

In California, a child cannot become mentally retarded in the public schools without an intelligence test individually administered by a trained person certified by the State. Certification by a legitimate labeler

Table 7: Exposure to Risk of Being Labeled Retarded in the Public Schools at Various Stages in the Labeling Process

Characteristics	Sample Public School Population (6–15 yrs age) (N = 1565) %	Referred by Principal to Pupil Personnel Department (N = 747) %	Tested by Psychologist (N = 865) %	Found Eligible for Placement IQ 79– (N = 134) %	Recommended for Placement (N = 81) %	Placed in Status of MR (N = 71) %
Sex						
Male	50.4	65.2	63.1	59.0	62.5	69.1
Female	49.6	34.8	36.9	41.0	37.5	30.9
Ethnic Group						
Anglo	81.0	82.7	82.9	47.4	37.9	32.1
Mexican-American	11.0	6.9	7.6	32.7	40.9	45.3
Black	7.9	10.3	9.5	19.8	21.2	22.6
Social Status						
Housing Decile (1–5)	36.1	39.4	38.8	70.7	72.7	74.6
Below Age-Grade Norm	4.0	27.2	27.3	57.4	51.9	52.9

is required by law before a child can achieve the status of mental retardate. There are three phases in the psychological labeling process: being selected for testing, failing the test, and being recommended for placement in special education. A child must pass through each of these phases in order to achieve the status of retardate.

Whom Does the Psychologist Select for Testing?

It is not usually possible for a school psychologist to administer an individual intelligence test to every child referred for evaluation. Therefore, each psychologist has to decide which children he will test. If he decides not to test a child, that child cannot hold the status of mental retardate in the public school.

There were 865 children in the referral study who had been administered an individual intelligence test by a school psychologist, 70.1% of the total. There were 369 (29.9%) of the referred children who were not tested. These children escaped the risk of being assigned the status of mental retardate. None of the variables presented in table 7 differentiated the characteristics of the children tested from the characteristics of the children referred by principals and teachers. The distribution by sex and ethnic group were almost identical, as were the average housing value and the percentage behind their age-grade norm. However, some characteristics not shown on table 7 did differentiate the children tested from those not tested. Source of referral and reason for referral were significantly related to the probability that a child would be tested ($p<.001$). Children referred by a principal-teacher team were tested in 76.6% of the cases, and those referred by a parent or relative were tested 63.6% of the time. If the child was referred by a community agency, there was a 33.3% probability he would be tested. If referred by a counselor or a dean, there was only a 19.4% chance that he would be tested.

Reason for referral also distinguished tested from nontested children. When the teacher or principal referred the child for evaluation for placement in a specific program outside the regular classroom, such as a class for the mentally retarded or for the gifted, the probabilities were approximately 9 in 10 that the psychologist would test him. If, however, he was referred because of academic difficulty with no reference to special education, the probability that he would be tested dropped to 7 in 10. If he was referred primarily because of behavior problems and the referral did not mention special placement or academic difficulty, his chances of being tested were only 4 in 10. Children who were tested were, on an average, significantly younger (mean age 9.8 vs 12.8 years), were in significantly lower grades (mean of 3.4 vs 6.3 grades), and were more likely to be from higher housing-value deciles (deciles 6.3 vs 5.9).

This pattern clearly demonstrates the key role of the teacher-principal in the labeling process. Not only did they decide which children would be sent for psychological evaluation and thus subjected to the risk of being identified as eligible for placement in the status of mental retardate but they also determined, to a large extent, which children would probably be tested by the psychologist. If they referred a child for evaluation for special education in a class either for the mentally retarded or for the gifted, there was a high probability he would be tested. If they referred him only for academic difficulties, there was a lower probability he would be tested. If they mentioned only behavior problems, he probably would not be tested.

Screening both for the "gifted" and the "mentally retarded" takes place very early in the child's career in the public school. Such referrals were most likely to be tested, hence the low grade level of the tested compared with the nontested children. The large number of children referred for placement in classes for the "gifted" during the referral year (378) also explains the relatively high socioeconomic level and Anglo background of tested as compared with nontested children. Those referred for the "gifted" program tended to come from significantly higher socioeconomic levels and Anglo homes.

Who Failed the IQ Test?

Although the school psychologist has some discretion in certifying which children are eligible for placement in the status of mental retardate, the general rule prior to 1971 was that children with an IQ below 80 were eligible for placement, while those with an IQ of 80 or above were not eligible. Once tested, a child's IQ becomes the most critical variable determining whether he retains the status of "normal" student or moves closer to the status of "mental retardate."

We compared the characteristicis of the 134 tested children who scored 79 or below on the intelligence test with those of the 731 children who tested 80 or higher. Boys who were tested failed the intelligence test at approximately the same rate at which they were referred, thus maintaining the surplus of males and making more males than females eligible for placement in special education. Fifty-seven percent of those who failed the IQ test were behind their age-grade norm. Significantly more Mexican-American and Black children failed the iintelligence test than Anglo children ($p<.001$). Only 47.4% of the children with IQ 79 or below were Anglos, while 32.7% were Mexican-American and 19.8% were Black. The children who scored 79 or below also came significantly more often from lower socioeconomic statuses as measured by the mean value of housing on the block on which they lived (p<.001).

This shift is most important. The 1,234 children referred to the Pupil Personnel Services were similar in ethnic distribution and socioeconomic status to the total population of the school district. This pattern continued until the point in the labeling process at which the intelligence test was administered. *As soon as the intelligence test was used, the higher failure rate of children from lower socioeconomic background and from minority homes produced the disproportions characteristic of classes for the mentally retarded.* Apparently, there is no ethnic or socioeconomic bias in the type of children referred by the principal-teacher team or tested by the school psychologist. The disproportionate number of low-status and minority children in special education classes first appears at the juncture in the referral process when standardized intelligence measures are used for diagnosis.

Children with an IQ of 79 or below were significantly more likely to have been referred primarily for placement in special education than to have been referred for low academic performance, behavior problems, or for other reasons. About one-half of those tested and found to have an IQ of 79 or below were referred, initially, as possible candidates for special education, while the other half of the failures were referred for other reasons. Only 4.1% of those with an IQ of 80 and over were referred for special education. Teachers were essentially conservative in their labeling.

Who Was Recommended for Placement?

Only 64.0% of the children with IQs of 79 or below in the year of the referral study were recommended by the psychologists for placement in special education. We compared the characteristics of the 53 children who were not recommended for placement, even though they were clinically eligible, with the 81 children recommended for placement.

The children who were eligible for placement but were not recommended by the psychologist and hence escaped the status of mental retardate were more likely to be Anglos (p<.01), to come from homes of higher socioeconomic levels (p<.05), and to have had teachers who referred them for some reason other than placement in special education (p<.001). *Their average IQ was not significantly higher than that of children who were recommended for placement* (71.4 vs 69.0). In fact, 20.0% of those not recommended for placement had IQs below 64.

On the other hand, those who were recommended for placement were more likely to be Mexican-Americans (40.9% of those recommended for placement vs 15.6% of those not recommended for placement), to be from low socioeconomic levels (mean housing decile 4.1

vs 5.2), and to have been referred by the teacher-principal team as a potential mental retardate (65.0% vs 25.5%). Once again, the teacher's recommendation emerges as a critical correlate of the psychologist's decision. A child who is eligible for the status of mental retardate on the basis of his IQ is significantly more likely to be recommended for placement in that status by the psychologist if the teacher originally referred the child to be evaluated for special education. If she referred the child for any other reason, he was significantly less likely to be recommended for placement, even though he was tested and was found clinically eligible.

Stage 6: The Labeling

Ten children were tested, had an IQ below 80, were recommended for placement by the psychologist, and still did not actually appear in the special education classes the year following the referral study. With this small number of cases, statistical comparisons are not feasible. The children who escaped the status of mental retardate, even at this late stage in the labeling process, tended to be young, Anglo females. Seventy percent of the children who were not placed were Anglos, and only 32.1% of those placed were Anglos. Eighty percent of those who escaped the label were under twelve years of age, while only 58.0% of those placed were this young. The average grade in school of the children who were placed was 4.3, compared with an average grade of 2.3 for those who were not placed.

We traced the ten children who escaped the mental retardate status to see exactly what had occurred in each case. We found that seven of these children escaped the status of mental retardate in Riverside when their families moved to another school district. We do not know whether these children were subsequently referred and labeled in their new schools.

The family of one seven-year-old girl enrolled her in Catholic school following the public school recommendation that she be placed in special education. She was not nominated by teachers in the parochial schools and did not hold the status of mental retardate in that system when we studied those schools. There were two Anglo girls in the third grade who remained in their regular classes in public school, even though they were recommended for placement by the psychologist. They were both originally referred by their teachers for behavior problems and academic difficulties but not for placement in special education. One had an IQ of 66, the other an IQ of 67. We do not know how it happened these girls retained their "normal" status. No parent conference was held in either case. The father of one girl held a high-level position in a local bank, and the other was a graduate engineer.

Stage 7: The Labeled

During the year of the referral study, there were 71 children who were recommended for placement and who actually appeared in special education classes the following year. Sixty-nine percent of these children were males, 74.6% were from homes in the lowest five deciles in housing value, and 61.7% were in kindergarten through fourth grade at the time of referral. Only 32.1% were Anglos, 45.3% were Mexican-Americans, and 22.6% were Blacks. The significance of these percentages is best understood when a comparison is made with the characteristics of the general population of the school district and the characteristics of children at various other stages in the labeling process as shown in Table 7.

If boys and girls were placed in the status of mental retardate in proportion to their percentage in the population, we would expect 36 boys and 35 girls to have achieved the status of mental retardate during the year of the referral study. Instead, 49 boys and 22 girls were placed, 36.0% more boys and 37.0% fewer girls than we would anticipate.

We found that 49.0% fewer Anglo children were placed in the status of mental retardate than would be expected from their proportion in the student population, and that the rate of placement for Mexican-American children was four times larger and for Black children three times larger than would be expected. These ethnic disproportions appear only at the point in the labeling process at which the IQ test is administered. Minority children are not referred by teachers at a higher rate than their percentage in the population, nor are they tested at a higher rate. *Following the intelligence test, ethnic disproportions continued to increase.* Although *47.4%* of those found eligible for placement were Anglos, only *37.9%* of those recommended for placement were Anglo and only *32.1%* of those placed were Anglo. On the other hand, the percentage of Mexican-American and Black children increased in subsequent stages. While *32.7%* of those eligible were Mexican-American, *40.9%* of those recommended and *45.3%* of those placed were of Mexican heritage. Black children made up *19.8%* of those eligible, *21.2%* of those recommended for placement, and *22.6%* of those actually placed.

Children from low-status homes (housing deciles 1–5) run twice the risk of being labeled as mentally retarded as do children from higher status homes. This disproportion also appears only at the point in the labeling process when the intelligence test is administered, and it continues to rise at each stage thereafter until 74.6% of the children placed are from the five lowest deciles, twice as many as appear in the general population. Clearly, children of nonmodal sociocultural backgrounds are exposed to the greatest risk of being labeled as mentally retarded in the public schools.

Children who are behind the age-grade norm are referred by teachers at a rate seven times greater than would be expected, and this disproportion jumps to thirteen times greater when the IQ test is administered. In the year of the referral study, over half the children placed were behind their age-grade norm.

Since it was possible that the year of the referral study was atypical, we examined the characteristics of the 271 children in the central case register who were still enrolled in special education classes at the time of the study of formal organizations. This file represents the cumulative effect of many years of referrals and placements. In this file, males were overrepresented but not so markedly as in the referral study (52.0% male vs 48.0% female). Ethnic disproportions were of approximately the same magnitude as in the referral study (31.5% Anglo, 50.1% Mexican-American, and 18.2% Black). Children from less affluent neighborhoods still predominated. Seventy-four percent of the children in special education were living on blocks in the lowest five deciles in housing value. We concluded that the labeling process is relatively stable and the characteristics of the children who were placed during the year of the referral study were not significantly different from those placed in other years.

Stage 8: Vacating the Status of Retardate

Any status in the public schools is time limited. Eventually everyone moves on to other social systems either by graduation, dropping out, or being excluded or expelled. How do the mental retardates in the public schools vacate that status?

There were 108 persons nominated as mentally retarded by the public schools who were no longer holding the status of mental retardate in the schools at the time of the agency study. Twelve of them (11.1%) had graduated from the program, 25 of them (23.1%) had dropped out of school without completing the program, 50 of them (46.3%) had been excluded from the school program or placed in other types of programs or institutions, and 21 of them (19.4%) had been returned to the regular class. The average tenure in special education for children who graduated was significantly longer (6.6 years) than that for children in the three groups who did not remain in special education (range 1.9 to 2.9 years). None of the social characteristics that differentiated persons during the labeling process were significant in the unlabeling. Children who followed the four different exit routes from the retardate status did not differ significantly in sex, ethnic group, or socioeconomic status.

However, we did find that students who dropped out of special education were significantly older when they were first referred and those who were sent to other programs and institutions were significantly younger when they were first referred than students who returned to regular class or graduated. Perhaps older children are more aware of the negative valuation placed on special education and are more prompt in rejecting the role and dropping out of school, and children who are placed when they are younger are more likely to accept the role and adapt to it.

Children who were eventually excluded from the program and placed in other programs or in other institutions spent an average of 1.9 years in special education in the public school. They differed most from the three other groups. According to information in their school files, those excluded had more physical disabilities and more interpersonal problems than children in the other three categories. A significantly larger percentage of them were rated as having a very short attention span, being poorly adjusted, being emotionally disturbed, and having a stronger possibility of neurological involvement than any other group.

Children who were returned to the regular classroom also had distinctive characteristics. In addition to having significantly higher average IQs than other groups, a significantly smaller percentage of them were rated as having possible neurological involvement. Their emotional adjustment and interpersonal relations ratings were similar to those of the children who graduated or dropped out of the program. They appeared to be the most "normal" clinically of the four categories. There were no significant differences between the group who graduated and the group who dropped from the program on any of the behavioral or clinical characteristics studied.

To summarize, the route followed by a pupil in the unlabeling was related not to his social characteristics but to his clinical and behavioral characteristics. Those who returned to the regular class had higher IQs and a lower probability of neurological involvement. Those who were sent to other programs or other institutions had more physical disabilities and were more likely to be rated as poorly adjusted, emotionally disturbed, creating interpersonal problems, or having possible neurological damage. The children who dropped out of school or remained for graduation fell between the two extremes.

Conclusion

We found that becoming a mental retardate in the public schools is a complex social process, which hinges on a series of crucial decisions made by teachers, principals, and psychologists. Some children are exposed to a much higher risk of achieving the status of mental retardate than others. The higher proportion of children from lower socioeconomic levels and minority groups in special education classes does not appear to be the result of higher overall rates of referral by teachers or higher rates of testing. Rather, it appears to be the result of the clinical diagnosis itself, a diagnosis that relies almost exclusively on an IQ test. Those who failed the IQ test were disproportionately from lower socioeconomic levels and ethnic minority groups. Children recommended for placement and those actually placed were even more disproportionately from ethnic minorities and lower socioeconomic levels. Children whose backgrounds do not conform to the modal sociocultural configuration of the community are exposed to a higher risk of being labeled mentally retarded.

Once placed in the retardate status, a child may vacate it by graduating, dropping out, being transferred to some other program or institution, or returning to regular classes. The course which he follows depends largely on his behavioral and clinical rather than his social characteristics.

Institutionalized Anglocentrism: Labeling Mental Retardates in the Community

Anglocentrism, institutionalized and legitimated by the diagnostic procedures used in the formal organizations of the community, appears to be the most pervasive pattern in labeling the mentally retarded in the community.

Anglocentrism is a specific form of ethnocentrism. Ethnocentrism refers to the tendency, common to all societies, for persons to believe that the culture of their own group is superior to that of other groups. Ethnocentrism leads people to act as if the language, history, life style, and values of their own group are the "right" and "good" standards by which the behavior of all other persons ought to be measured. As a consequence of ethnocentrism, people are prone to devalue the performance of others who do not completely share their cultural orientations, and may place them in less esteemed statuses in the society or may even ban them completely from participation in the society.

Anglocentrism is a form of ethnocentrism in American society. In the United States, the cultural patterns of the segments of the population consisting of white, Anglo-Saxon Protestants has been the dominant influence since colonial times and had never been seriously threatened (Gordon, 1964). English language, English literature, Anglo-American political and social systems, and Anglo-American history make up the major portion of the public school curriculum. Training in a language other than English and learning about the history and culture of other societies comes late in the educational sequence and has never been a primary concern in American life. Historically, most immigrants from other cultures have entered the American social system at the lowest socioeconomic levels and have gradually climbed into the middle classes and gained entry to the mainstream of American life through learning the English language and adopting the life style of the Anglo core culture. Anglo conformity has been the measure of success. Historically, this Anglocentrism has relegated non-Anglos to marginal social statuses. The Anglocentrism of the labeling process as practiced by formal organizations in the community was demonstrated by four of the major findings of the social system epidemiology of mental retardation.

First, disproportionately large numbers of persons from low socioeconomic levels and non-Anglo backgrounds are holding the disesteemed status of mental retardate in the community. This overrepresentation of non-Anglos is particularly pronounced in those public institutions established for the purpose of promulgating and enforcing the public norms of the core culture: the public schools, law enforcement agencies, welfare and vocational rehabilitation agencies. Anglocentrism is not so pronounced in the labeling processes in private organizations.

Second, the Anglocentrism of the labeling process is further demonstrated by the finding that Mexican-Americans and Blacks holding the status of mental retardate are less deviant than Anglos holding that status. Non-Anglos labeled as mentally retarded have higher IQs and fewer physical disabilities than labeled Anglos. Thus, when clinical characteristics are held constant, non-Anglos are exposed to a greater risk of being labeled mentally retarded.

Third, the Anglocentrism of formal organizations is shown by the finding that "situational" retardation is more common among non-Anglos. This means that more of the labeled non-Anglos were labeled by only one or two formal organizations. Their retardation was specific to a particular social system, primarily the public schools, and was not a comprehensive status which they held in many different groups.

Fourth, we found that Anglocentrism in labeling the mentally retarded is primarily a pattern found in formal organizations. The evidence for this conclusion rests on the finding that lay persons questioned in the household survey did not nominate disproportionately large numbers of non-Anglos as mental retardates. The ethnic and socioeconomic characteristics of persons labeled as mentally retarded by neighbors and acquaintances did not differ significantly from the ethnic and socioeconomic characteristics of the community. The overrepresentation of non-Anglo groups was characteristic only of nominees from formal organizations.

Two findings support the conclusion that Anglocentrism in labeling results primarily from the diagnostic procedures used in formal organizations, mainly an IQ test based on a statistical definition of "normal." In the study of the normative structures of formal organizations, those organizations that relied most heavily upon the statistical definition of "normal," the IQ test, were the organizations with the greatest overrepresentation of low socioeconomic and minority ethnic groups among the labeled retarded. On the other hand, retardates labeled by organizations that also used the medical-pathological model and included a medical diagnosis in the labeling process were more representative of the total community. In addition, those organizations labeling the least deviant persons, in terms of IQ test score and physical disabilities, were also labeling the most non-Anglo retardates. The diagnostic procedures used and the level of the norms applied by formal organizations were clearly related to whether that organization was nominating a disproportionate number of non-Anglos.

In the study of the labeling process in the Public Schools, Anglocentrism first appeared at the stage in the referral process when the IQ test was administered. Although teacher-principal teams referred Mexican-American and Black children and children from lower socioeconomic levels at about the same rate as their percentage in the school population, about three times more Mexican-American and Black children and about twice as many children from lower socioeconomic levels appeared among those failing the intelligence test as would be expected from their proportion in the population of the school district. Subsequently, this disproportion increased. Four times more Mexican-American and three times more Black children were placed in special education classes than would be expected from their percentage in the district, because proportionately more Mexican-American and Black children with low IQs were recommended for placement and were ultimately placed. It was at the point in the referral process when the intelligence test was administered that the sharp ethnic disparities first appeared.

We conclude, therefore, on the basis of our social system epidemiology of mental retardation in the community, that institutionalized Anglocentrism is a recurring pattern in the labeling process, a pattern that is closely linked with the statistical definition of "normal" and the IQ test.[1]

[1] The findings in this chapter reflect labeling procedures as they existed in the 1960s prior to the passage of California Senate Bill 33 in the 1971 legislative session which now requires procedures similar to those suggested in Chapter 17 of this study.

Part III

THE CLINICAL EPIDEMIOLOGY

Chapter 8

DEFINING MENTAL RETARDATION FOR THE CLINICAL EPIDEMIOLOGY

In the social system epidemiology, it was clear that the most significant group of labelers in the community were clinicians trained in the clinical perspective. Of special importance were those clinicians schooled in the statistical model of "normal" and using the IQ test. We learned that the clinical perspective and the professional labelers who are the culture bearers for that perspective compose the most significant social group in the community in relation to mental retardation. They, and they alone, have official responsibility for defining subnormals. They are the legitimate labelers.

If we are to understand the labeling process, we must place ourselves in the role of the professional clinician in order to study the ramifications of the clinical perspective. Consequently, in the clinical epidemiology, we approach the study of mental retardation as if we were professional labelers. We operate strictly from the clinical perspective. For this portion of the study, we accept the assumptions and definitions of the statistical model, analyze the population of Riverside from this viewpoint, and then try to understand what the implications of this perspective are when applied to a multiethnic society. For this reason, there is a distinct, conceptual disjuncture between part 2 and part 3 of this volume. We will try to reconcile these discontinuities in part 4.

Assumptions of the Clinical Epidemiology

All of the epidemiologies of mental retardation in the literature are based on the clinical perspective. This was true not only of epidemiologies using field surveys but also of epiemiologies that used nominations from informants. In this part of our study, we will proceed according to the assumptions of the pathlogical-statistical model of normal and assume (1) that mental retardation is individual pathology; (2) that mental retardation has characteristic symptoms, which can be identified in any segment of the population using standardized diagnostic instruments administered by adequately trained diagnostians; (3) that the diagnostic instruments employed by clinicians are valid and reliable instruments for measuring symptoms in all population segments; (4) that normal persons are those who fall within one standard deviation above or below the mean of the population as determined statistically and that subnormals are those who fall below one standard deviation; (5) that a case of mental retardation may exist, undetected, by persons in the community and can be screened out and diagnosed in the course of a field study.

The aim of our field survey was to screen all the individuals living in a representative sample of the housing units in Riverside to determine whether they "had" the symptoms of mental retardation. The validity of such a clinical epidemiology is determined by the effectiveness with which diagnostic procedures used in a clinical setting can be adapted for use in fieldwork so that findings from the field screening closely approximate the results that would have been obtained if every person screened had been examined in a clinic by a certified diagnostician.

A clinical epidemiology begins with the abstract verbal definition of pathology to be studied. Consequently, the first step in the field survey was to define precisely the symptoms of mental retardation and the level of severity required before an individual was to be classified as pathological. In constructing this definition, we wished to use the definitions and terms most generally accepted by professional clinicians so that we could examine the implications of assuming a clinical perspective in the field of mental retardation.

Among the most influential definitions of mental retardation are those of A. F. Tredgold; E. A. Doll; A. F. Tredgold and K. Soddy; C. E. Benda; L. Kanner; the English Mental Deficiency Act of 1927 and the Mental Health Act of 1959; the Group for the Advancement of Psychiatry; the American Association on Mental Deficiency; the President's Panel on Mental Retardation; and the statutory definitions contained in the laws of various states. Some of these constructs have been elaborated in great detail and will not be reproduced in full. However, ten summary quotations, arranged in chronological order, reveal the primary elements of these definitions and the point at which they differ.

> Mental defectiveness means a condition of arrested or incomplete development of mind existing before the age of eighteen years, whether arising from inherent causes or induced by disease or injury (Mental Deficiency Act of 1927, Section 1, Paragraph 2).

> [Mental deficiency is] a state of incomplete mental development of such a kind and degree that the individual is incapable of adapting himself to the normal environment of his fellows in such a way as to maintain existence independently of supervision, control, or external support (Tredgold, 1937, pp. 4–5).

We observe that six criteria by statement or implication have been generally considered essential to an adequate definition and concept. These are (a) social incompetence, (b) due to mental subnormality, (c) which has been developmentally arrested, (d) which obtains at maturity, (e) is of constitutional origin and (f) is essentially incurable (Doll, 1941, p. 215).

A mentally defective person is a person who is incapable of managing himself and his affairs, or being taught to do so, and who requires supervision, control, and care for his own welfare and the welfare of the community (Benda, 1954, p. 1115).

Mental deficiency or amentia, then, is a condition in which mind has failed to reach complete or normal development. . . . The essential purpose of mind is that of enabling the individual so to adapt himself to his environment as to maintain an independent existence. . . . From the biological and social aspect the one who can do this is to be regarded as normal, while the one whose mental development does not admit of this is to be regarded as defective (Tredgold and Soddy, 1956, pp. 1–2).

Two widely differing types of people have been lumped together by an all-inclusive nomenclature:

(1) The one type consists of individuals so markedly deficient in their cognitive, emotional, and constructively conative potentialities that they would stand out as defectives in any existing culture. . . .

(2) The other type is made up of individuals whose limitations are definitely related to the standards of the particular culture which surrounds them . . . in our midst their shortcomings, which would remain unrecognized and therefore, nonexistent in the awareness of a more primitive cultural body, appear as soon as scholastic curricula demand competition in spelling, history, geography, long division, and other preparations. . . . It is preferable to speak of such people as intellectually inadequate rather than mentally deficient (Kanner, 1957, pp. 70–71).

Severe subnormality is a state of arrested or incomplete development of mind which includes subnormality of intelligence and is of such a nature and degree that the patient is incapable of leading an independent life or of guarding himself against serious exploitation, or will be so incapable when of an age to do so (Mental Health Act of 1959, Section 4, Paragraph 2).

Mental retardation is a chronic condition present from birth or early childhood and characterized by impaired intellectual functioning as measured by standardized tests. It manifests itself in impaired adaptation to the daily demands of the individual's own social environment. Commonly these patients show a slow rate of maturation, physical and/or psychological, together with impaired learning capacity (Group for the Advancement of Psychiatry, 1959, p. 7).

Mental retardation refers to subaverage general intellectual functioning which originates during the developmental period and is associated with impairment in adaptive behavior (Heber, 1961, p. 3).

The mentally retarded are children and adults who, as a result of inadequately developed intelligence, are significantly impaired in their ability to learn and to adapt to the demands of society (President's Panel on Mental Retardation, 1962, p. 1).

Intellectual subnormality and subnormal adaptive behavior are two symptoms which appear in all of these definitions. Three additional symptoms appear in more than one definition: that the condition appear during the developmental period; that there be biological involvement; and that the condition be chronic. Each of these symptoms will be discussed in turn and a working definition of mental retardation will be developed for the field survey.

The Symptom of Mental Subnormality

Every definition explicitly or implicitly states that defective intellectual functioning is a symptom of mental retardation. Wording varies, but all have the same general intent: "incomplete mental development," "incomplete development of mind," "mental subnormality," "mind has failed to reach complete and normal development," "deficient in their cognitive . . . and constructively conative potentialities," "subnormality of intelligence," "impaired intellectual functioning," "subaverage general intellectual functioning," and "inadequately developed intelligence."

These phrases refer to symptoms that clinicians have traditionally measured by intelligence tests. Such tests have helped establish the dominance of the clinical perspective in the field of mental retardation. For many professional diagnosticians, mental subnormality means poor performance on a standardized intelligence test administered and interpreted by a qualified person.

Beyond this general agreement, however, there is considerable variation in exactly where different authorities draw the line between normal and subnormal performance on an intelligence test. The highest upper limit has been set by Kanner and Heber. Kanner considers an intelligence quotient of 85 to be the top limit for the category he calls "intellectually inadequate" (Kanner, 1957). Heber defines "subaverage intellectual functioning" as performance on a measure of general intellectual functioning that is greater than one standard deviation below the population mean (Heber, 1961). This means that a person with an IQ of 84 or below on the Stanford-Binet LM Form or the Wechsler scales would be rated as intellectually subnormal. By this criterion, approximately 16% of the population would qualify as intellectually subaverage.

Educational usage generally places the dividing line somewhat lower. The highest IQ for placement in a class for the educable mentally retarded ranges between 75 and 79, depending on local usage.

Test designers propose a considerably lower demarcation line. Wechsler classifies persons with an IQ of 69 and below in the defective category, as do Terman and Merrill, creators of the Stanford-Binet LM Form (Wechsler, 1958; Terman and Merrill, 1960). This lower limit corresponds more closely with traditional definitions. Tredgold and Soddy state that "a person whose IQ is below 70 is probably mentally deficient" (Tredgold and Soddy, 1956), and the Group for the Advancement of Psychiatry agrees (GAP Report No. 43, 1959).

Given this wide variation in opinion, our clinical epidemiology refrains from adopting any one of these positions, and we will report findings using all three cutoff points.

Thus, our working definition of intellectual subnormality contains three levels: A person will be defined as intellectually subnormal at the 16% level (AAMD criterion) when his performance on a recognized, standardized intelligence test administered and interpreted by a qualified clinician is an IQ of 84 or below; at the 9% level (educational criterion) with an IQ of 79 or below; and at the 3% level (traditional criterion) with an IQ of 69 or below.

The Symptom of Subnormal Adaptive Behavior

An individual's ability to perform social roles appropriate for his age and sex is the most ancient and durable basis for classifying persons as fools or geniuses, dullards or prodigies, witless or wise, retarded or gifted. Long before standard measures were invented, men passed judgment on the performance of other men and separated the savants from the simpletons.

Eight of the ten definitions of mental retardation refer directly or indirectly to the inability of the mental retardate to play his social roles competently. Again, varied phrases have the same general intent: "incapable of adapting himself to the normal environment of his fellows," "social incompetence," "incapable of managing himself and his affairs," unable to "adapt himself to his environment as to maintain an independent existence," "incapable of leading an independent life," "impaired adaptation to the daily demands of the individual's own social environment," "impairment in adaptive behavior," "impaired in their ability . . . to adapt to the demands of society."

We will follow the lead of Heber and call this symptom "adaptive behavior," treating other terms as close synonyms.

Legal definitions of mental retardation place even greater emphasis on social performance as a criterion of mental deficiency than do clinical definitions. The following excerpts from statutory provisions of four states illustrate the tenor of legal definitions of mental deficiency (Lindman and McIntyre, 1961).

"Mentally deficient persons" means those persons, not psychotic, who are so mentally retarded from infancy or before reaching maturity that they are incapable of managing themselves and their affairs independently, with ordinary prudence, of being taught to do so, and who require supervision, control, and care for their own welfare, or for the welfare of others, or for the welfare of the community (California Code Ann., 5250, 1952).

The words "feeble-minded person," shall mean any person afflicted with mental defectiveness from birth or from an early age, so pronounced that he is incapable of managing himself and his affairs and of subsisting by his own effort, or of being taught to do so, or that he requires supervision, control, and care for his own welfare, or for the welfare of others, or for the welfare of the community, and who cannot be classified as an insane person (Nebraska Rev. Stat. 83–219, 1958).

The term "feeble-minded" as used in this title shall be so construed as to include all individuals, except the "insane," who by reason of mental deficiency are incapable of doing the work of the grades in the public schools in a reasonable ratio to their years of life; or who by reason of mental deficiency and other associated defects are incapable of making the proper adjustments to life for one of their chronological age (So. Dakota Code 30.0402, 1939).

"Mental deficiency" is a state of subnormal development of the human organism in consequence of which the individual affected is mentally incapable of assuming those responsibilities expected of the socially adequate person such as self-direction, self-support, and social participation (Washington Rev. Code 72.33.020, 1958).

The only law that defines mental deficiency in terms of mental test scores is that of the state of Virginia, which designates "a maximum mental age of three years according to the Binet or other approved mental tests" as one measure of deficient mentality.

The most complete verbal description of adaptive behavior appears in a monograph supplement to *The American Journal of Mental Deficiency* (Heber, 1961). In this monograph, Heber includes most of the elements of "social adjustment" covered in other definitions and specifically addresses the issue of the need for different criteria in assessing young children, school-age children, and adults. His definitive statement currently forms the conceptual foundation for the clinical evaluations being made by many clinicians and has been a primary reference point in our definition of adaptive behavior. The dimension of *Adaptive Behavior* refers primarily to the effectiveness with which the individual copes with the natural and social demands of his environment. "It has two major facets: (1) the degree to which the individual is able to function and maintain himself independently, and (2) the degree to which he meets satisfactorily the culturally imposed demands of personal and social responsibility" (Heber, 1961, p. 61).

According to Heber, impaired adaptive behavior can be assessed by evaluating three aspects of adaptation: (a) maturation, (b) learning ability, and/or (c) social adjustment. Those aspects of adaptation important in making an evaluation of performance vary with age.

Maturational processes are the most crucial aspects of adaptive behavior in the evaluation of infants and young children. Heber defines maturation as "the sequential development of self-help skills of infancy and early childhood such as: sitting, crawling, standing, walking, talking, habit training, and interaction with age-peers." Thus, the early assessment of adaptive behavior is almost completely in terms of sensory-motor development.

Learning ability is more critical during the school years. In Heber's definition, this refers to individual skill and ease in gaining knowledge through experience. Learning difficulties usually become most obvious in the academic situation, and consequently this aspect of adaptive behavior is difficult to assess in the preschool years.

Social adjustment refers to the manner in which the child relates to his parents, his peers, and other adults during preschool and school age. For the adult, social adjustment is the ability to function independently, to be engaged in gainful employment, and to meet and conform to other personal and social responsibilities.

Heber makes subnormal adaptive behavior mandatory for a diagnosis of mental retardation. He concludes: "The inclusion of criteria of impaired adaptive behavior in the definition (of mental retardation) demands that objective measures of general intelligence be supplemented by evaluation of the early history of self-help and social behavior, by clinical evaluation of present behavior, and by whatever measures of academic achievement, motor skills, social maturity, vocational level, and community participation are available and appropriate" (Heber, 1961, p. 4).

A Working Construct of Adaptive Behavior

Our working construct of adaptive behavior corresponds closely to that of Heber but incorporates the sociological concept of the social role as a unifying focus. When clinicians speak of social adjustment, social maturity, or social competence, they refer to an individual's ability to perform successfully in the social roles considered appropriate for his age and sex. Therefore, we are conceptualizing adaptive behavior as an individual's ability to play ever more complex social roles in a progressively widening circle of social systems. As a person matures, the behavioral standards of society become more demanding and the number and complexity of social roles that he is expected to play increases. His ability to cope with these increasing expectations for social-role performance constitutes his adaptive behavior.

The individual's success in learning the roles expected of him in the family, neighborhood, peer group, school, and community is the basis on which judgments of his social adequacy are made by persons playing reciprocal roles in those systems. It is this sort of judgment that is implied in legal codes describing a feebleminded person as one who is "incapable of managing himself and his affairs," as one who cannot make "proper adjustments to life for one of his chronological age," or as one who is not able to assume "those responsibilities expected of the socially adequate person." It is this kind of judgment, made informally and unsystematically, that is systematized in our clinical epidemiology.

In a relatively undifferentiated society, children may progress from child roles to adult roles with few discontinuities. An adult may be able to master the full complement of roles available to one of his age, sex, and social position. Having once achieved adult status and mastered the appropriate roles, he seldom may be required to learn additional roles. However, in a pluralistic, urban society characterized by geographic and social mobility, adults frequently find themselves in new social systems and must learn new roles and internalize new values. In American society, socialization to unfamiliar social roles is a lifelong process.

Identifying a typical role-learning sequence would be easier in a less differentiated society. However, the clinical perspective assumes that even in a complex, industrial society there is a basic sequence of social roles that are typically learned and internalized by a majority of the population. It also assumes that there is a broad consensus as to what constitutes socially acceptable role performance at various age levels and, consequently, that adaptive behavior can be measured, using the statistical model of "normal" (see chapter 1).

Infancy: Birth through Two Years

The family is the primary social system for the child under two. He does not play roles in the strict sense of taking the role of the "other" and acting back toward himself from the perspective of the other. Therefore, measures of adaptive behavior cannot actually evaluate role performance in children this young. However, it is possible to identify certain developmental and maturational abilities and certain embryonic social skills that must be achieved and that are the building blocks from which later social-role performance is formed. Among the more important of these developmental accomplishments are self-locomotion, sitting, toileting, eating, and acquiring the rudiments of speech. The young child also learns rudimentary social skills as he begins to interact with other persons by smiling, making noises, and reaching toward them. By the last half of the first year of life, he ordinarily can recognize a stranger, respond to his own name, cooperate when being dressed, repeat acts when people laugh, offer toys to others, and otherwise demonstrate his growing awareness of self and others.

Preschool:Three through Five Years

Immediately preceding school entrance, the child is ordinarily expected to assume more responsibility for his own cleanliness and toileting; for dressing and undressing himself; for being able to distinguish harmful and dirty objects from edible ones; for using tools such as crayons, watercolors, and scissors without harming himself and others; and for performing simple household tasks and running errands. He is expected to be able to move about his home and neighborhood with minimal supervision, to follow simple directions, and to cooperate with other children by playing games according to rules. This greater independence assumes that he can manage most of his social interactions with minimal adult direction, can relate events that have happened to him, and can communicate his desires to others.

School: Six through Fifteen Years

School adds a new, complex social system to the life space of the child. He now must comprehend a social structure containing unfamiliar roles such as teacher, principal, secretary, custodian. He must learn to play a new and demanding role himself—that of pupil. The child must locate himself not only vis-à-vis the teacher, principal, custodians, and other pupils in his class, but also in relation to those "big" pupils who have special prerogatives and responsibilities different from his own. He must learn the roles and values of his peers and simultaneously meet the ever increasing demands of the teacher. If he is to be promoted and to avoid placement in special classes, the child must learn to count and read, to write, to sing songs, to draw and build, and a multitude of other intricate skills.

At the same time that he is learning new roles in school, the child is expected to perform more complex family roles and to learn many new roles in the community: the role of customer in a store, handling his own money and making his own selections; of pedestrian on the street, obeying traffic lights and crosswalk markings; of driver of wheeled vehicles, whether they be bikes, or scooters, or skateboards; of babysitter, tending younger children; of employee, earning money by selling newspapers, gardening, or doing household tasks; and so forth.

The Adult: Sixteen and Over

For the adult, the primary new role is occupational. Except for housewives and students, an adult is expected to play a productive occupational role and to be financially self-sufficient. Indeed, self-support is directly or indirectly indicated as a criterion of "social adequacy" in most of the legal definitions of mental deficiency cited earier.

Community roles of various types are part of the role matrix of the majority of American adults. Forty-two percent of Riverside adults report attending church once a week or more, and 82% attend at least occasionally. Playing the role of citizen by voting and signing petitions is also common. In Riverside, 60% of the population over 21 are registered to vote and 33% have signed one or more petitions for a referendum or a proposition (Mercer and Butler, 1967). Sixty-eight percent of the persons in our study reported visiting friends once a week or more, and 52% reported visiting co-workers that often. Seventy-eight percent of the adults reported participating in one or more formal organizations. Sixty-one percent of the adults in our study reported visiting neighbors once a week or more, and 55% reported visiting relatives frequently. The pattern of social roles expands with age, and the adult participates in a more complex and differentiated network of social systems than the child. For adults, adaptive behavior is measured both by the number of roles the adult is playing and by his level of performance in those roles.

The Working Definition of Adaptive Behavior

The working definition for abnormal adaptive behavior, like that for intelligence, is based on a statistical model of "normal," uses three criteria levels, and varies in content with the age of the person being evaluated:

> Adaptive behavior is evaluated on the basis of community-wide norms in which each individual is compared with his age peers and subnormality is defined on three levels: the lowest 16%, the lowest 9%, and the lowest 3%.
>
> Adaptive behavior in the young child is the extent to which he has acquired the self-help and social skills upon which more complex role performance can be built—such skills as sitting, crawling, standing, walking, talking, toilet training, and responding to other persons.

Adaptive behavior for the older child and adult is the extent to which that person is playing a full complement of social roles appropriate for his age and is performing in those roles in a manner comparable to that of other persons of his age in the society.

Appearance of Symptoms during the Developmental Period

Six of the ten definitions of mental retardation require that subnormalities in intellectual and adaptive behavior originate during the developmental period. The Mental Deficiency Act of 1927 specifically states that mental defect is a "condition of arrested or incomplete development of mind existing before the age of 18 years." The Mental Health Act of 1959 retains the original wording except that it drops reference to a specific age limit. Doll's third criterion states that the mentally subnormal are "developmentally arrested." Tredgold implies that the disability appears during the developmental period when he speaks of "incomplete mental development." The AAMD definition contains the most precise current statement of this criterion. It clearly states that the condition is to "originate during the developmental period" and then specifies that, although the upper limit of the developmental period cannot be precisely specified, "it may be regarded, for practical purposes, as being at approximately sixteen years" (Heber, 1961).

This requirement is included indirectly in our working construct of mental retardation. Adaptive behavior questions asked of persons past sixteen years of age include several retrospective items on school performance, which cover the developmental period.

Biological Impairment as a Symptom of Mental Retardation

Two of the ten definitions explicitly state that mental retardation has a biological base, others imply organic involvement, while still others do not mention any physiological criterion. This unresolved issue has a long history.

Some take the position that all mental retardation has a biological base. Two of Doll's six criteria reflect this position. He believed that retardation "is of constitutional origin" (Doll, 1941). When Tredgold and Soddy discuss the etiology and classification of mental defect, they write as follows: "In our view this imperfection of mind is invariably accompanied by defective development of brain, but this may arise from different causes." In a table presenting their conception of the etiological classification of the amentias, "simple aments" are regarded as the lower range of normal intelligence with possible genetic factors involved. All other varieties of amentia are related to biological abnormalities resulting from genetic, deprivative, traumatic, or infective sources (Tredgold and Soddy, 1956). The English Mental Deficiency Act of 1927 defines mental defectiveness as "arising from inherent causes or induced by disease or injury," terminology echoed by Jervis who defines it as "caused by disease or genetic constitution" (Jervis, 1954).

Knobloch and Pasamanick have accumulated impressive evidence for their hypothesis that a continuum of reproductive casualty exists and that many children from disadvantaged homes suffer from organic injury, which makes their adjustment to the heavy social and psychological demands of their environment doubly difficult (Knobloch and Pasamanick, 1959; Pasamanick and Knobloch, 1958).

In contrast, there are those who argue that psychological and cultural factors may produce mental retardation without biological implications. The Mental Health Act of 1957 refrains from reiterating the biological stand of the earlier law. Masland, Sarason, and Gladwin, in their exhaustive review of research on psychological and cultural factors in retardation, demonstrate the large number of psychological and cultural factors that are sufficient in themselves to explain subnormal mental development without recourse to biological explanation. They propose that professionals differentiate between individuals who have demonstrable central nervous system pathology that interferes with normal social and intellectual functions, and individuals who do not have demonstrable central nervous system pathology. They suggest that the term *mental deficiency* be applied to the former and *mental retardation* to the latter (Masland, Sarason, and Gladwin, 1958). The World Health Organization urges a similar distinction. It suggests that those who are organically damaged be called *mentally defective* while those who suffer only from learning disabilities be termed *mentally retarded* (World Health Organization Technical Report Series, 1954). Kanner proposes that the term *intellectually inadequate* be used for persons who are able-bodied and would be regarded as normal in cultures less complex than that of modern American and that the designation *mentally deficient* be reserved for persons "so markedly deficient . . . they would stand out as defective in any existing culture" (Kanner, 1957). In another place he suggests that the labels *relative feeblemindedness* and *absolute feeblemindedness* be used for recognizing these differences (Kanner, 1949*b*).

In view of these divergent viewpoints, we decided that biological abnormality should not be a mandatory criterion for mental retardation. In the working definition for the field survey, mental retardation may have biological components, but evidence of organic involvement is not required for a diagnosis of retardation. Those with organic involvement are classified as Type 1 retardates and those with no evidence of serious organic involvement are classified as Type 2 retardates.

Chronicity as a Symptom of Mental Retardation

There are also divided opinions on whether mental retardation is a chronic condition and, hence, essentially incurable. Itard's attempt to educate the "Wild Boy of Aveyron" proceeded over Pinel's prognosis that the condition was irreversible. Sequin's work was greeted with skepticism by Esquirol. For a time, Guggenbuhl's enthusiastic belief that Cretinism could be cured through proper diet, baths, massage, physical exercises, and certain types of medication was applied to all types of feebleminded children (Kanner, 1964).

Binet was quite optimistic about the possibility of changing the intellectual capacity of children and devised a system for this type of instruction. However, when eugenicist H. H. Goddard became the champion of mental testing in the United States in the early 1900s, there was a decided shift toward the belief that mental subnormality is biological in nature and essentially incurable (Tuddenham, 1962).

The preliminary report of the Committee on Mental Retardation of the Group for the Advancement of Psychiatry defines mental retardation "as a chronic condition present from birth or early childhood" (Group for the Advancement of Psychiatry, 1959). This is a restatement of the position taken twenty years earlier by Doll when he proposed that mental retardation is "essentially incurable" (Doll, 1941). Much of the literature dealing with "pseudoretardation" also implies that "real" retardation is a chronic condition.

Tredgold and Soddy, however, have taken direct issue with Doll. They point out that certain types of retardation, notably Cretinism, have been successfully treated and that it is "illogical to jettison a diagnosis made on clinical grounds for the sole reason that a cure has been found" (Tredgold and Soddy, 1956).

With the emergence of evidence that cultural and social forces are factors in producing the symptoms of mental retardation in normal-bodied persons, others have opposed the idea that all forms of mental retardation are irreversible. The American Association on Mental Deficiency definition explicitly focuses diagnosis on present performance and is not concerned with predicting future behavior or with attempting to discover intellectual potential not manifested in current performance (Heber, 1961). In our working definition, we have taken the position that diagnosis does not depend on prognosis but is based on current intellectual performance and adaptive behavior.

A Working Definition of Mental Retardation for the Field Survey

This overview reveals general agreement on two major symptoms: (1) the mental retardate is one who is impaired in his ability to meet the demands of the social world, and (2) the mental retardate is intellectually subnormal. We have accepted Heber's two-dimensional symptomatology of mental retardation because it appears to represent the area of agreement in current clinical concepts. Heber states:

> An individual must demonstrate deficiencies in both *Adaptive Behavior and Measured Intelligence* in order to meet the criteria of mental retardation. *Measured Intelligence* cannot be used as the sole criterion of mental retardation since intelligence test performances do not always correspond to level of deficiency in total adaptation. *Adaptive Behavior* cannot be used as the sole criterion of mental retardation since deficiencies in adaptation are frequently a function of personal-social or sensory-motor factors independent of inadequacies in intellectual functioning *per se* (Heber, 1961, p. 55–56).

The working definition of mental retardation used in the field survey, therefore, was as follows: A mental retardate is an individual who is subnormal in intellectual functioning, using three levels for defining subnormality: the lowest 16% or IQ 84 and below (AAMD criterion); the lowest 9% or IQ 79 and below (educational criterion); and the lowest 3% or IQ 69 and below (traditional criterion). He is subnormal in adaptive behavior, using three levels for defining subnormality: the lowest 16% of the population his age (AAMD criterion); the lowest 9% of the population his age (educational criterion); the lowest 3% of the population his age (traditional criterion). The mental retardate may show evidence of biological impairment, but this is not mandatory to a diagnosis of mental retardation.

Chapter 9

OPERATIONALIZING THE MENTAL RETARDATION CONSTRUCT

After defining the symptoms that characterize the pathology being studied, the epidemiologist proceeds to develop a categorical system by which he can classify the population at risk and a set of operations for making the actual classifications.

Typology of Mental Retardation

The working typology of mental retardation that is presented in table 8 was developed for the clinical epidemiology. Our definition of clinical retardation includes two primary symptoms: subnormal intellectual performance and subnormal adaptive behavior. It also includes one optional symptom: evidence of organic involvement or physical disability. The instrument used to operationalize the concept of intellectual performance was an intelligence test. Adaptive behavior was operationalized using scales based on the concepts presented in chapter 8. Physical disability was operationalized with a scale containing questions about organic involvement.

Mental Retardates

Mental retardates, as operationally defined for the clinical epidemiology, are persons in types 1 and 2, those who fail both intellectual performance and adaptive behavior. Type 1 mental retardates, the physically disabled, fail all three measures. We hypothesized that they would have relatively low IQs and would be persons who would qualify as severely, profoundly, or moderately retarded if diagnosed in a clinic. Some would be "trainable" mental retardates if diagnosed in a school system. Into this class would fall the "organics."

Type 2 mental retardates are those who fail both the intellectual and the adaptive behavior dimensions but have few physical disabilities. We hypothesized that these normal-bodied individuals would probably fall in the moderate, mild, or borderline intellectual range and would be likely to be diagnosed as "familial" or "undifferentiated" in a clini-

Table 8: Typology of Mental Retardation

	Failure Mandatory for a Diagnosis of Mental Retardation		Failure Optional for a Diagnosis of Mental Retardation	Clinical Types (Hypothesized)
Type	Intellectual Performance	Adaptive Behavior	Physical Disability	
Mental Retardates				
1	Fail	Fail	Fail	Severely and Profoundly Retarded—TMR
2	Fail	Fail	Pass	Moderately and Borderline Retarded "Familial and Undifferentiated"—EMR
One-dimensional Retardates				
Intellectual Failures: Quasi-retarded				
3	Fail	Pass	Fail	Theoretical Type—No Cases Anticipated in Epidemiology
4	Fail	Pass	Pass	Persons Not Socialized in the Modal Sociocultural Configuration of the Community
Adaptive Behavior Failures: Behaviorally Maladjusted				
5	Pass	Fail	Fail	The "Physically Disabled" Who Are Also "Handicapped"
6	Pass	Fail	Pass	Behaviorally Maladjusted
Nonretarded				
7	Pass	Pass	Fail	The "Physically Disabled" Who Are Not "Handicapped"
8	Pass	Pass	Pass	"Normal" Population

cal setting. In an educational setting, they would likely qualify as "educable" mental retardates.

One-dimensional Retardates

The quasi-retarded are those who are subnormal in intelligence but normal in adaptive behavior. They are persons likely to be diagnosed as mentally retarded by community agencies because they fail the intellectual measure, but they are not mental retardates when a two-dimensional definition is used, because they pass the adaptive behavior measure. The quasi-retarded are one-dimensional retardates because they have only one of the mandatory symptoms, low intellectual performance. Type 3 quasi-retardates fail the physical disability scale in addition to the intellectual measure, while Type 4 persons are normal-bodied. It was hypothesized that few persons in the community would qualify as Type 3 quasi-retardates because it seems unlikely that anyone who fails an intelligence test and also has physical disabilities will be performing his social roles at a level comparable to his peers.

Type 4 contains quasi-retardates who are normal-bodied. We hypothesized that most of these normal-bodied persons who fail an intelligence test but have adequate adaptive behavior would be persons who lack the skills and knowledge needed to pass an intelligence test because they have not been socialized in families that conform to the sociocultural mode for the community. However, they reveal their ability to cope intelligently with life's problems in nonacademic role performance.

Types 5 and 6 are also "one-dimensional" retardates because they are adaptive behavior failures who have normal IQs. Type 5 consists of persons who not only are subnormal in adaptive behavior but also have physical disabilities. They are the physically disabled who are also "handicapped" because their disabilities interfere with normal role performance.

Persons who have normal intellectual ability and no physical disabilities yet fail adaptive behavior are classified as Type 6, the behaviorally maladjusted. We hypothesized that this type of one-dimensional retardate would consist of persons who show evidence of emotional maladjustment or disturbance, which would account for their inability to fulfill role expectations even though they have statistically normal intelligence and no visible organic dysfunctions.

The Nonretarded

Types 7 and 8 pass both the intellectual measure and the Adaptive Behavior Scale. They are the nonretarded. Type 7 persons have physical disabilities but, nevertheless, fill a normal complement of social roles and hence are "physically disabled" but not "physically handicapped." Type 8, those who pass all the scales, are the clinically normal. We anticipated that this clinical category would contain between 75% and 80% of the persons in the community.

In chapter 8 we discussed the three cutoff points used by clinicians and workers in the field of mental retardation: the lowest 16% of the population, the lowest 9%, and the lowest 3%. We are calling these cutoffs the AAMD criterion, the educational criterion, and the traditional criterion, respectively.

The aim of the clinical epidemiology is to approximate evaluations made by professional diagnosticians. Therefore, we will present our findings using all three of the cutoff levels used by clinicians, and will report the characteristics of persons diagnosed as clinically retarded when intellectual performance and adaptive behavior both fall in the lowest 16% of the population, in the lowest 9% of the population, and in the lowest 3% of the population. Proceeding in this fashion makes it possible to assess the differential impact of each cutoff level on the characteristics of persons defined as subnormal.

Operationalizing Intellectual Performance

The selection of the intelligence test to be used in evaluating intellectual performance was based on three considerations. Because we wished to estimate accurately which individuals in the population would have been labeled as mentally retarded if they had all been evaluated by professional diagnosticians, it was essential that the test be a standard measure, widely used by clinicians. In addition, we needed a test that would discriminate at lower performance levels and not simply group all low scorers together in an undifferentiated aggregation. Finally, a test was needed that would evaluate all age groups from infancy through the adult years, in order to increase comparability over the entire age span being studied.

The Stanford-Binet Form LM met all three requirements. It is the oldest and most studied standard intelligence test and is used extensively in clinical practice. It discriminates well at the extremes of the normal distribution, making it possible to differentiate the very low performer from the moderately low performer. The Kuhlmann-Binet, a downward extension, can be used to test young children and the severely retarded.

Operationalizing Adaptive Behavior

Although adaptive behavior is the most ancient basis for judging individual competence, it has never been measured systematically. Empirical referents for a "socially adequate person" are largely unspecified, and clinical judgments depend primarily on unstandardized, intuitive evaluations. Although Heber recommends that the clinician evaluate an individual's early history of self-help and social behavior in assessing adaptive behavior, he notes the lack of suitable measures and suggests categorizing adaptive behavior on four levels, using a table prepared by Sloan and Birch to illustrate these four levels for three age groups (Sloan and Birch, 1955). "Though useful data would be obtainable from separate classification of the various aspects of *Adaptive Behavior,* the lack of suitable measurement techniques prohibits the development of a complex multifaceted classification at this time" (Heber, 1961).

Lack of a standardized measure of adaptive behavior is one of the primary criticisms of the AAMD classification system (Sheerenberger, 1965). The lack means that the dimension has not been extensively used in clinical diagnosis.[1] However, there are two scales that are widely used in clinical practice to rate infants and young children, and these scales include items related to adaptive behavior: the *Vineland Social Maturity Scale*[2] and the *Gesell Developmental Scales*[3] (Doll, 1965; Gesell, 1948 *a, b,* 1956).

[1] The Parsons' Adaptive Behavior Project (5-RO1 MH 14901) has published through the American Association on Mental Deficiency, 1969, an Adaptive Behavior Scale, which is designed for rating hospitalized populations. The Cain-Levine Social Competency Scale was developed as a method for measuring the social competence of trainable mental retardates. It is published by Consulting Psychologists Press, Palo Alto, California, 1963.

[2] Administration of the *Vineland Social Maturity Scale,* first published in 1935, consists of a guided interview with a respondent who is familiar with the behavior of the individual being evaluated. The 117 items in the scale are sequentially arranged by chronological age level from birth to adulthood. Items focus on eating, dressing, locomotion, communication, social relations, and occupation. They indicate the individual's growing capacity for self-help and increasing participation in activities leading to independent adult behavor.

Item scoring is subjective. The final raw score, based on the number of items passed, may be converted to a Social Age, which, in turn, may be used to derive a Social Quotient. The Vineland Scales were normed on 620 subjects, 10 "normal" persons of each sex from birth to 30 years of age. Frequently used in clinical assessments of young children, the Vineland is seldom used in the clinical evaluation of adolescents and adults. Heber regards it as "the best single measure of *Adaptive Behavior* currently available," but does not recommend that it be used as the sole determinant of adaptive behavior particularly for adolescents and adults. Clinicians are advised to supplement test data with clinical observations and information about the person's everyday behavior (Heber, 1961, pp. 62–63; Buros, 1965).

[3] *The Gesell Developmental Schedule* is a measure of adaptive behavior, which has been especially popular with pediatricians and neurologists. First appearing in 1925, the scales provide a detailed description of infant and child behavior from four weeks to six years of age, based on the observations of the clinician. There are ten subtests, each containing age-appropriate items concerned with the child's postural, prehensory, perceptual, adaptive, and language-social behavior. The scale was normed by repeated testing of 49 boys and 58 girls at each of twenty age levels from four weeks through five years. All children were Caucasian and were selected from a homogeneous middle-class background in a restricted locality. Other scales have subsequently been developed or are in the process of being developed.

Neither could be incorporated directly into field screening procedures because they are designed for use in a clinical setting. The Vineland requires an extensive clinical interview, which allows the examiner considerable discretion in the wording and ordering of the questions. The Gesell scales are based on actual observation and testing of the subject. However, the content of both scales was a valuable source of material for developing many of the standard questions finally used in the Adaptive Behavior Scales of our clinical epidemiology.

We followed Jastak's lead and used his two social criteria: school achievement for older children and adults, and occupational achievement for adults (Jastak, MacPhee, and Whiteman, 1963). However, we did not feel that these two criteria were sufficient or that any of the existing measures for young children were comprehensive enough for our purposes. Therefore, we proceeded to develop additional items covering other facets of adaptive behavior, especially for older children and adults, and pretested our own procedures. In the pretest, we combined adaptive behavior and physical disability items into one index and used a multilevel screening procedure. Experience with the pretest convinced us that there should be separate scales for adaptive behavior and physical disability items and that multistage screening was less desirable than age-graded sets of items.

We conceptualized adaptive behavior as an expanding, age-graded dimension in which the individual gradually increases the number of social systems in which he participates and the number and complexity of the roles he plays in those systems. His ability to cope with these increasing demands and to play social roles comparable to others of his age and sex constitute his adaptive behavior. The scales were based on six principles.

Conformity to Current Clinical Practice and Definitions Insofar As Possible

The Vineland and Gesell scales are used extensively by clinicians. Wherever feasible, we modified items and materials from those scales for use in the field survey, always preserving their basic intent (Doll, 1965; Gesell, 1948 *a, b* and 1956). Items from both scales are phrased as direct structured questions asked of each respondent in a specified order. Other questions were added to cover the major categories of adaptive behavior described by Heber, Sloan and Birch, and Jastak (Heber, 1961; Sloan and Birch, 1955; Jastak, MacPhee, and Whiteman, 1963). In addition, some of the content of the scales for older age groups were drawn from studies of the social adjustment of adult retardates living in the community (Kennedy, 1948; Saenger, 1957; Windle, 1962).

Age-graded Content Reflecting the Increasing Number and Complexity of Social Roles

The items in the Adaptive Behavior Scales mirror the changing pattern of expectations which a person meets in the course of his life. The item content for each of the scales can be seen in Appendix B.

Questions for children under six years of age were adapted almost entirely from the work of Doll and Gesell. Of the nineteen items in each scale, six are from the Vineland, ten are modifications of Gesell items, and three are from our own earlier research on retarded children. For the infant, the scales emphasize developmental skills such as locomotion, self-help, the use of language, and response to social stimuli. The questions for preschool children cover the child's increasingly complex role performance around the home, with his peers, and in the neighborhood.

Scales for school-age children contain thirty-one questions. Six are modifications from the Vineland, ten are adapted from Gesell, and fifteen deal with specific role performances in the school, family, and community. These ask whether the child has had trouble learning; whether he has repeated grades; whether his grade placement is appropriate for his chronological age; and whether he has difficulty getting along with teachers, friends, neighbors, and other family members. Questions also focus on other social skills, such as behavior at the dinner table, comprehension of time concepts, handling money, competing in class and on the playground, participating in clubs and on teams, working without supervision, and so forth.

For persons 16 through 49 years of age, the scales contain twenty-nine questions. Eight are adapted from Vineland items and the remaining questions cover five general areas: home, neighborhood, education, occupation, and community participation. Specifically, questions were asked about participation in various community roles; participation in formal organizations; participation in religious activities; leisure time activities; voting behavior; and interaction with friends, neighbors, and co-workers. In addition to educational and occupational items, adults were asked about participation in the collective culture through reading books, magazines, and newspapers; attending movies; and watching adult-type television programs.

Calibrated with the Pace of Social Development

Social development, like physical and intellectual development, proceeds at a more rapid rate in the early years of life than in later years. For this reason, the item content of the scales changes every three months for persons under two years of age, every six months for persons in their third year of life, and every year for persons 3 through 15 years of age. There is one set of questions for persons 16 through 19 years of age, and separate scales for persons 20 through 29, 30 through 39, and 40 through 49.

Maximum Discrimination in the Negative End of the Distribution

The clinical epidemiology is focused on pathology and does not aim to differentiate superb performers from the average. Consequently, the adaptive behavior items are designed to identify persons who fall well below the average, and contain questions that will be passed by most persons being screened. The low ceiling clusters the scores of most persons in the general population in an undifferentiated group of "normals," while the scores of persons in the lowest 16% are highly differentiated. However, the scales are scored on the assumption that adaptive behavior is normally distributed in the general population and would have been normally distributed in the survey sample if more difficult items had been included and the scale ceiling had been higher. The fieldwork revealed, as was expected, that the actual distribution of scores on the scales is skewed negatively. Performers with few failures cluster at the positive end of the distributions, and poor performers spread out in a negative tail.

Items already normed by Doll or Gesell were placed in the age-graded scales so that the items at any age level were those which had been normed for persons of that age or for the age level immediately below that of the individual being screened. We did not ask any questions normed for age levels above the chronological age of the persons being screened. For example, three of the six items from the Vineland that are in the six-year-old scale cover behavior normal for a five-year-old child and three cover behavior normal for a six-year-old child. As a result of this procedure, adjoining age scales have some questions in common. That is, the six-year scale contains some items that are in the five-year scale and some that are in the seven-year scale. The amount of overlap varies somewhat from age group to age group.

The highest and lowest age levels are special situations in which this principle cannot be followed precisely. Originally, we attempted to screen children six months of age and younger but found that the behavioral floor made it difficult to find appropriate items at a level of difficulty low enough so that the screening would be roughly equivalent to the relative level of difficulty of items used for older children. In addition, behaviors with a social content were virtually nonexistent. For these reasons, the adaptive behavior scales do not screen persons under seven months of age.

In the adult years, increased age brings relatively little change in role expectations. Beyond 16 years of age, scale content stabilizes, and all items adapted from the Vineland Scale for adults are behaviors normal for a 12-year-old. Items in the Adaptive Behavior Scales developed specifically for the study are placed at age levels appropriate to the expanding role careers of individuals in American society.

Adapted for Administration in a Household Interview with One Respondent Speaking for Other Members of the Family

The nature of the respondent and the field situation had to be taken into account in the development of the scales. In general, information about children was supplied by a parent, usually the mother, unless some other adult was regularly responsible for the child's care. Information about adults could be supplied by the adult himself, but was frequently supplied by some other member of the family: a spouse, a parent, or a grown son or daughter living in the household. The most common situation of this kind was for a wife to answer questions about her husband. Consequently, scales had to be limited to the kinds of information which the respondent would be likely to know about other adult family members and would be willing to report.

Respondents to field interviews include the entire spectrum of the general population. Immigrants with no formal education and little comprehension of English were asked the same questions as college-educated persons active in the academic and intellectual life of the community. Questions had to be stated simply enough to be understood by the least educated and yet not offend more sophisticated respondents. Consequently, questions were designed to refer to observable behavior that can be described clearly in basic English and can be readily translated into Spanish, such as, "How old is———? What grade is ——— in school?" and so forth.

In general, questions were phrased to deal with current rather than past behavior because responses to retrospective questions are less reliable. The few retrospective questions that do appear in the adult scales relate only to education and occupation.

Items Are Selected and Scored to Give More Weight to More Important Roles

Adaptive behavior is judged on two counts. Is the person filling a full complement of roles typical for persons of his age? Is he performing his roles at a level congruent with social expectations for persons of his age and sex? Both facets of performance were important in the selection and scoring of items, especially for the school-age and adult scales.

More important role complexes, such as the pupil role for school children and educational and occupational roles for adults, are covered by more than one question. Multiple questions weight these roles more heavily in the total social-role performance score and give a more differentiated evaluation of level of performance.

Educational Roles. The pupil role is the most important role in determining how a school-age child will be judged by others. Therefore, this role is weighted more heavily than other roles in the school-age scales by having three questions focused on academic performance. The three items are designed to represent different degrees of difficulty with the pupil role.

There were five educational items in the adult scale. It was necessary to develop a scoring scheme for adult educational achievement that would differentiate those who had never had an opportunity to go to school from those who attempted school and failed, because 9 percent of the adults of Mexican American descent had never attended school, since they were reared in Mexico and did not have this opportunity.

Occupational Role. The occupational role presented some complexities because of sex differences and because it was necessary to take the student role into account in the scoring. Sex differences in occupational role expectations are ubiquitous. A female who is a housewife automatically passes three of the five occupational items. Even if she has never filled an occupational role at any time in her life, she will score only one failure if she is currently a housewife. If she has ever held a job, regardless of its level, and she is a housewife at the time of the interview, she will be rated as fulfilling all occupational social-role expectations. A man, on the other hand, must be currently employed in a job that rates above the third decile to be fulfilling modal expectations. Thus, it is easier for a woman to pass the occupational items than it is for a man. Although this seems an inequity, the scoring scheme does reflect social realities. In American society, a woman can meet society's occupational role expectations by becoming a housewife. This is less demanding than the role expectations for males, but is the modal pattern for adult females.

A second consideration in the scoring scheme is that of adjusting to the role of "student," a socially acceptable alternative to an occupational role. About 10 percent of the adults in our sample were still in school. As with the housewife, a student who has never held a job is penalized one point on the occupational items but passes the other items. Again, this scoring reflects social realities. Although the status of student is a transitory one, it is a socially acceptable way of postponing the demands of the occupational world. Who is to say whether being a student is more or less difficult than holding a job rated at the fourth decile or above? Society suspends judgment and so must we.

Operationalizing Physical Disability

Although organic involvement is not required by our definition of mental retardation, the incidence of physical disability is high among the clinically retarded, and biological abnormalities are frequently used in arriving at differential, medical diagnoses concerning specific types of mental retardation. Physical abnormalities make mental retardates more visible, tend to be particularly evident among the more severely retarded, and often are the primary symptoms used to diagnose retardation in the very young.

Although the field interview could not include any type of physical or medical examination, the interview schedule did contain a series of questions designed to identify persons with obvious disabilities. Several items were adapted from the patient census and preadmission questionnaires developed at Pacific State Hospital, Pomona, California. These questions asked about ambulation, speech, vision, hearing, sleeping, and arm-hand use in dressing and eating. In addition, retrospective questions about seizures, accidents, operations, and illnesses that might have had central nervous system involvement were included. The response error to the physical disability items would tend to be in the direction of underreporting, especially on questions about older children and adults requiring long-term recall of illnesses, operations, and accidents.[4] As phrased and coded, the responses to the items represent judgments which lay persons are able to make with a relatively high level of reliability. As in the case of the adaptive behavior scales, the physical disability scales vary in content by age group. The scales for preschool children contain questions about complications of pregnancy and birth injury, while scales for older children and adults focus mainly on current functioning. Appendix C contains the items in the scales for each age group.

A person's score on the scale is the number of items he fails. The rate of failure on any given physical disability item for the population as a

[4] There is no way to assess the amount of underreporting to retrospective questions. The National Health Interview Survey compared medical records with reports given in interviews and found no significant difference in reporting by sex, race, education of head of household, family income, or number of persons in the household. They found reporting just as accurate when another family member is responding as when a person is responding for himself. The longer the time lapse between interview and episode, the greater the underreporting. Overreporting was negligible (National Center for Health Statistics, 1965).

whole is very low, and scores are only a rough estimate of gross biological impairment. They give some indication of the extent to which physical disabilities, visible to a lay respondent, exist in the general population. As with adaptive behavior, persons in the lowest 16%, 9%, and 3% of the population were rated as subnormal at the AAMD, educational, and traditional criterion levels.

The Screening Interview

The research design for the study called for a first-stage screening of a large sample of the population, using the adaptive behavior and physical disability scales, and then a second-stage testing of a subsample, using an intelligence test. We will call these samples the screened sample and the tested subsample, respectively. (Details of the methodology appear in Appendix A.)

Sample Design for the Screened Sample

A stratified area probability sample of 3,198 housing units was selected from the City of Riverside so that all geographic areas and socioeconomic levels in the city would be represented in their proper proportion. Census tracts were used as the basis for geographic stratification, and the average dollar value of housing units on each census block, as reported in the United States Census, was used as the basis for socioeconomic stratification. The census blocks were divided into ten equal groups by average value of housing so that decile 1 contained the least expensive dwellings and decile 10 the most expensive dwellings. Each housing unit was assigned the housing-value decile for its block, a socioeconomic measure that is frequently used in all our analyses.

Fieldwork

Introductory letters addressed to each householder by name were sent before the arrival of the interviewer assigned each housing unit. All 46 interviewers were college educated, and 36 were teachers. Spanish-speaking interviewers were assigned to all households with Spanish surnames, Black interviewers were assigned to interview in housing units located in predominantly nonwhite blocks, and Anglo interviewers were randomly assigned the remainder of the households.

In each household, one adult member, usually the mother, served as respondent and provided information about all other members of the household to whom she was related. Servants, lodgers, or other unrelated individuals living in the same housing unit were individually interviewed. The average interview lasted approximately one hour and fifteen minutes. There were 275 vacant housing units, leaving 2,923 occupied housing units to be contacted. There were 2,696 interviews completed in 2,661 housing units, an overall response rate of 90.7%.

Scoring the Adaptive Behavior and Physical Disability Scales

Altogether, 6,907 persons were screened using the adaptive behavior and physical disability scales: 1,026 preschool children (7 months through 5 years of age), 1,875 school-age children (6 through 15 years of age), and 4,006 adults (16 through 49 years of age). An item analysis was done on each scale to determine which questions best distinguished persons who failed a large number of questions from persons who failed fewer items. The least effective questions were eliminated. The final adaptive behavior scales contained 15 items for preschool children, 23 items for school-age children, and 27 items for adults. The final physical disability scales contained 12 items for preschoolers 7 months through 24 months of age, 16 items for preschoolers 25 through 71 months of age, 11 items for school-age children, and 15 items for adults. The school-age and adult adaptive behavior and physical disability scales contained a larger number of items that differentiated persons with a large number of failures from persons with a small number of failures at a statistically significant level than did the scales for preschool children.

The adaptive behavior score for each individual was calculated by counting the number of items failed. Preschool children with 7 or more failures fell into the lowest 3% of that age group (the traditional criterion), school-age children with 9 or more failures fell into the lowest 3% for that age group, and adults with 8 or more failures fell into the lowest 3% of adults. Failing scores at the 9% cutoff (educational criterion) were 5 or more failures for preschoolers, 7 or more failures for school-age children, and 6 or more failures for adults, while failing scores at the 16% cutoff (AAMD criterion) were 5 or more failures, 6 or more failures, and 5 or more failures, respectively.

Since questions in the Physical Disability Scales cover major, visible disabilities, 2 or 3 failures indicate relatively serious impairment. Therefore, it required fewer physical disability failures to fail the 3 criterion levels on the Physical Disability Scales than on the Adaptive Behavior Scales. Preschool children failed the traditional criterion with 5 or more failures, the educational criterion with 4 or more failures, and the AAMD criterion with 3 or more failures. Only two cutoffs could be distinguished for school-age children. They failed the traditional criterion with 2 or more failures and the AAMD criterion with 1 or more failures. Adults failed the traditional criterion with 3 or more disabilities, the educational criterion with 2 or more disabilities, and the AAMD criterion with 1 or more disabilities. Chapter 10 describes the sociocultural characteristics of persons who failed the Adaptive Behavior Scales.

Chapter 10

CHARACTERISTICS OF PERSONS FAILING THE ADAPTIVE BEHAVIOR SCALES

Having established the raw score cutoff points for the AAMD, educational, and traditional criteria for subnormal adaptive behavior, we investigated the characteristics of persons who were statistically subnormal in adaptive behavior when norms were based on a sample of the total community. We analyzed two biological variables, sex and physical disabilities; and two sociocultural variables, socioeconomic status and ethnic group. Persons who failed at each criterion level were compared with persons who passed to determine if differentials in adaptive behavior are related to these four characteristics. Preschool, school-age, and adult persons have been analyzed separately because the content of the Adaptive Behavior Scales differs for each of the major age categories.

Differentials in Adaptive Behavior by Sex

Among the 1,026 preschool children from 7 through 71 months of age, significantly more boys than girls failed the Adaptive Behavior Scale at the educational criterion, the lowest 9% (70.1% vs 29.8%, $p<.01$) and the AAMD criterion, the lowest 16% (63.4% vs 36.5%, $p<.01$). At the traditional criterion, lowest 3%, there also were more male failures (67.7% vs 32.3%), but the number of cases in the failing group ($N=31$) was too small to yield statistical significance. The correlation between sex and adaptive behavior score was .12 ($p<.01$).

Sex differences were also pronounced among the 1,875 school-age children. At all three criterion levels, males were significantly more likely to fail than females ($r = .15$, $p<.01$). The percentage of failures that were males were 69.4%, 72.1%, and 69.5% at the three criterion levels. We examined the sex differences to determine if higher male failure was characteristic of all ethnic groups and found that failure rates for the two sexes were approximately the same for Mexican-American and Black school-age children but significantly different for Anglo school-age children. Thus, the sex differences found for the total population result from Anglo boys having significantly more adaptive behavior failures than Anglo girls.

We analyzed each of the items appearing in more than one of the age scales for school-age children and found that 10 of the 29 items were failed significantly more often by boys than girls ($p<.01$). Boys were more likely to have trouble learning (25.9% vs 14.1%); were less likely to write letters to friends (26.4% vs 7.7%); were more likely to repeat grades in school (16.0% vs 7.4%); were more likely to have trouble with the police (8.6% vs 1.4%); were less likely to go to the store by themselves (23.6% vs 9.1%); were less likely to read to themselves (28.0% vs 17.1%); were less likely to be interested in their clothes (21.5% vs 9.1%); were less likely to use the dictionary (11.3% vs 3.1%); were more likely to be behind their age-grade norm (9.0% vs 4.9%); and were less likely to work without supervision (7.7% vs 1.1%). There were no items failed significantly more often by girls. The number of children for whom there was information on each question varied from 357 to 1,873 because most questions appeared in some age scales but not in others.

The most striking characteristic of the list was the number of school-related items failed more frequently by boys. Six of the ten items that differentiated the sexes were related to performance in school or to skills that were acquired in school such as reading, writing, and using the dictionary. Of the non-school-related items failed more frequently by boys, one involved difficulties with the police, another had to do with working without supervision, and two were linked to cultural characteristics of sex roles—going to the store by oneself and being interested in clothes. In American society, girls probably are more likely to go to the store to help with household shopping and are more preoccupied with their clothes than are boys.

Among the 4,006 adults, sex differences were small and statistically insignificant when the group was treated as a whole ($r = .01$, NS). However, when each ethnic group was examined separately, there was a tendency for Anglo males to fail the Adaptive Behavior Scales at a higher rate than females, but there was no difference in the performance of Mexican-American and Black males when compared with Mexican-American and Black females.

Four of the items failed more frequently by men were related to school performance and were very similar to items failed more frequently by school-age boys. Men were more likely to have had trouble learning in school and to have repeated grades ($p<.001$). They were less prone to write letters and to read books ($p<.001$). When sex differences between adult Anglos were analyzed within four age groups (16–19, 20–

29, 30–39, 40–49), differences on these items were consistent over all age levels.

There was a differential pattern of visiting, which was probably linked to cultural characteristics of the sex roles. Women were more likely to visit neighbors. They were less likely to visit co-workers, probably because many did not work. The co-workers they would be visiting would be those of their husbands. The differential responses by sex to these questions tended to balance each other.

Men were also more likely to fail the occupational-level item and the item asking if they were currently working. These items were easier for females to pass than males because women may pass either of them by being a housewife. It was the higher failure rate for males 16 through 29 that produced the overall difference. In the age group 30–49, more females failed the occupational items than males, but the trend was not large enough to be statistically significant. The only adaptive behavior items failed more often by Anglo women were visiting co-workers, participation in games and sports, and traveling alone.

Differentials in Adaptive Behavior by Physical Disability

School-age children and adults who failed the Adaptive Behavior Scales had significantly more physical disabilities than persons who passed the Adaptive Behavior Scales ($r = .22$ and $.18$, $p<.001$). Differences were significant for preschool children at the AAMD criterion, and the trend was clear at the less stringent levels.

Six questions accounted for the differences in school-age children, and these questions were all related to school roles. Children with more physical disabilities were more likely to be behind their age-grade norm, to have problems learning in school, to have repeated one or more grades, to have had trouble with their teachers, to be unable to work without supervision, and to have trouble with school friends ($p<.001$). Parents of children with physical disabilities did not report significantly more difficulty with interpersonal relations in the family or neighborhood, nor were there differences in other types of non-school-related roles.

Significantly more of the 221 adults with two or more physical disabilities failed almost every item on the Adaptive Behavior Scale ($p<.001$). The occupational items were of particular interest. Physically disabled adults were more likely to be unemployed (2.5% vs 14.9%), were more likely to be dependent on others for support (3.1% vs 12.2%). were more likely to have an occupation in the lowest three deciles

(7.5% vs 16.2%), were more likely to need supervision when they work (4.1% vs 10.4%), and were more likely never to have held a job (2.6% vs 5.4%).

Adults with physical disabilities were also more educationally restricted. A higher percentage of the physically disabled have completed eight or fewer years of formal education (4.5% vs 13.6%), have had trouble learning in school (8.2% vs 19.4%), have dropped out of school because of academic or discipline problems (3.6% vs 9.0%), and have attended classes for the mentally retarded (.2% vs 1.4%).

Adults with physical disabilities were also reported to live much more restricted social and intellectual lives than than persons with fewer disabilities. More of the disabled never participated in sports (16.5% vs 29.4%), never read newspapers (11.1% vs 19.5%), never went to movies (13.0% vs 24.4%) never read magazines (7.9% vs 13.1%), never attended church (14.9% vs 26.5%), never visited friends (2.4% vs 7.2%), never played competitive games (4.9% vs 19.8%), and never went to the store alone (1.3% vs 8.6%). They were less likely to discuss the local news and sports and to write letters. Physical disability was clearly related to adaptive behavior for adults.

Differentials in Adaptive Behavior by Socioeconomic Level

Duncan's Socioeconomic Index rating of the occupation of the head of the household was one measure of socioeconomic status used in the study (Reiss, 1961). This index was based on census data and incorporates the educational level, income level, and prestige rating of various occupations into an index with scores having a possible range from 0 to 99.

The socioeconomic status of preschool and school-age persons who failed the Adaptive Behavior Scales did not differ significantly from that of those who passed ($r = -.05$). Indeed, at the traditional criterion, the lowest socioeconomic group (0–19) was slightly underrepresented. At the educational and AAMD cutoff points, the socioeconomic level of those who failed the scales was almost identical to that of those who passed.

Differences in adaptive behavior by socioeconomic level were very marked for adults ($r = -.29$, $p<.001$). Only 20% of the passing adults lived in households ranked between 0 and 19 on the socioeconomic index, but 40% of the adults failing the Adaptive Behavior Scales lived in such households. Persons from households ranked 40 and above were consistently underrepresented at all criterion levels. This was especially true in the socioeconomic range 80–99. Although 12% of the general adult population fell into this category, only 3% of those who failed the Adaptive Behavior Scale came from households of high rank.

Low-status adults failed almost every item in the Adaptive Behavior Scales significantly more often than high-status adults. Educational roles and activities related to education were failed significantly more often by lower-status adults. More lower-status persons have completed eight years or less of schooling; never read books, newspapers, or magazines; dropped out of school for academic or discipline problems; had trouble learning; and repeated grades. Lower-status adults also lead a much more restricted social life. Significantly more of them never participated in formal organizations, sports, and competitive games; report no leisure activities; never vote; and never visit friends, relatives, or co-workers. Higher-status persons fill more social roles at a higher level of complexity. The only activities that did not differentiate low- and high-status persons were attendance at movies and church, watching television, and visiting neighbors.

Socioeconomic Status within Ethnic Group

Because persons from lower socioeconomic levels in Riverside tend to belong to ethnic minorities, ethnic and socioeconomic factors are confounded in these findings. How much does socioeconomic status influence adaptive behavior scores when ethnic group is held constant?

When Anglo adults who had passed and failed the Adaptive Behavior Scales were compared by socioeconomic status, the differences were very large. Almost three times more adults from lower socioeconomic ranks failed the Adaptive Behavior Scales at the traditional cutoff than would be expected from their percentage in the Anglo adult population, and over twice as many failed at the 9% and 16% cutoff levels. Thus, socioeconomic level is highly related to adaptive behavior in the Anglo population.

Although there are few white-collar workers or professionals among Mexican-Americans and the total socioeconomic range is relatively narrow, Mexican-American adults from lower socioeconomic levels also failed the Adaptive Behavior Scales at a higher rate than higher-status Mexican-Americans. Approximately 20% more persons in the failing group came from the lowest socioeconomic rank than would be expected by their percentage in the adult Mexican-American population. Only half as many as would be expected appeared in the middle ranges. These differences were statistically significant for the 9% and 16% cutoffs, but the number of cases was too small to produce statistical significance at the 3% criterion.

There were no differences by socioeconomic status for the adult Black population. In fact, at the 3% cutoff, there were fewer failing adults in lower socioeconomic categories than would be expected. Expected percentages and observed percentages were almost identical at the two other cutoff levels.

Differentials in Adaptive Behavior by Ethnic Group

There is no tendency for preschool children (r = .02) or school-age children (r = .05) of one ethnic group to fail adaptive behavior more frequently than children in other ethnic groups. Differences of considerable magnitude, however, emerged for adults regardless of the criterion level used (r = .28, $p < .001$). Mexican-American adults constituted approximately 6% of the population passing the Adaptive Behavior Scales, but made up over 25% of those who failed at the 16% level, 28% of those failing at the 9% level, and 38% of those failing at the 3% level. In other words, five times as many Mexican-American adults failed the Adaptive Behavior Scales as would be expected from their proportion in the population. Although Black adults failed the Adaptive Behavior Scales at approximately twice the expected rate at the 16% and 9% criterion levels, they did not contribute disproportionately to the failures at the 3% cutoff.

We compared ethnic group, while holding socioeconomic status constant, in order to determine the extent to which ethnic differences may be related to socioeconomic differences. Low status is defined as a Duncan Socioeconomic Index score of 0–29, while middle status is defined as a score of 30–69. There are too few Mexican-American and Black adults holding statuses ranked at 70 or above to permit analysis at that level.

When socioeconomic level is held constant, Blacks are no longer overrepresented in failing categories. Mexican-Americans, however, continue to be significantly overrepresented and Anglos significantly underrepresented. Two and one-half times more low-status Mexican-Americans fail the Adaptive Behavior Scales than would be expected, while only two-thirds as many Anglos fail as would be expected. Differentials tend to disappear for middle-status persons, reaching statistical significance only at the AAMD criterion. As minority adults become upwardly mobile, the differences between their adaptive behavior and that of the majority population tend to disappear.

The Nature of Ethnic Group Influences on Adaptive Behavior

Both socioeconomic status and ethnic group are significantly related to adaptive behavior in adults. When either is held constant, the other still has an effect.

The higher rate of failure for persons whose backgrounds do not conform to the modal configuration for the community is not surprising. When a statistical model of "normal" is used to evaluate behavior influenced by environmental factors, persons from nonmodal backgrounds will appear as "abnormal" when compared with a general population composed primarily of Anglo, middle-class persons (see chapter 1). This difference is more marked in the case of adults than children.

Two factors probably contribute to the accentuation of differences in adults. As persons grow older, there are more groups in which they participate, and the roles they play expand. Therefore, adult behavior is more differentiated than that of children. Unlike children, adults are not required to participate in the public school system or in other social institutions which have a homogenizing effect on role behavior. They participate in a variety of distinct social groups, neighborhoods, and work locations, and develop their own distinctive role configurations.

Second, items in the Adaptive Behavior Scales for adults focus almost entirely on social-role behavior, while scales for children have more maturational items that are related primarily to physical development and are not so influenced by sociocultural factors. We studied those items more frequently failed by Mexican-American and Black adults than by Anglo adults for four age groups: 16–19, 20–29, 30–39, and 40–49.

In all, Mexican-American adults failed 14 of the 29 items in the adult scales more often than Anglo adults ($p<.001$). A higher percentage of Mexican-American adults of all ages completed less than eight years of formal education. This difference was as true for Mexican-American teenagers as for older persons. More Mexican-American adults dropped out of school because of academic or discipline problems, and significantly more had repeated grades in school than Anglos of the same age. Other items related to educational skills also were failed significantly more often. They were less likely to read magazines, to read newspapers, to read books, and to write letters.

Three occupational items also differentiated Mexican-American adults from Anglo adults. For all age levels except 20–29, Mexican-American adults were significantly less likely to have current employment and, for all age levels, were significantly more likely to have occupations ranked in the lowest three deciles. Mexican-American teenagers and adults over 40 were also significantly more likely to be dependent on others for economic support.

A third major category in which the role behavior of Mexican-American adults was significantly different from that of Anglo adults was participation in formal organizations and participation in games. Mexican-American adults of all ages were significantly less likely to participate in formal organizations, and, except for teenagers, less likely to play competitive games such as cards and checkers. Finally, Mexican-American adults 20–29 and 40–49 were less likely to vote and participate as citizens.

The list of items that did not differentiate between Anglo and Mexican-American adults is instructive. It consists almost entirely of behaviors that take place in an informal social setting: visiting friends, attending movies, visiting neighbors, visiting co-workers, visiting relatives, traveling to nearby towns, reading and talking about local news, going to the store and shopping for clothing, working with little or no supervision, watching adult television programs, and participating in religious activities.

Mexican-American adults participated significantly less often in the institutional structures of the dominant society: the educational system, the occupational world, and the formal organizations of the community. They were less structurally integrated into the total community, and their adaptive behavior scores reflected this sociocultural difference. We compared Mexican-American adults who failed the Adaptive Behavior Scales at the AAMD criterion with Mexican-American adults who passed to determine what, in addition to socioeconomic disadvantage, was related to differential role performance among Mexican-American adults. The effect of socioeconomic status was held constant by comparing only those Mexican-Americans in the lowest housing deciles (1–3) with each other and those in the higher deciles (4–10) with each other.

The impact of sociocultural variables was striking, especially for low-status Mexican-Americans. Mexican-American adults from the lowest three deciles who failed the Adaptive Behavior Scales were more likely to come from homes in which the spouse of the head of household had never held a job and had less formal education. The head of household in families of those who failed had an average of two-and-one-half years less formal education than in the families of those who passed, and was less likely to be participating in any formal organizations. Failures were also more likely to come from households with many children and from households where English was seldom spoken. Seventy-four percent of the failing adults came from homes where English was spoken half the time or less, while 47% of those passing came from predominantly Spanish-speaking homes. Only 1% of the families of failing persons spoke English all the time.

Although Anglo adults who failed were more likely to be male and to have physical disabilities, these two biological variables were insignificant for low-status Mexican-American adults. Sociocultural variables had an overriding impact.

Sociocultural variables were not as statistically significant for higher-status Mexican-Americans, but trends were identical with those found for lower-status adults. There were 101 Mexican-American adults in deciles 4–10 and 31 who failed the Adaptive Behavior Scales at the 16% cutoff level. Most of the spouses of higher-status households have worked at some time in their lives, and all the heads of households participated in at least one formal organization. Therefore, these characteristics did not differentiate. It was the education of the spouse of head which emerged as the key cultural variable. Fathers of those who passed had about the same amount of education as the fathers of those who failed—10.9 years, compared with 10.0 years. The spouse of head in households of those who failed, however, had significantly less education—an average of 8.3 years, compared with 10.2 years. Higher-status Mexican-American females were also more likely to fail the Adaptive Behavior Scales. This seems to indicate that most higher-status Mexican-American men were more educated and, hence, more acculturated to Anglo society than their wives. In this situation, the level of the adaptive behavior performance of family members becomes more contingent on the spouse's education than on that of the head.

Families of those who failed also tended to be larger and to speak English less often in the home, but these differences did not reach statistical significance. The families of 75% of the passing persons speak English most of the time or all the time, while only 45% of the families of failing persons speak English that often. As with lower-status persons, higher-status Mexican-American adults who failed adaptive behavior had no more physical disabilities than persons who passed.

We conclude that sociocultural characteristics were primary variables in differentiating Mexican-American adults who passed the Adaptive Behavior Scales from those who failed. The level of education of the spouse in the family was the single most important factor; but education of the head, participation of the head in formal organizations, size of the household, working experience of the spouse, and use of English in the home were also related. Physical disabilities were not a significant factor.

Multivariate Analysis of Differentials in Adaptive Behavior

It is apparent from the analysis of biological and sociocultural factors that they not only were significantly related to performance on the Adaptive Behavior Scales but were also related to each other. In order to assess interrelationships and to determine the amount of variance in adaptive behavior that can be accounted for by these variables, taken singly and together, we performed a stepwise multiple regression for preschool children, school-age children, and adults. In this regression analysis, sex, physical disability, ethnic group, and socioeconomic level were treated as independent variables, and adaptive behavior as the dependent variable.

Although the two biological characteristics, sex and physical disability, were significantly correlated with adaptive behavior in preschool and school-age children ($R = .15$ and $.26$, $p<.001$), together they accounted for only 2.3% of the variance in adaptive behavior in preschool children and 6.8% of the variance in the adaptive behavior scores of school-age children. The addition of ethnic group and socioeconomic level only increased the amount of the explained variance to 2.9% for preschool and 7.3% for school-age children.

For adults, the situation was reversed and the sociocultural variables were more significant. Socioeconomic level was the primary explanatory variable ($r = .29$), with ethnic group running a close second ($r = .28$). R was increased from .29 to .36 by adding ethnic group to socioeconomic status. The amount of variance in adaptive behavior explained by these variables was larger than for children. Eight percent of the variance was explained by socioeconomic status alone, rising to 13.0% with the addition of ethnic group and to 16% with the addition of physical disabilities ($R = .40$).

We conclude that adaptive behavior was more closely tied to the biological factors of sex and physical disabilities for children and to the sociocultural factors of socioceonomic status and ethnic group for adults. For all age groups, however, the amount of variance in adaptive behavior explained by a combination of these four factors was modest. Over 92% of the variance in adaptive behavior in children and 84% of the variance in adaptive behavior for adults was not explained by the four factors studied in this analysis. Although performance on the adult scales was significantly influenced by socioeconomic status and ethnic group, the total impact of these variables was less than might be anticipated, considering the fact that items were selected to measure role behaviors most typical of the Anglo core culture and there were significantly higher rates of failure among low-status persons and persons from ethnic minorities.

Chapter 11

CHARACTERISTICS OF PERSONS FAILING THE INTELLECTUAL DIMENSION

It was not possible to administer an intelligence test to everyone who was in the screened sample. Therefore, a subsample was selected for testing. The tested subsample was a disproportionate, stratified selection of cases from the larger sample of persons screened in the household survey. Each subsample person was weighted according to the number of individuals of the same age, ethnic group, socioeconomic level, score on the combined Adaptive Behavior–Physical Disability Scale, and sex (for Anglos) which he represented in the screened sample. All of the statistics presented in this chapter are based on data from the 186 preschool children, 292 school-age children, and 182 adults in the tested subsample multiplied by their sampling weights to reproduce an estimate of the distribution of intelligence test scores in the screened sample.

As in the analysis of the Adaptive Behavior Scales, we will examine two biological variables—sex and physical disabilities—and two sociocultural variables—socioeconomic status and ethnic group.

Sex and Physical Disability as Factors in Subnormal Intellectual Performance

There were no significant sex differences in performance on the intellectual measures. There also was no significant difference in the percentage of preschool children with low IQs who had no physical disabilities and the percentage of children with high IQs who were not disabled at any criterion level ($r = .05$). On the other hand, differences were very significant at every criterion level for school-age children ($r = -.21$, $p<.001$). Eighty-eight percent of the school-age children with an IQ below 70, 34% of those with an IQ under 80, and 31% of those with an IQ under 85 had one or more physical disabilities ($p<.001$).

Forty percent of the adults with an IQ below 70 and 43% of the adults with IQs under 80 had one or more physical disabilities ($p<.001$). There were no differences when the AAMD criterion was used. However, the linear correlation between IQ and physical disability score was a negligible −.05 for adults. Although physical disabilities characterized a significant number of adults who had very low IQs, physical disability was not highly related to intelligence along the entire range of IQ test scores.

Differentials in Intelligence Test Scores by Socioeconomic Level

Preschool and school-age children were combined for the analysis of socioeconomic level. Low socioeconomic status is a distinguishing characteristic of both children and adults with low IQs at all criterion levels. Results are similar regardless of the socioeconomic measure used.

Only 25% of the children in the community come from homes in which the occupation of the head of household has a socioeconomic index score of 0–19, but 84% of the children with an IQ of 69 or below, 76% of those with scores under 80, and 55% of those with scores under 85 come from such homes. When the occupation of the head is classified into two categories—blue-collar vs white-collar—differences are even more marked. Between 40% and 45% of the children with high IQs come from blue-collar homes, but 95% of those with an IQ under 70 and 93% of those with an IQ under 80 come from blue-collar homes! Even at the AAMD criterion, 87% of the children failing the IQ dimension are from blue-collar homes. The mean housing-value decile for the blocks on which low IQ children lived ranged from 3.5 to 3.9, depending on the criterion level used. The mean housing decile of children with clinically normal IQs ranged from 6.1 to 6.5. These differences are all significant ($p<.001$). Education of the head of household as a fourth index of socioeconomic level reveals differences comparable to the other three measures. About 25% of the children with clinically normal IQs come from homes in which the head has less than a high school education, but almost 75% of the children with low IQs come from such homes ($p<.001$).

When adults are compared using the same variables, differences follow the same pattern as that for children, except that they are even more extreme at traditional and educational criterion levels. Adults with low IQs are even more likely than children to come from homes in which the occupation of the head rates between 0 and 19 on the Duncan Index. They, too, are more likely to come from blue-collar homes, from homes located in neighborhoods with low housing value, and from homes in which the head has not graduated from high school.

When all age groups were combined and those having an IQ below 85 were compared with those having an IQ of 85 or higher, we found that the mean socioeconomic index score of the heads of households in which the low group were residing was 20.0, compared with a mean score of 50.5 for persons with high scores ($p<.001$). The average years of education for the heads of household in the low group were 8.3, compared with 12.9 for the high group ($p<.001$). The linear correlation between IQ and socioeconomic level was .38 for preschool children, .35 for school-age children, and .45 for adults, indicating that 12% to 14% of the variance in children's IQs and 20% of the variance in adults' IQ can be accounted for by socioeconomic index score alone.

Because most Mexican-American and Black families are concentrated in lower socioeconomic statuses, a meaningful contingency table analysis of socioeconomic status within ethnic group is not feasible for these two groups. However, among Anglos, the low-scorers on intelligence tests are definitely concentrated in lower socioeconomic levels: 45.8% of the Anglos with an IQ of 85 and above are from homes rated 60 or above on the Duncan Index, while only 7.5% of those with low IQs come from families in this category ($p<.001$).

Differentials in Intelligence Test Scores by Ethnic Group

Ethnic group and socioeconomic status are highly correlated ($r = .39$ for children and .34 for adults).[1] Therefore, we would anticipate a heavy concentration of persons from ethnic minorities among low-scorers on intelligence tests if only because many persons from ethnic minorities have low socioeconomic status.

We found that over half of the children 7 months through 15 years of age who had low IQs, regardless of the criterion cutoff used, were of Mexican-American heritage, while only 7.1 to 11.4% of those passing the intelligence tests were from this group. Similarly, over 25% of the children receiving failing scores were Black, while only 8.1% of the children in the passing population were Black. Although 79.6% of the children in the study were Anglo, only 12.5% of those with an IQ below 85 were Anglo. The correlation between ethnic group and IQ was not significant for preschool children ($r = .13$) but was significant for school-age children ($r = .40$, $p<.001$).

The correlation was even greater for adults ($r = .53$, $p<.001$). Seventy percent of the adults with an IQ below 70 were of Mexican heritage. Sixty-six percent of those with an IQ below 80 were Mexican-Americans. The disproportion is not so large when the IQ cutoff is 84, but even then, 53.1% are Mexican-Americans, a figure four-and-one-half times higher than would be expected from their percentage in the general population. Black adults are also slightly overrepresented in

[1] These correlations were computed on the tested subsample, using the weights assigned to each case as described in Appendix A. A similar correlation computed for the entire screened sample was .43.

the low-scoring category. Thirteen percent of those with IQs below 69 were Black, compared with 6% of those with higher scores. However, Black adults are not overrepresented at the AAMD criterion. Conversely, Anglo adults are underrepresented at all three criterion levels. Although they make up approximately 88% of those passing the intelligence tests, they make up only 16.8% of those with scores below 70, 22.1% of those with scores below 80, and 40.3% of those with scores below 85.

We combined all ages and compared the ethnic group of persons with an IQ below 85 with that of persons having a score of 85 or above. While Anglos comprise 92.7% of those with IQs above 84, they make up 26.7% of those with low scores. Conversely, Mexican-Americans make up 3.8% of the persons in the population with an IQ above 84, but constitute 55.9% of those in the low category. Blacks make up 3.5% of the persons with high IQs, but 17.4% of those with low IQs. The correlation between ethnic group and IQ was .43 ($p<.001$).

Do these ethnic differences persist when socioeconomic status is held constant? To answer this question, we selected only persons from households in which the occupation of the head was rated between 0 and 29 on the Duncan Index and compared the ethnic composition of the group with IQs above 84 with the group with scores of 84 and below. Ethnic differences persist at approximately the same magnitude as when socioeconomic status was not held constant ($p<.001$). There are about five times more Mexican-Americans in the below 85 group than in the high IQ group, almost twice as many Blacks, and only one-fifth as many Anglos. The low group contained 14.8% Anglo, 62.3% Mexican-American, and 22.9% Black, while comparable percentages in the high IQ group were 74.1%, 13.1%, and 12.8%. There were too few high-status Mexican-American and Black adults in the tested subsample to make meaningful comparisons within the high-status group.

We conclude, therefore, that persons from minority groups are more likely to fail an intelligence test even when socioeconomic status is held constant. The disproportionately larger number of persons from ethnic minority groups in low IQ categories is even more significant because we estimate that the tested subsample may slightly underestimate the number of minority adults with low IQs.

Relative Impact of Sociocultural Variables on IQ and Adaptive Behavior

A stepwise multiple regression analysis was conducted to investigate the interrelationships between sex, physical disability, ethnic group, and socioeconomic status in predicting IQ, using the weighted frequencies in the tested subsample. Preschool children, school-age children, and adults were analyzed separately and then the three age groups were combined.

When we compare the findings on adaptive behavior reported in chapter 10 with the findings on IQ reported in this chapter, a clear pattern emerges. Although performance on both the intelligence tests and the Adaptive Behavior Scales is related to socioeconomic status and ethnic group, the relationship between these sociocultural variables and IQ is consistently greater with IQ than adaptive behavior. This is especially true for children. Socioeconomic status is not correlated with adaptive behavior at all in preschool and school-age children (r = .05) but is highly correlated with IQ (r = .38 and .35). Both IQ and adaptive behavior are related to socioeconomic status for adults, but the relationship is slightly greater for IQ (r = .45) than it is for adaptive behavior (r = .29). Between 40% and 45% of the adults failing adaptive behavior were from households rated 0–19 on the Duncan Index, but 67% to 97% of those failing the intelligence test were from such homes.

Ethnic group was not correlated with performance on the adaptive behavior scales for preschool children (r = .02) or school-age children (r = .05), but IQs for children were highly related to ethnic group (r = .13 for preschool and .53 for school-age children). More minority adults scored low on both adaptive behavior and IQ, but again ethnic disparities were greatest on the intelligence test. Between 25% and 38% of the adults failing adaptive behavior were Mexican-American, while 38% to 70% of the adults failing IQ were Mexican-American (r = .28, compared with r = .53).

When socioeconomic status is controlled by comparing only low-status persons (Duncan Index of 0–29), both adaptive behavior and IQ are still more frequently failed by Mexican-American adults, but again the differentials are greater for IQ than adaptive behavior. Between 38% and 47% of the low-status persons who failed adaptive behavior at the three criterion levels were Mexican-American, while 62% of the low-status persons with an IQ below 85 were Mexican-American.

Comparison of the multiple regressions also demonstrates the higher relationship between sociocultural variables and IQ than between sociocultural variables and adaptive behavior. Ethnic group and socioeconomic level account for 15% to 20% of the variance in IQ for children but almost none of the variance in adaptive behavior. Ethnic group accounted for 37.2% of the variance in IQ for adults but only 13% of the variance in adaptive behavior. When all age groups are combined, the sociocultural variables explain 25% of the variance in IQ but less than 5% of the variance in adaptive behavior.

We must conclude that sociocultural factors do influence both adaptive behavior and intellectual performance, but are a more important influence on intellectual performance than on adaptive behavior as it is measured by our scales. This is especially noteworthy when we consider that the Adaptive Behavior Scales were explicitly designed to measure social-role performance as typified by the core culture. Apparently, social-role performance is more generalizable across socioeconomic and ethnic lines than the cognitive and intellectual skills measured by the IQ. These relationships illustrate graphically the limitations of the clinical perspective and statistically normed diagnostic instruments when dealing with phenomena related to sociocultural variables.

Chapter 12

CHARACTERISTICS OF THE CLINICALLY RETARDED— THE ELIGIBLES

Having examined the characteristics of those who scored as subnormal in adaptive behavior or intelligence, we are now prepared to combine the measures to identify those in the field survey who were subnormal in both intellectual performance and adaptive behavior. These are two-dimensional retardates—the clinically retarded—according to the operational definition adopted for the field survey. We will report the findings by presenting statistical comparisons of the social characteristics of persons who appeared in each major category of the typology, the clinically retarded, quasi-retarded, behaviorally maladjusted, and the "normal."

Family Background Characteristics of the Clinically Retarded

We found that socioeconomic status and ethnic group were highly related to both adaptive behavior score and IQ. Therefore, we would expect that these two social characteristics and others associated with them would differentiate persons in the four major groups.

Table 9 compares the clinically retarded, the quasi-retarded, the behaviorally maladjusted, and the "normal" on socioeconomic factors, parental education, family structure, living conditions, and ethnic origins. These are the variables that formed the modal sociocultural configuration for the community in chapter 3. All frequencies are derived from the tested subsample, and all comparisons are made using weighted frequencies from that sample. The AAMD criterion was used.

The Clinically Retarded (Type 1 + 2)
Compared with the Quasi-retarded (Type 3 + 4)

Persons who failed both adaptive behavior and IQ were more socioeconomically disadvantaged than those who failed only IQ. A larger percentage of the clinically retarded came from homes in which the head of household has an occupation ranked 0–29 on the Duncan Socioeconomic Index. The occupation of the spouse in households of the clinically retarded is also more likely to be ranked 0–29 on the

Table 9: Family Background Characteristics of the Clinically Retarded Compared with the Quasi-retarded, Behaviorally Maladjusted, and "Normals"

Characteristic	Clinically Retarded (Type 1 + 2) (Nw = 243)	Quasi-retarded (Type 3 + 4) (Nw = 267	Behaviorally Maladjusted (Type 5 + 6) (Nw = 681)	"Normal" (Type 7 + 8) (Nw = 5,619)	Significance Level: 1 + 2 vs 3 + 4	1 + 2 vs 5 + 6	1 + 2 vs 7 + 8
Socioeconomic Variables							
% SES Index Head 0–29	86.3	65.5	34.4	25.5	<.001	<.001	<.001
% SES Index Mother 0–29	66.5	54.7	35.7	20.8	<.001	<.001	<.001
% Housing Decile 1–3	64.6	43.4	28.8	18.2	<.001	<.001	<.001
Education of Parents							
% Head High School Graduate	17.7	42.9	70.1	82.1	<.001	<.001	<.001
% Mother High School Graduate	22.4	44.1	67.8	72.0	<.001	<.001	<.001
% Head Repeated Grades	19.3	30.7	21.5	9.6	<.01	NS	<.001
Family Size and Structure							
% Head Divorced, Separated, Widowed	16.1	5.2	15.2	8.7	<.001	NS	<.001
Mean Persons in Household	5.3	5.9	4.8	4.6	<.001	<.001	<.001
Living Conditions							
% Deteriorating or Dilapidated Housing	30.4	14.1	19.6	9.2	<.01	<.001	<.001
% Moved 2+ Times in Last 10 Years	50.0	66.2	70.3	72.9	<.001	<.001	<.001
% Renting	37.4	15.7	37.1	24.9	<.001	NS	<.001
Ethnic Origins							
% Speaks English All the Time	35.4	54.3	93.3	93.4	<.001	<.001	<.001
% Head Foreign Born	21.0	16.8	1.5	1.2	NS	<.001	<.001
% Head Born in South	29.8	58.6	8.6	13.2	<.001	<.001	<.001

NOTE: The typology based on the 16% criterion was used. All differences were tested using the chi-square test of the significance of difference between independent samples. The statistical significance of differences among all four groups for the entire sample was tested and found significant prior to internal comparisons.

Duncan Socioeconomic Index. More clinical retardates live in neighborhoods in which the housing value ranks in the lowest three deciles.

Education of adults is significantly lower in the families of the clinically retarded than in those of the quasi-retarded. While almost half the heads of households in families of the quasi-retarded have graduated from high school, only 18% of those in the families of the clinically retarded are high school graduates. The same situation exists for spouses. Only half as many spouses in the homes of the clinically retarded graduated from high school as in the homes of the quasi-retarded. This finding is especially interesting because more heads of households in families of the quasi-retarded actually repeated grades in school than the heads of the families of clinically retarded. The heads of household in the families of the quasi-retarded were more persistent in pursuing their education.

Families of the quasi-retarded are larger in size; families of the clinically retarded are more likely to have a head of household who has been divorced, separated, or widowed. More of the clinically retarded than quasi-retarded are living in deteriorated or dilapidated dwellings. Although more of the families of the clinically retarded are renting their homes, they are significantly less geographically mobile than the families of the quasi-retarded. Only 50% of them have moved two or more times in the past ten years, compared with 66% of the quasi-retarded.

A most interesting configuration in family background appeared in the three measures for ethnic origin. Approximately the same number of heads of households in the two groups were foreign born, but significantly more families among the clinically retarded speak Spanish at home. It appears that the foreign-born heads of households in the families of the quasi-retarded have made an effort to learn English and speak it at home and that this is not so true in families of the clinically retarded. A large percentage of the heads of households of both groups were born in the southern states, but significantly more of the quasi-retarded than clinically retarded came from such families.

In brief, the clinical retardate comes from a more socioeconomically and educationally disadvantaged home environment than the quasi-retarded. Persons with low IQs who pass adaptive behavior come from homes more similar to the modal sociocultural configuration for the community.

The Clinically Retarded (Type 1 + 2) Compared with the Behaviorally Maladjusted (Type 4 + 5)

In table 9, the family backgrounds of the clinically retarded are also clearly differentiated from those of the behaviorally maladjusted. Those who failed adaptive behavior but passed the intelligence measures come from socioeconomic backgrounds significantly higher than those of the clinically retarded and the quasi-retarded, but lower than that of the "normals." The clinically retarded have the highest percentage of persons living under disadvantaged circumstances. The quasi-retarded have the next highest percentage, followed by the behaviorally disturbed, and the "normals."

Adult education shows the same linear pattern. The percentage of heads of households and spouses who are high school graduates increases significantly from the clinically retarded to the behaviorally maladjusted. The percentage of heads of households who have repeated grades is approximately the same. There is approximately the same percentage of broken homes in both groups, but the families of the behaviorally maladjusted are smaller in size. In these respects, the behaviorally maladjusted are more like the clinically retarded and the quasi-retarded and less like the "normals."

The families of the behaviorally maladjusted are more mobile than those of the clinically retarded. They are equally likely to be renting, but less likely to be living in dilapidated housing. Most families of the behaviorally maladjusted speak English all the time in the home, and few heads of households are foreign born or from southern states. In these respects, they are almost identical to the "normals" and least like the clinically retarded. In general, they come from less stable, lower-status Anglo families.

The Clinically Retarded (Type 1 + 2) Compared with "Normals" (Type 7 + 8)

The clinically retarded differ from the "normals" on every family background variable that was studied. The "normals" come from significantly more affluent backgrounds. They come from homes with better-educated adults. Their families are significantly smaller and less likely to have been broken by divorce, separation, or death. The "normals" change dwellings more frequently than the clinically retarded, but are less likely to be renting or to be living in deteriorated housing. Most of them come from English-speaking families in which the head of household was born in the United States, outside of the South.

To summarize, the family background characteristics of persons in the four major types defined in the field survey form a linear pattern from socioeconomic and educational disadvantage to socioeconomic and educational advantage. Persons from families whose characteristics are most like the modal sociocultural configuration for the community are most likely to be clinically "normal," while those from nonmodal backgrounds are most likely to be categorized as clinically retarded.

Personal Characteristics of the Clinically Retarded

Table 10 compares the personal characteristics of the clinically retarded with those of the quasi-retarded, behaviorally maladjusted, and the "normals," using the AAMD criterion. In part 2 of this volume, we reported that significantly more school-age persons and more males were labeled as retardates by most formal organizations in the community. This was not true for persons screened as clinically retarded in the household survey. There was no surplus of school-age persons in any of the four types screened in the fieldwork. The average age for all groups is approximately twenty-two years. There were significantly more males among the behaviorally maladjusted (63.4%), but the male–female ratio for the clinically retarded and quasi-retarded did not differ significantly from that for the "normals" in the community.

Ethnic disproportions, however, were even more pronounced than those found in the community labeling study. Only 22.9% of the clinically retarded and 30.1% of the quasi-retarded were Anglos. Over 66.2% of the clinically retarded and 46.6% of the quasi-retarded were Mexican-American, while 10.8% of the clinically retarded and 23.3% of the quasi-retarded were Black. The behaviorally maladjusted and "normals" were predominantly Anglos and reflected the ethnic distribution in the community.

The clinically retarded were more physically disabled than any other group, but differences were statistically significant only when they were compared with the quasi-retarded or the "normals." The behaviorally maladjusted had a mean disability score only slightly lower than that for the clinically retarded.

Social-Role Performance of the Clinically Retarded

School-age Children

We compared the performance of the clinically retarded school-age child with that of the quasi-retarded, behaviorally maladjusted, and "normal" on specific items in the Adaptive Behavior Scales. Although the clinically retarded tended to do less well on most adaptive behavior questions, the differences were statistically significant only for five school-related items when the clinically retarded were compared with the quasi-retarded and the "normal." The clinically retarded school-age child is significantly more likely to be behind the grade expected for

Table 10: Personal Characteristics of the Clinically Retarded, the Quasi-retarded, the Behaviorally Maladjusted, and "Normals"

Characteristic	Clinically Retarded (Type 1 + 2) (Nw = 243)	Quasi-retarded (Type 3 + 4) (Nw = 267)	Behaviorally Maladjusted (Type 5 + 6) (Nw = 681)	"Normal" (Type 7 + 8) (Nw = 5619)	Significance Level		
					1 + 2 vs 3 + 4	1 + 2 vs 5 + 6	1 + 2 vs 7 + 8
Sex							
% Male	48.1	51.3	63.4	46.5	NS	<.001	NS
Ethnic Group							
% Anglo	22.9	30.1	84.2	88.9			
% Mexican-American	66.2	46.6	8.3	5.4	<.001	<.001	<.001
% Black	10.8	23.3	7.5	5.6			
Mean Physical Disability Score	.91	.43	.71	.34	<.001	NS	<.001

NOTE: The typology based on the 16% criterion was used. All differences were tested using the chi-square test of the significance of difference between independent samples.

his age in school (51.2%, compared with 3.1% and 2.8%); to have repeated one or more grades (68.3%, compared with 13.8% and 6.3%); to be reported by his mother as having trouble learning in school (92.7%, compared with 47.2% and 7.8%); to be in remedial or other special school programs (66.9%, compared with 7.5% and 8.7%); and to be having "problems" in school (85.4%, compared with 33.3% and 26.8%). However, the clinically retarded differed significantly from the behaviorally maladjusted on only two items, being behind their age-grade norm (51.2% vs 26.1%) and having repeated grades (68.3% vs 41.8%). On the other three characteristics, differences were not statistically significant.

There were no statistically significant differences in the performance of the four groups on community and family-role items, but there was a persistent pattern in the responses, which should be noted. More of the behaviorally maladjusted were reported to have had difficulty in every area relating to interpersonal relations. More of the behaviorally maladjusted had had trouble with the police. On the other hand, a high percentage of the clinically retarded were reported to get along "very well' with teachers (68.6%), friends (71.4%), mother (84.2%), father (82.3%), sisters (41.9%), and brothers (38.2%). The only area in which the clinically retarded had more interpersonal difficulties than the behaviorally maladjusted was in the neighborhood. This consistent pattern confirms, to some extent, the validity of calling this group, who have normal IQs but subnormal adaptive behavior scores, the behaviorally maladjusted. We would expect just this kind of pattern in social-role performance in persons of normal intelligence who are having emotional problems.

Thus, clinical retardation is highly related to academic-role performance in school for school-age children. However, the clinically retarded cannot be differentiated systematically from the quasi-retarded, the behaviorally maladjusted or the "normals" in their performance in community and family roles. This important finding parallels findings reported in Chapter 6. Much mental retardation is a "school specific" condition. Academic roles were the only roles that caused difficulty for many persons who were identified as clinical retardates in the field screening and who were holding the status of mental retardates in some community social systems. It is surprising that such a "school specific" pattern should emerge so clearly in a field survey not directed at a study of social institutions in the community. Clinical retardation does not greatly influence an individual's interpersonal relations at home or in the community, but it definitely influences his adjustment in one social institution—the school.

Table 11: Social-role Performance of Adult Clinical Retardates Compared with Behaviorally Maladjusted and "Normal"

Characteristics	Clinically Retarded (Type 1 + 2) (Nw = 175)	Behaviorally Maladjusted (Nw = 397) (Type 5+ 6)	"Normal" (Nw = 3294) (Type 7 + 8)	Significance Level 1 + 2 vs 5 + 6	Significance Level 1 + 2 vs 7 + 8
Education-Intellectual Roles					
% Failed One or More Grades	27.3	35.5	12.6	NS	<.001
% Some Trouble Learning	45.1	43.6	6.5	NS	<.001
% High School or More	13.1	53.9	76.3	<.001	<.001
% Dropped—School Problems	69.7	26.9	4.0	<.001	<.001
% Never Reads Books	58.3	45.3	5.4	<.01	<.001
% Never Reads Magazines	49.7	29.9	3.5	<.001	<.001
% Never Reads Newspapers	46.3	5.3	1.6	<.001	<.001
Occupational Roles					
% Never Worked at a Job	26.3	5.0	4.0	<.001	<.001
Occupational Level When Working					
% Partially or Wholly Dependent	25.7	10.8	.5	<.001	<.001
% White-collar	15.2	40.1	68.5		
% Skilled or Semiskilled	38.4	34.8	23.0	<.001	<.001
% Unskilled	46.4	25.1	8.5		
Family Roles					
% Head of Household or Spouse of Head	75.4	84.9	79.7	NS	NS

General Community Roles					
% Active Member of a Club	29.1	48.8	95.7	<.001	<.001
% Never Votes	69.6	35.7	5.8	<.001	<.001
% Never Goes to Movies	28.6	34.3	7.8	NS	<.001
% Works with Little Supervision	93.7	96.4	99.8	NS	<.001
% Never Goes to Store Alone	13.1	18.2	.1	NS	<.001
% Never Travels Alone	12.6	12.7	1.0	NS	<.001
Informal Community Roles					
% Never Participates in Sports	56.6	38.3	13.4	<.001	<.001
% Never Goes Dancing	56.0	22.6	21.1	<.001	<.001
% Never Plays Parlor Games	41.1	31.4	1.1	NS	<.001
% Never Visits Relatives	28.2	40.6	25.8	<.001	NS
% Never Visits Co-workers	18.2	46.4	15.4	<.001	NS
% Never Writes Letters	21.1	39.5	.8	<.001	<.001
% Never Attends Church	22.9	46.7	16.2	<.001	NS
% Never Visits Neighbors	17.7	27.0	8.1	NS	<.001
% Never Visits Friends	13.1	16.6	2.5	NS	<.001

NOTE: The AAMD criterion was used (16%). Chi-square test was used to test significance of differences (2 df) and then partitioned.

Adults

Performance in educational and intellectual roles differentiated the clinically retarded adult from the behaviorally maladjusted adult even more clearly than it differentiated school-age children. Approximately equal proportions of both groups failed one or more grades in school, and were reported to have had "trouble learning." In spite of this similarity, significantly more of the behaviorally maladjusted graduated from high school (53.9%, compared with 13.1%) and fewer dropped out of school because of academic or discipline problems or lack of interest. Present intellectual activities clearly distinguished them from each other. The clinically retarded were more likely never to read books (58.3%, compared with 45.3%), magazines (49.7%, compared with 29.9%), or newspapers (46.3%, compared with 5.3%).

Occupational roles also distinguished the two groups. Twenty-six percent of the clinically retarded adults had never held a job of any kind, and 25.7% were partially or wholly dependent on others for financial support. The occupational level of the clinical retardate who had worked was also significantly lower than that of the behaviorally maladjusted. Only 15% of the clinically retarded had had white-collar jobs, compared with 40% of the behaviorally maladjusted, while 46% of the clinically retarded were unskilled laborers, compared with 25% of the behaviorally maladjusted.[1]

Table 11 also compares family and community roles as revealed in interview responses. Here the comparisons are less clear-cut. There was no difference in the percentage of the two groups who were heads of households or spouses of heads of households. Fewer of the retarded were active members of a club or voted in elections, but there were no differences in the percentage of those who attended movies, traveled alone, worked without supervision, or shopped by themselves. A large percentage of the clinically retarded never went dancing, participated in sports, or played parlor games; but the latter difference did not reach statistical significance.

On questions dealing specifically with interpersonal relations, the same pattern emerged as that which we found for school-age children. More clinically retarded adults participated in informal social exchanges than did the behaviorally maladjusted. Four of the six comparisons are significant ($p<.001$), and all comparisons are in the direc-

[1] White-collar jobs are those classified in the U.S. census as professional, technical, and kindred workers; managers, officials, proprietors (nonfarm); clerical and kindred workers; sales workers. Blue-collar jobs are those classified as craftsmen, foremen, and kindred workers; operative and kindred workers; private household workers; service workers; farm owners, managers, foremen, and laborers; and laborers (nonfarm).

tion of less participation by the behaviorally maladjusted. Significantly more of the behaviorally maladjusted never attended church or wrote letters and never visited relatives or co-workers. Slightly more never visited neighbors or friends. These findings further confirm the validity of the operational distinction between the clinically retarded and the behaviorally maladjusted.

Every educational and occupational comparison between the clinically retarded and the "normals" is large ($p<.001$) and of sufficient magnitude to be both statistically and socially significant. While 76% of the "normals" have graduated from high school, only 13% of the "clinically retarded" have a high school diploma. Less than 7% of the "normals" had some trouble learning in school, but 45% of the clinically retarded had difficulties. Their current reading habits were strikingly different. Only 5.4% of the "normals" never read books, compared with 58% of the clinically retarded. Of the "normals," 3.5% never read magazines, compared with 49.7% of the clinically retarded, and 1.6% of the "normals" never read newspapers, compared with 46.3% of the retarded.

Adult occupational roles were also very different. While less than 1% of the "normal" adults were partially or wholly financially dependent, 25.7% of the clinical retardates were partially or wholly financially dependent and were not housewives or students. Just 4% of the "normal" population had never held a job, compared with 26% of the clinically retarded. While 68% of the "normals" were white-collar workers and only 8.5% were in unskilled occupations, the comparable percentages for the clinically retarded were 15.7% and 46.5%, respectively.

There is no difference between clinical retardates and "normals" in the percentage of those who were heads of households or spouses of heads of households; nor the percentage of those who visited relatives, visited co-workers, or attended church. However, performance in every other community role was significantly different. The clinically retarded participated less in all aspects of the life of the community, both formal and informal. Comparisons between the social-role performance of the clinically retarded and the quasi-retarded adults will be presented in a later chapter.

In interpreting the findings presented in this section, it is important to remember that those classified as clinically retarded because they failed IQ and the adaptive behavior scales were persons predominantly from lower socioeconomic backgrounds, from socially disadvantaged circumstances, and from ethnic minority groups. Their family backgrounds differed markedly from the sociocultural mode of the community. Many of the differences in their role performance were accentuated by these differences. Thus, behavioral differences between persons in the four types should not be interpreted as due solely to clinical variables.

Part IV

CURRENT ISSUES IN THE CLINICAL PERSPECTIVE

In parts 2 and 3 of this book we have examined the meaning of mental retardation in Riverside from both a clinical and a social system perspective. We have found numerous points at which clinical and social systems diverge and have also noted points at which they tend to converge. We have found that who is defined as mentally retarded depends on who is doing the defining and the procedures and norms he is using. Some persons are defined as mentally retarded by all definers and all procedures. Others are defined as mentally retarded by some definers and some procedures but not by others.

In part 4 we will discuss current issues in the clinical perspective, as revealed in this epidemiology, and identify those modifications in the clinical perspective that would maximize convergences between clinical and social system definitions of mental retardation.

Chapter 13

A ONE- OR A TWO-DIMENSIONAL DEFINITION?

Throughout the fieldwork, we operationalized mental retardation using a two-dimensional definition. Persons had to be subnormal in measures of both intellectual performance and adaptive behavior before they were classified as clinically retarded. This definition was used because most of the documented definitions of mental retardation refer to both intelligence and social adjustment. The AAMD definition specifically states that mental retardates are those who are subnormal in both intelligence and adaptive behavior, even while it deplores the fact that there are no standardized measures of adaptive behavior and that clinical judgments about adaptive behavior must rest on subjective evaluations.

Even though the AAMD nomenclature advocates a two-dimensional definition, for all practical purposes the definition follows a one-dimensional statistical model. It proceeds to specify five levels of mental retardation in terms of only one dimension—the IQ. The five levels of retardation are delineated by standard deviation units along a theoretical normal distribution of IQs.

When there is evidence of organic impairment, it is possible to use the pathological model in addition to the statistical model of "normal," and the credibility of the diagnosis is strengthened. Yet, in many cases, there is no evidence of biological dysfunction, and in actual clinical practice a diagnosis of mental retardation may be reached entirely on the basis of performance on an intelligence test.

We do not regard the term *quasi-retarded* as synonymous with *pseudoretarded.* "Pseudo retardation" refers to those situations in which a person who is intellectually normal appears to be subnormal during clinical diagnosis because of factors extraneous to his intellectual ability, which temporarily depress his performance. This apparent intellectual subnormality may result from temporary handicaps produced by hunger, fatigue, illness, emotional problems, anxiety in the test situation, unfamiliarity with the test situation, and so forth. Quasi-retardates, on the other hand, are not persons suffering from temporarily depressed performance or extraneous, handicapping conditions; they are individuals who reliably test as subnormal on an IQ test and normal in adaptive behavior.

Clinicians who conceptualize mental retardation solely in terms of intellectual performance would not identify the quasi-retarded as a separate group. This group emerges as a logical category only within a two-dimensional definition of retardation. Thus, we anticipate that some of the persons classified as quasi-retarded in the field epidemiology may have been labeled as mentally retarded by agencies that give primary weight, when making clinical judgments, to performance on an IQ test and do not systematically evaluate adaptive behavior.

Because clinical practitioners actually use a one-dimensional model rather than a two-dimensional model, the typology developed in the Riverside epidemiology diverges significantly from the day-to-day decision-making of clinicians. Therefore, we must determine whether our measures meet the assumptions of a two-dimensional model and then examine the consequences of the two-dimensional model by comparing our results with those we would have found if we had used a definition based entirely on IQ.

It is possible that adaptive behavior and intelligence are so closely correlated that they are not really independent measures. If they are essentially interchangeable, then an individual's IQ will suffice for a "diagnosis," and there is no need for the cumbersome, two-pronged definition developed in the survey. Therefore, our first task is to determine if our measures of adaptive behavior and intelligence are tapping different kinds of behaviors and skills.

Are Intelligence and Adaptive Behavior Independent Dimensions?

The first and simplest line of evidence is pragmatic—the schema worked. Sizable numbers of persons appeared in each of the eight categories of the typology. For example, when the AAMD criterion is used, there are 72 disabled and 171 nondisabled clinical retardates (Type 1 + 2); 63 disabled and 204 nondisabled quasi-retarded (Type 3 + 4); 182 disabled and 502 nondisabled behaviorally maladjusted (Type 5 + 6); and 978 disabled and 4,641 nondisabled "normals" (Type 7 + 8). If adaptive behavior, IQ, and physical disability were not varying independently, some of the categories would have been empty. Even Type 3, the physically disabled with low IQ and "normal" adaptive behavior, contained 63 persons. This was the one category we had hypothesized might not contain any cases.

A second and more precise analysis was made using correlations to determine the amount of the variance in each measure that could be accounted for by the others.[1] The correlation between IQ test score and adaptive behavior was —.29 for preschool children, —.31 for school-age children, —.18 for adults, and —.20 for all ages combined. These correlations indicate that IQ and adaptive behavior are least correlated for adults. Adaptive behavior can account for only about 3.2% of the variance in IQ in this age group. The school-age adaptive behavior scales contain several school-related items that inquire about academic performance and are more highly correlated with IQ, accounting for about 9% of the variance in IQ. For all age groups, adaptive behavior accounts for only 4% of the variance in IQ test score.

Scores on the physical disability scales were less correlated with IQ test scores than adaptive behavior. The correlation between IQ and physical disability was —.07 for preschool children, —.31 for school-age children, —.01 for adults, and —.04 for all ages combined. These correlations were insignificant except for school-age children, when physical disabilities could account for about 9% of the variance in IQ. Correlations between scores on the physical disability scales and the adaptive behavior scales were generally higher, .12 for preschool children, .35 for school-age children, .18 for adults, and .26 for all ages combined. Thus, physical disability score accounted for over 12% of the variance in adaptive behavior score for school-age children and almost 7% of the variance in the adaptive behavior scores of all ages combined.

Although the correlations between adaptive behavior and IQ test scores were statistically significant ($p<.001$), adaptive behavior does not actually account for a sufficiently large percentage of the variance in IQ to conclude that the IQ test can, simultaneously, serve as a measure of both intellectual performance and social-role performance. Nor can physical disabilities be ignored as a separate dimension. The three dimensions appear to be sufficiently independent to warrant separate measures and a two-dimensional definition.

The Impact of the Two-dimensional Definition on Prevalence Rates

The first principle that must be clearly understood in dealing with prevalence rates based on two behavioral dimensions is that the 3%

[1] Two separate analyses were made, one based on the tested subsample when each case had been multiplied by its sampling weight, and the other based on the unweighted subsample. The purpose of this duplicate calculation was to determine the effect, if any, of using the weighted rather than the unweighted scores. Differences

criterion does not mean that 3% of the persons in the population will be defined as retarded; the 9% criterion does not mean that 9% of the population will be retarded; nor does the 16% criterion mean that 16% of the population will be defined as retarded. When two dimensions are used, a person must be in the lowest 3% on *both* dimensions in order to be clinically retarded. Some people will be in the lowest 3% in IQ but not in adaptive behavior, and some will be in the lowest 3% in adaptive behavior and not IQ. These people will not be defined as retarded. Thus, when a 3% criterion is used, prevalence rates will always shrink to considerably less than 3%. The same principle also holds for the 9% and 16% criteria.

In Riverside, the 3% criterion produced a crude prevalence rate in the general population of 9.7 per 1,000 (.97%); the 9% criterion produced a general population rate of 18.9 per 1,000 (1.89%); and the 16% criterion produced a general population rate of 34.7 per 1,000 (3.47%). Increase in these rates is not proportionate to increase in criterion and, of course, will vary with the characteristics of the population being studied.

Table 12 shows precisely how this principle operates in the case of crude prevalence rates for the City of Riverside. We found, from the tested subsample, that there were an estimated 150 persons in the screened sample who had an IQ of 69 or below. This number would produce a crude prevalence rate of 21.4 per 1,000 using a one-dimensional definition. However, 82 of those with IQs 69 or below passed the Adaptive Behavior Scales. This left 68 persons defined as retarded, a shrinkage of 54.7%. Similarly, at the 9% level there were 258 persons with an IQ of 79 or below; but 126 of these passed the Adaptive Behavior Scales, leaving 132 defined as clinically retarded. This was a shrinkage of 48.8%. Comparable shrinkage at the AAMD criterion was 52.3%. At the 3% level, 82 persons, who would have been designated as mentally retarded under a one-dimensional system relying entirely on IQ, were not classified as retarded in the field survey. There were 126 such persons using the educational criterion and 267 such persons using the AAMD criterion. We have called these persons the quasi-retarded.

The same situation occurs with adaptive behavior, but is not shown in the table. At the 3% criterion, 293 persons failed adaptive behavior, but 225 of them had an IQ above 69, leaving only 68 as clinically retarded. This is a shrinkage of 76.8%, a greater shrinkage than occurs for

between correlations produced by the weighted subsample and those produced by the unweighted subsample were negligible. We concluded that it made little difference whether the relationships between adaptive behavior, IQ, and physical disability are calculated from the weighted or unweighted subsample.

Table 12: Prevalence Rates for Clinical Retardation per 1,000 for Selected Subgroups Comparing the Rates Using a One-dimensional with Those Using a Two-dimensional Definition

	Number Fail IQ	Rate per 1,000 Fail IQ	Number Fail IQ Pass A-B	% Shrinkage	Number Fail IQ Fail A-B	Rate per 1,000 Fail IQ Fail A-B
Traditional Criterion (IQ 69- and Adaptive Behavior, Lowest 3%)						
Total Population	150	21.4	82	54.7	68	9.7
Anglo	25	4.4	0	0	25	4.4
Mexican-American	100	149.9	60	60.0	40	60.0
Black	22	44.9	20	90.9	2	4.1
Deciles 1–3 (Low)	125	78.7	69	55.2	56	35.2
Deciles 4–7 (Middle)	20	7.0	11	55.0	9	3.1
Deciles 8–10 (High)	5	2.0	2	40.0	3	1.2
Educational Criterion (IQ 79- and Adaptive Behavior, Lowest 9%)						
Total Population	258	36.8	126	48.8	132	18.9
Anglo	48	8.4	13	27.1	35	6.1
Mexican-American	161	241.4	76	47.2	85	127.4
Black	49	100.0	38	77.5	11	22.4
Deciles 1–3 (Low)	188	118.3	86	45.7	102	64.2
Deciles 4–7 (Middle)	59	20.6	36	61.0	23	8.0
Deciles 8–10 (High)	11	4.3	4	36.4	7	2.8
AAMD Criterion (IQ 84- and Adaptive Behavior, Lowest 16%)						
Total Population	510	72.8	267	52.3	243	34.7
Anglo	135	23.5	80	59.2	55	9.6
Mexican-American	283	424.3	124	43.8	159	238.4
Black	88	179.6	62	70.5	26	53.1
Deciles 1–3 (Low)	273	171.8	125	45.8	158	99.4
Deciles 4–7 (Middle)	146	50.9	76	52.1	70	24.4
Deciles 8–10 (High)	91	35.8	75	82.4	16	6.3

NOTE: The total for the ethnic groups does not add up to the total population because there were a few persons classified as "Other Ethnic Group" not reported in this table.

IQ failures. Comparable shrinkage in adaptive behavior failures was 79.4% at the 9% criterion and 73.7% at the 16% criterion. Of course, the shrinkage in adaptive behavior failures is of little practical concern at present because adaptive behavior has never been systematically used as a single criterion for diagnosing mental retardation.

Does shrinkage occur proportionately in various subgroups of the population or are some groups more affected than others? Table 12 presents the prevalence rates for selected subgroups, using a one-dimensional definition, and compares them with rates using a two-dimensional definition.

Impact on Ethnic Rates of a Two-dimensional Definition

Looking first at ethnic group at the traditional criterion, 100 of the 150 persons with IQs below 70 were Mexican-American, 22 were Black, and 25 were Anglo. If rates are calculated simply from IQ, the rate for Anglos would be 4.4 per 1,000 population, 149.9 per 1,000 for Mexican-Americans, and 44.9 per 1,000 for Blacks. When adaptive behavior is also taken into consideration, none of the Anglos with an IQ below 70 pass the adaptive behavior scale. Therefore, the prevalence rates for Anglos are not influenced by the introduction of the adaptive behavior measure. On the other hand, 60% of the Mexican-Americans and 90.9% of the Blacks with low IQs pass adaptive behavior. When those who pass adaptive behavior are eliminated from the prevalence rates, it leaves 25 Anglos, 40 Mexican-Americans, and 2 Blacks diagnosed as clinically retarded. Using the traditional criterion, the prevalence rates per 1,000 then become 4.4, 60.0, and 4.1 respectively—a very significant reduction in rates for Mexican-Americans and Blacks.

At the educational criterion there is more divergence between adaptive behavior and IQ for the Anglo group, but it is still much less than for minority persons. Twenty-seven percent of the Anglos with an IQ below 80 have adequate adaptive behavior and are not screened as clinically retarded, while 47.2% of the Mexican-Americans and 77.5% of the Blacks are coping satisfactorily with their social roles. The rate of mental retardation, using a one-dimensional definition, would be 241 per 1,000 among Mexican-Americans and 100 per 1,000 among Blacks, but shrinks to 127 and 22 respectively, when adaptive behavior is also considered.

When the AAMD criterion is used, there is a great divergence between IQ and adaptive behavior for all groups. Fully 59% of the Anglos who have an IQ of 84 and below pass the adaptive behavior scale, reducing the one-dimensional rate from 23.5 per 1,000 to 9.6 when adaptive behavior is also evaluated. Mexican-American rates, using only the IQ test, are greatly inflated when an AAMD criterion is used. Fully 424 per 1,000 of the Mexican-American population would be evaluated as clinically retarded! The rate is cut in half by evaluating adaptive behavior but is still very large, 238 per 1,000. Black rates reach 180 per 1,000 when only the IQ test is used but shrink to 53 when adaptive behavior is also considered. From 70% to 90% of the Blacks who fail the IQ test at various levels pass the adaptive behavior scales at those levels.

As would be expected, a similar pattern appears for socioeconomic status but is less pronounced than in the case of ethnic group. At the traditional criterion, using a one-dimensional definition based only on IQ, the prevalence rates for housing deciles 1–3 is 78.7 per 1,000 but drops to 35.2 per 1,000 when a two-dimensional definition is used. The reduction in rates for deciles 4–7 and 8–10 is small, 7.0 to 3.1 per 1,000, and 2.0 to 1.2 per 1,000 respectively. Evaluating adaptive behavior has little effect on the diagnosis of middle- and high-status persons, but greatly affects the diagnosis of low-status persons.

Using only IQ, persons from low-status families have rates eleven times higher than the rates for middle-status persons and thirty-nine times higher than rates for high-status persons. If only the IQ test is used, we would expect 118 per 1,000 of the low-status persons in Riverside to have an IQ of 79 or below and 172 per 1,000 to have an IQ of 84 or below, while only 4.3 per 1,000 of the high-status persons would have an IQ of 79 or below, and 35.8 per 1,000 would have an IQ of 84 or below. Addition of adaptive behavior to the evaluation reduces all the rates by about half, but the socioeconomic difference remains. However, a 50% shrinkage has a more significant impact at the lower- than at the higher-status levels because rates are higher initially. A reduction of the rate from 118 per 1,000 to 64 is of more substantive significance than a reduction from 4.3 per 1,000 to 2.8, even though both are about equivalent in terms of overall percentage reduction.

The most important aspect of these figures is the finding that the Anglo rates, at the traditional criterion, were not affected at all by the addition of the adaptive behavior dimension, while rates for Mexican-Americans and Blacks were greatly reduced. An evaluation of adaptive behavior when screening Anglos at the traditional criterion level contributes little additional information to that provided by the IQ test. Those who fail IQ also tend to fail adaptive behavior. There has been no pressing need to develop diagnostic instruments to evaluate adaptive behavior for the Anglo population.

The addition of an adaptive behavior measure is important in evaluating persons from ethnic minorities and lower socioeconomic statuses —persons from backgrounds that do not conform to the modal pattern for the community. Many of them may fail the intelligence test mainly because they have not had the opportunity to learn the cognitive skills and to acquire the knowledge needed to pass such tests. Their deficiencies are limited primarily to performance in formal test situations.

When their adaptive behavior outside of an academic setting is evaluated, they demonstrate by their ability to cope intelligently with problems in other areas of life that they are not mentally deficient. Today, such abilities are not systematically assessed in determining a person's level of mental functioning. Persons whose backgrounds do not conform to the community mode are penalized by the one-dimensional definition.

On the other hand, when a two-dimensional definition is used, persons from minority backgrounds and lower socioeconomic status are given credit for their ability to cope intelligently with their social roles in nontest situations. This more global assessment eliminates a majority of them from consideration as comprehensively subnormal.

Social-role Performance of the Quasi-retarded

Chapter 12 compared the family background characteristics of the quasi-retarded and the clinically retarded and reported that the quasi-retarded come from a higher socioeconomic level; from homes in which the adults have more education; from homes that are less frequently broken by divorce, separation, or death; from homes that are less geographically mobile; and from backgrounds that are similar to the modal configuration of the community. They have had more opportunities to acquire the adaptive behaviors generally typical of American society. They have demonstrated their ability to assimilate these behaviors by having an average of only 2.1 adaptive behavior failures, compared with an average of 8.3 failures for those who are clinically retarded. Indeed, their adaptive behavior is very similar to that of the "normal" population, which has an average of 1.6 failures. Physically, the quasi-retarded do not enjoy any special advantage over the clinically retarded. About 14% of the clinically retarded have three or more physical disabilities, but 7.5% of the quasi-retarded are similarly disabled. The differences are not statistically significant.

Chapter 12 presented an analysis of the role behavior of the quasi-retarded school-age child and compared his performance with that of the clinically retarded child. Individuals in both groups have an IQ below 85, but the differences in their social-role performance in school were remarkable ($p<.001$). Significantly more of the clinically retarded have had trouble learning (92.7% vs 47.2%), are below age-grade norm (51.2% vs 31.1%), have repeated grades (68.3% vs 13.8%), and have been enrolled in remedial or special programs (66.9% vs 7.5%). There is no difference in their performance in family and community roles. It is clear that the primary difference between the clinically retarded and quasi-retarded school-age child is that the quasi-retardate, in spite of his low IQ, has somehow managed to cope with his school roles. He has avoided repeating grades, getting behind in his class, and being placed in remedial or special programs. His parents are less likely to mention that he has had problems in school. Undoubtedly, his family background, which includes more highly educated parents, a more stable home, and a higher socioeconomic level, has contributed to his skill in mastering the role demands of the school.

For the adult, occupational roles present the major challenge. Achieving financial independence, finding a place in the world of work, and being able to manage one's own affairs are the primary tests of social competence in the adult.

Unfortunately, the number of adults in our tested subsample who failed IQ but passed adaptive behavior was too small for reliable, statistical analysis, but an overview of their social-role performance is still informative. An estimated 80% of the quasi-retarded adults graduated from high school; they all read books, magazines, and newspapers; all have held jobs; 65% have white-collar positions; 19% have skilled or semiskilled positions, while 15.7% are unskilled workers. All of them are able to work without supervision; participate in sports; travel alone; go to the store by themselves; and participate in informal visiting with co-workers, friends, and neighbors. The quasi-retarded are participating more fully in the life of the community than the clinically retarded. The only member of the group who is partially dependent on others for support is an unmarried, 20-year-old girl still living with her parents.

Qualitative View of the Quasi-retarded

We have selected some cases from the field survey to serve as examples of the kinds of persons who would have been classified as mentally retarded under a one-dimensional definition but who are reclassified as quasi-retarded when a two-dimensional definition is used. Closer scrutiny of some of the school-age children and adults who have IQ test scores below 70 but have normal adaptive behavior provides an opportunity to make some qualitative judgments about the validity of regarding these persons as quasi- rather than comprehensively retarded.

Juan, a twelve-year-old Mexican-American boy, illustrates the school-age quasi-retardate who fails the traditional criterion intellectually (IQ 54), but presents no problem in his own social milieu and passes adaptive behavior with only five failures. The youngest of three children, Juan started school later than usual and is below the age-grade norm. He has had some trouble learning in school and has attended remedial reading classes; however, he has never been placed in special classes for the mentally retarded. He has never had a serious illness, accident, or operation, but does have some difficulty hearing. Juan failed only those adaptive behavior items which require reading: he does not read books, newspapers, or magazines for his own enjoyment; does not enjoy doing arithmetic problems; nor does he follow the funnies in the newspaper.

Like many Mexican-American children, Juan comes from a family that is not very familiar with Anglo society. His fifty-three-year-old father was reared in Mexico, but has lived in the United States for twenty-six years. He received no formal education in rural Mexico and is currently an unemployed orange-picker and field laborer, receiving unemployment insurance. Juan's mother was also reared in Mexico and left school after the third grade. At one time she worked as a housekeeper in private homes, but is now a full-time housewife. The family speaks Spanish most of the time at home and understands little English. They do not subscribe to a daily newspaper or to any magazines nor do they have any books in the home. They have many informal contacts with relatives, friends, neighbors, and co-workers, and watch all kinds of television programs. Juan's older sister has had no serious difficulties in school, but his older brother, age fourteen, repeated the third grade and is now below the grade-norm for his age. The brother has had some trouble learning in school, especially in reading. With a tested IQ of 69 and an adaptive behavior score of 4, he, too, would be classified as a quasi-retardate.

Dolores is one of three Puerto Rican children adopted by an Anglo couple. She has an IQ of 64, 4 adaptive behavior failures, and no physical disabilities. She is currently in special education classes in the public school, but the only adaptive behavior items which she failed were school-related. She has had some trouble learning in school, and has had special difficulties with reading. Although she does need help with her homework, her role performance outside of school was quite typical of a fifteen-year-old. She likes to play competitive games that require following rules; she goes to the store to buy minor articles of clothing; she is active in a social club with children her age; she is able to work around the home with little or no supervision; she is concerned about her appearance; she keeps her room in order; and so forth. Her nineteen-year-old brother is also in special education classes, although he manages a paper route and participates actively in sports. Like his sister, he seldom reads or writes.

Two mothers, one Mexican-American and the other Black, illustrate the characteristics of adults who are likely to be classified as quasi-retarded at the 3% criterion.

Maria, a forty-four-year-old Mexican mother of five, scored 65 on the intelligence test, 5 on the adaptive behavior scale, and had no physical disabilities. She was reared in New Mexico and her father was a fruit picker. After they moved to California, Maria completed the ninth grade and subsequently worked as a fruit packer. She reports no serious illnesses, operations, or accidents, regularly attends the Roman Catholic Church, and leads an active informal social life visiting friends, family, and neighbors. Although the family speaks English most of the time, the interview was conducted in Spanish. The

family enjoys watching Spanish-language television broadcasts and listens to the daily news in Spanish.
Maria's husband completed only the ninth grade and now works as a truck driver. Their twenty-five-year-old son is presently preparing to be a pharmacist. The twenty-one-year-old daughter graduated from high school and now works as a beauty operator. A second son graduated from high school the spring before the interview and will be attending college in the fall. He hopes to major in accounting and has worked as a mechanic's helper in a garage, as well as having worked in a supermarket. The two younger children are still in high school and will graduate next year. Although Maria scored low on the intelligence measures, there is nothing about her style of life nor the characteristics of her children that would indicate inadequacy in parental or other social roles.

The second woman failed both IQ and physical disabilities at the 3% level but manages to support her four children and participate in the social world of her neighbors, friends, and co-workers.

Betty is a twenty-six-year-old Black woman with an IQ of 59, an adaptive behavior score of 4, and a physical disability score of 3. She is separated from her husband and is rearing her four children, ranging in age from nine months to four years. Betty reported having had some trouble learning in school, but did graduate from high school and is currently working thirty hours a week as a maid in a motel to support her children. She receives no financial support from either public or private sources. Betty has had no serious accidents, operations, or illnesses with central nervous system implications but reports having some difficulty hearing, talking, and sleeping. She reports reading the newspaper and *True Story* magazine. She enjoys games and sports and goes dancing frequently, but does not participate much in formal organizations. In her spare time, Betty watches television; listens to music; and visits neighbors, friends, and co-workers frequently. On the WAIS, Betty did not know why people should pay taxes or where rubber comes from. She could name only three men who had been President of the United States. She said there were sixty weeks in a year and thought that the average woman was "six or seven feet tall." According to her, dark clothes are warmer than light-colored clothes because "they are a heavier fabric."

These persons and others who were quasi-retarded, using the traditional criterion, would be ranked as moderately or mildly retarded if a one-dimensional definition based solely on IQ performance were used. As we have seen, some of the school-age children are in special education classes. Yet, the adaptive behavior of these school-age children in nonacademic roles appears normal and they manage relatively complex role-sets outside of school. The adults fulfill the roles of parent, neighbor, relative, and friend, and many participate in the occupational and organizational structure of the larger society. However, as is clearly shown in Betty's case, they may not have the kind of information needed to pass an intelligence test and are exposed to the risk of being labeled mentally retarded.

Summary

A clinician cannot assume that with the IQ measure alone he can evaluate an individual's ability to cope with his social environment, especially if he is evaluating someone from a background that does not conform to the sociocultural mode for the community. If only IQ is used to diagnose mental retardation and the clinician does not concern himself with evaluating other facets of behavior, then many persons from minority groups and lower socioeconomic status who are coping intelligently with social situations and interpersonal relations may be diagnosed as mentally retarded. The addition of adaptive behavior as a second evaluative dimension in the diagnosis of mental retardation has relatively little impact on rates for Anglos or middle- and high-status persons but significantly reduces both Mexican-American and Black rates.

We conclude, therefore, that a two-dimensional definition of mental retardation, which requires that a person fail both adaptive behavior and IQ before being diagnosed as mentally retarded, is justified. The lack of a systematic means for assessing adaptive behavior in the home, neighborhood, school, and community has undoubtedly been one reason why clinicians have tended to rely almost entirely on intelligence tests in making diagnoses. The two-dimensional definition needs to be operationalized, and a more adequate means should be devised for evaluating an individual's ability to cope intelligently with social situations and interpersonal relations.

Chapter 14

WHICH CRITERION?

Throughout this volume, we have reported findings from the field survey using all three of the criteria currently used by various social agencies to define mental retardation: the AAMD criterion, which defines those persons in the lowest 16% of the scoring distribution as subnormal; the educational criterion, which defines those in the lowest 9% as subnormal; and the traditional criterion, which defines those in the lowest 3% as subnormal. As shown in the analysis of the clinical case register, there is little consensus on the part of the clinicians as to the criterion to be used. There is a sharp decline in the rate at which additional persons are labeled as mentally retarded by community organizations as IQs increase above 70. To confound the situation further, 8% of those nominated as mentally retarded by clinical organizations had an IQ above 85 and a few had IQs above 100. A person may be labeled as mentally retarded by one agency and not by another, depending on the criterion used in that agency.

Binet wrote over half a century ago, "It will never be to one's credit to have attended a special school. We should at the least spare from this mark those who do not deserve it" (Binet and Simon, 1905). This is no less true today. There are those who are protected by the label of mental retardate because they cannot manage their own affairs. They need nurturance and supervision. There are others for whom the label retardate is a burden and a stigma, depriving them of an opportunity for a full education and plaguing them as they strive to find a place for themselves in adult society. A critical issue in mental retardation is that of distinguishing those for whom the label is a shield from those for whom it is an impediment. Central to this issue is the question "Which criterion?"

We postulate that the decision about the appropriate criterion should be based on four considerations: (1) What is the criterion on which there is the highest level of consensus among professionals in the field of mental retardation? (2) How does the choice of criterion affect the total number of persons who will be diagnosed as clinically retarded? (3) How is the choice of criterion related to the sociocultural characteristics of persons screened as clinically retarded? (4) Which criterion best identifies those who need nurturance without stigmatizing, unnecessarily, persons who are likely to fulfill adult role expectations? In short, at what criterion is there convergence between clinical and social system definitions?

What Is the Criterion on Which There Is the Highest Level of Consensus?

Comparing the Rate of Eligibility with the Rate of Labeling

Table 13 compares rates for labeled retardation with rates for eligibility, based on the field survey. The crude prevalence rates for the eligibles is consistently higher than the crude rate for the labeled, and rates becomes increasingly divergent as the criterion level is raised. The gap between the rate of eligibility and the rate of actual labeling for the total population increased from 4.6 per 1,000 using the traditional criterion, to 11.1 using the educational criterion, to 26.6 using the AAMD criterion. The gap widens about equally for both males and females and for persons with and without physical disabilities. However, the gap between the rate of eligibility and the rate of labeling widens much more for persons from lower socioeconomic status than it does for higher-status persons. The difference between the rate of eligibility and the rate of labeling is 25.1 per 1,000 persons in housing-value deciles 1 through 3 at the traditional criterion, but rises to 48.4 per 1,000 at the educational criterion and to 83.2 per 1,000 at the AAMD criterion. The gap is much less for persons in housing deciles 4 through 7: minus 1.2 at the traditional criterion, rising to 1.7 at the educational criterion and to 17.8 at the AAMD criterion. There is no significant widening of the gap for persons in deciles 8 through 10. The rate for labeling is slightly higher than the rate of eligibility at the traditional and educational criteria, and the gap is a negligible 1.5 at the AAMD criterion. This indicates that there are few clinically eligible high-status persons who are not also labeled, and that there are many more low-status persons eligible than are actually labeled. The discrepancy gets greater as the criterion becomes more stringent.

Comparing ethnic groups, we find a close correspondence between eligibility and labeling for the Anglos. The gap is small and does not increase very greatly as the criterion is raised. For Blacks, the rates of eligibility and the rates for labeling correspond relatively closely at the traditional and educational criteria, but the gap becomes 38.4 per 1,000 if the AAMD criterion is used. For Mexican-Americans, the rates for eligibility, using a strictly clinical definition, are much higher than the rates of labeling, and the differences widen from 40.4 per 1,000 at

Table 13: Rates per 1,000 Comparing the Labeled with the Field of Eligibles, Using All Three Criteria Levels

	Traditional Criterion (IQ 69–)			Educational Criterion (IQ 79–)			AAMD Criterion (IQ 84–)		
	Eligibles	Labeled	Difference	Eligibles	Labeled	Difference	Eligibles	Labeled	Difference
Crude Prevalence	9.7	5.1	4.6	18.9	7.8	11.1	34.7	8.1	26.6
Total Population									
Male	11.0	5.3	5.7	13.3	8.7	4.6	33.8	9.3	24.5
Female	8.5	4.9	3.6	24.3	7.0	17.3	35.7	7.2	28.5
Housing Decile									
1–3	35.2	10.1	25.1	64.2	15.8	48.4	99.4	16.2	83.2
4–7	3.1	4.3	−1.2	8.0	6.3	1.7	24.4	6.6	17.8
8–10	1.2	2.9	−1.7	2.8	4.5	−1.7	6.3	4.8	1.5
Ethnic Group									
Anglo	4.4	3.1	1.3	6.1	4.5	1.6	9.6	4.7	4.9
Mexican-American	60.0	19.6	40.4	127.4	30.5	96.9	238.4	31.3	207.1
Black	4.1	7.5	−3.4	22.4	13.9	8.5	53.1	14.7	38.4
Decile 1–3 (Low Status)									
Anglo	16.8	3.2	13.6	19.2	4.6	14.6	25.3	4.7	20.6
Mexican-American	87.1	22.2	64.9	174.3	35.1	139.2	281.0	35.7	245.3
Black	7.1	8.8	−1.7	21.3	15.1	6.2	24.9	15.8	9.1
Decile 4–7 (Middle Status)									
Anglo	3.3	3.5	−.2	5.3	4.9	.4	7.8	5.1	2.7
Decile 8–10 (High Status)									
Anglo	1.2	2.3	−1.1	2.4	3.6	1.2	6.1	3.6	2.5
Physical Disability									
0	6.9	2.9	4.0	15.2	5.2	10.0	31.2	5.4	25.8
1+	19.1	12.8	6.3	32.5	17.2	15.3	49.0	17.9	31.1

the traditional criterion to 96.9 at the educational criterion and 207.1 at the AAMD criterion. When socioeconomic status is held constant by looking only at rates by ethnic group for persons in deciles 1 through 3, discrepancies between eligibility and labeling become even more marked for Mexican-Americans and Anglos, but are somewhat reduced for Blacks.

Two patterns are quite clear. For middle- and high-status persons and for Anglos, rates of eligibity and rates of labeling are roughly parallel. There are few persons in these categories who are clinically eligible who are not labeled. This holds true regardless of the criterion level that is used. In addition, the prevalence rate for retardation does not increase markedly as the criterion is raised for these groups. Consequently, resolving the ambiguities about the criterion level used in defining subnormality is not so critical a matter for these groups as for lower-status persons and persons from ethnic minorities.

For low-status persons and persons from ethnic minorities, especially the Mexican-Americans, there is a big gap between eligibility and labeling, which becomes greater as more stringent criteria are employed. Consensus on whom should be labeled as mentally retarded breaks down for these groups and is especially lacking when the educational and AAMD criteria are employed. This same pattern of increasing divergence occurs for both sexes, all ethnic groups, and for persons with or without physical disability.

There was a greater correspondence between the field survey and the actual labeling practices of clinicians in the community when the field survey rates were calculated using the traditional criterion. There was less agreement between field survey rates and clinical case register rates when the educational criterion was used, even though the public schools are the largest single contributor to the clinical case register. While the public schools employ an IQ of 79 or below as a general cutoff, teachers do not refer every child who has an IQ below 80 for testing, and school psychologists do not label every child with an IQ below 80 as mentally retarded. They are much more likely to refer and to label persons with IQ below 70 as mentally retarded. Divergences are very large using the AAMD criterion. There are very few clinicians in the community systematically using one standard deviation below the mean as their criterion.

Multiple Nominations as a Measure of Consensus

There were 361 persons nominated as labeled retardates who had an IQ of 69 or below and thus failed at the traditional criterion. There were 215 persons nominated with an IQ between 70 and 84. They would qualify as "borderline retardates" if we assume that clinicians made some assessment of adaptive behavior, however informal. The traditional retardates were nominated by an average of 2.36 agencies. Forty-five percent of them were nominated by two or more agencies, and 31% of them were nominated by six or more agencies. On the other hand, the "borderline retardates" were nominated by an average of 1.49 agencies. Only 28% were nominated by two or more agencies, and none of them were nominated by five or more agencies ($t = 5.36$, $p < .001$). This discrepancy in number of nominations indicates that there is significantly more clinical consensus and more duplication of identification by clinicians in different social agencies when a person fails the traditional criterion than when he is "borderline." Evidently, persons labeled as clinically retarded using a traditional criterion are more likely to be perceived as subnormal by many significant others in their social environment than persons failing only at the educational or AAMD level.

The traditional criterion also corresponds most closely to the perception of lay nominators. The mean IQ of persons nominated as mental retardates by respondents in the field survey, i.e., the neighbor nominees, was 55.0. The estimated mean IQ of persons who were screened as clinically retarded in the field survey using a traditional criterion was 55.6. When the educational criterion was used, the estimated mean IQ was 64.2, and with the AAMD criterion the estimated mean IQ was 66.1. The evaluations of nonclinical nominators tend to converge with the evaluations of the clinical epidemiology when the traditional criterion is used.

Comparison with Other Epidemiologies

A third, more indirect method for measuring the criterion on which there is greatest consensus is to compare the rates secured in the Riverside field survey with rates secured in other epidemiological studies. Although these studies used many different research designs and diagnostic procedures, it is still possible to ascertain which criterion level in the Riverside field survey produces a rate most similar to rates reported in other studies.

Crude prevalence rates are much less useful than subgroup specific rates when comparing the amount of clinical retardation in populations that differ greatly from each other in ethnic composition or socioeconomic status. Unfortunately, most prevalence rates reported from other epidemiological studies of mental retardation have been in the form of crude rates rather than subgroup specific rates, except for a few that give age-specific rates. Jastak reports only for persons 10 through 64;

Leighton includes only persons over 18; Richardson reports for persons under 21; the Scottish Council rates are based on 11-year-olds; and Riverside rates are based on persons 7 months through 49 years of age.

Table 14 presents a comparison of the crude prevalence rates from the Riverside field survey with the prevalence rates from some other major epidemiologies. The size of the universe and the number of persons selected for study varies greatly from one investigation to the next. Lin screened the largest number of persons, 19,931, while Leighton studied the smallest number, 1,010. Most of the epidemiologies in the table were based on some form of survey sample or census, with or without the use of informants.

Even more critical than differences in sample size and survey proceures are differences in the diagnostic methods used. Some rates are based on medical or psychiatric examination without intelligence testing, while others include intelligence testing and medical diagnosis. Except for the Riverside survey, only Jastak's study makes systematic use of social-role performance as well as intellectual measures. He evaluated educational and occupational achievement.

Such varaitions in research design make it impossible to interpret differences in prevalence rates as differences in the amount of clinical mental retardation in the populations being compared. Crude rates range from 3.4 per 1,000 in Taiwan to 90.0 per 1,000 in Alamance County, North Carolina. Does this mean that there are 27 times more mental retardates in North Carolina than in Taiwan? Does Stirling County in Canada have six times more mental retardates per 1,000 than rural Tennessee and three times more than the urban slums of Baltimore? It is impossible to say from the evidence at hand. Differences in crude prevalence rates could as easily result from differences in methodology, diagnostic procedures, and definitions of mental retardation as from any actual differences in the characteristics of the populations studied.

The methodology, sampling, and definitional procedures of the Jastak study more closely approximate those of the Riverside field survey than any other of the epidemiologies reviewed in table 14. Crude rates from that study also coincide most closely with those of the Riverside survey. Jastak identified 3.8 mental retardates per 1,000 when he used a 2% cutoff, while the Riverside survey identified 9.7 per 1,000, using a 3% cutoff. Crude rates at the 9% level are almost identical for the two studies, 20.3 and 18.9. The Riverside survey, using the 16% cutoff, produces a rate of 34.7 per 1,000, while Jastak found a rate of 83.3 per 1,000 at a 25% cutoff. These differences are about what one would expect, given the differences in cutoff levels.

Table 14: Comparative Crude Prevalence Rates per 1,000 for General Population in Selected Epidemiologies

Investigator	Area	Year	Size of Universe	Number Persons Studied	Ages Studied	Method	Diagnostic Procedures	Rates per 1,000
Mercer-Dingman	Riverside, Calif. Urban	1963–64	73,550	6,889	7 mos to 49 yrs	Household Sample Survey	Adaptive Behavior and IQ Screening	
							Traditional Criterion (3%)	9.7
							Educational Criterion (9%)	18.9
							AAMD Criterion (16%)	34.7
Jastak	State of Delaware Urban and Rural	1954	—	2,117	10 to 64 yrs	Household Sample Survey	Social and Intellectual Measures	
							25% Level	83.3
							9% Level	20.3
							2% Level	3.8
Lemkau	Baltimore Urban	1936	55,129	3,337	All Ages	Census and Informants	IQ Score and Medical Diagnosis	6.8
Roth and Luton	Tennessee Rural	1938	22,845	1,721	All Ages	Census and Informants	IQ Score and Medical Diagnosis	8.2
Scottish Council Research in Education	Scotland	1947	80,000	1,215	11-year-olds	Census	Mental Tests 1936	6.0
							(IQ below 70) 1947	14.0
Primrose	Scotland Rural	1959	1,701	1,701	All Ages	Census	Medical Examination School Records	8.8
Essen-Moller	Rural Sweden	1956	2,500	2,500	All Ages	Census	Psychiatric Interview	10.0
Lin	Taiwan Urban and Rural	1946–48	19,931	19,931	All Ages	Census and Informants	Psychiatric Interview No Tests	3.4
Richardson et al.	Alamance County, North Carolina	1961–62	36,500	1,864	Under 21	Household Sample Survey	Parent Report Alone	79.0
							Clinical Examination	90.0
Leighton	Nova Scotia Rural County	1952	—	1,010	18 or more yrs	Household Sample Survey	Highest Grade Achievement and Comments of Doctor and Interviewer	48.0

Three studies appear to have used a statistical model and traditional criteria in defining mental retardation. Lemkau classified as retarded only persons with an IQ of 70 or below; Roth and Luton classified persons as "imbeciles, idiots, and morons"; and the Scottish Council reported intellectual performance for those "below 70." Rates for these studies closely approximate the rate of 9.7 per 1,000 found at the 3% criterion in the Riverside survey. Lemkau reports 6.8; Roth and Luton report 8.2; and the Scottish Council reported 6.0 in 1936 and 14.0 in 1947.

Primrose and Essen-Moller relied on psychiatric interviews and test information, when available. Using this combination of pathological and statistical definitions of normal, they also secured rates comparable to those at the traditional criterion in Riverside, 8.8 and 10.0, respectively.

Lin relied exclusively on psychiatric evaluation based on interviews and behavioral reports. Thus, his definition was based strictly on a pathological model without statistical criteria. He reports the lowest rate of any study, 3.4 per 1,000. This is about the rate found in Riverside for Type 1 mental retardates (the physically disabled) at the traditional criterion. Both studies that reported the highest rates relied on less formal screening procedures. Richardson used "parental reports" for field screening, and Leighton used a combination of the highest grade completed and the comments of doctor and interviewer as the basis for evaluation.

The studies in table 14 report rates ranging from 3.4 to 90.0 per 1,000, approximately the range between the traditional and AAMD criteria rates in the Riverside study. However, most other studies report rates closer to those secured at the traditional criterion in Riverside than rates secured at either the educational or AAMD criterion levels. There is a higher level of consensus on rates across the various major epidemiological studies when the traditional criterion is used.

Although a rate of 30.0 per 1,000 (3%) is frequently cited in the literature, there is little in the Riverside data or that of other studies to support such a figure. The rates for most studies fluctuate between 6.0 and 15.0 per 1,000 (0.6% and 1.5%). In Riverside, the 30 per 1,000 (3%) rate is reached only when the AAMD criterion is used. Traditional and educational criteria do not produce a prevalence rate this high.

How Does the Choice of Criterion Affect the Number of Eligibles?

Social problems are not self-defined. A particular condition is a social problem only as persons in a society regard it as problematic. In a very real sense, the issue of the choice of criterion for determining mental retardation is precisely that of defining the limits of a social problem in American society—a problem called mental retardation. If the criterion level is high, then the scope of the problem is greatly expanded. If the criterion level is low, relatively few persons will be rated as subnormal and the scope of the problem will shrink.

Obviously, the more stringent the norms, the more persons who will be eligible for the label of mental retardate. However, it is one thing to deal with rates in the abstract and quite another to look closely at the magnitude of the impact of one percentage point when projected to an entire nation.

In 1960, the United States Census estimated that there were 3,465,000 persons with Spanish surnames in the population of the states of Arizona, New Mexico, Texas, Colorado, and California.[1] If the field survey rate for Mexican-Americans based on the traditional criterion is used, we would estimate that 60.0 per 1,000, or 207,900 of the persons in the Spanish-surname population were eligible as clinical retardates at that time. According to the rate based on the educational criterion, the estimated number would rise to about 441,400. If the rate is based on the AAMD definition, the estimated total rises to 826,000.

More recent estimates are available for whites and nonwhites. According to population estimates made by the census bureau for January 1, 1969, there were about 177,482,000 white persons in the population of the United States.[2] This figure includes persons of Spanish surname. If we estimate that the Spanish-surname population may have grown to about 5,000,000 by then, we would surmise that the Anglo population (white population minus Spanish-surname population) was approximately 172,500,000 persons. Applying the Anglo rates based on the traditional criterion, an estimated 759,000 Anglos would be clinically retarded. If rates based on the educational definition are used, then 1,052,200 Anglos would qualify as retarded. If the AAMD criterion is used, 1,656,000 persons in the Anglo population would be eligible as clinical retardates.

In the 1969 population estimate the census bureau reported the nonwhite population as approximately 22,547,000. Using the traditional definition, we would estimate that about 92,400 persons in the

1 *United States Census of Population, 1960 (2) IB, Persons of Spanish Surname,* Table I, 2.

2 *United States Census Bureau, Current Population Reports. Population Estimates of the Population of the United States and Components of Changes, 1940 to 1969,* Series P-25, Number 418 March 14, 1969. Table 2, Estimates of the Total Population of the United States, Including Armed Forces Overseas, by Race, and Sex, April 1, 1940, to January 1, 1969, 11.

nonwhite population would qualify as clinically retarded, if the educational standard is used, 505,000 would qualify; if the AAMD definition is used, the estimate would rise to 1,200,000 persons.

The totals for the three subpopulations give a rough estimate of the total size of the "social problem" of mental retardation in the United States when it is defined by the three different standards now used by clinicians. Using the traditional definition, we would estimate that there are approximately 1,059,300 clinical retardates. If we include all those eligible under the usual educational standards, then the total rises to 1,998,600. When the AAMD criterion is used, the "problem" population expands to 3,682,000.

These are estimates based on a two-dimensional definition of mental retardation. If we had used rates based on a one-dimensional definition using only IQ, without taking adaptive behavior into account, then estimates for persons who are not members of the Anglo core culture would approximately double, and Anglo estimates would also increase.

These approximations are presented primarily to illustrate the tremendous difference which the clinical definition makes in determining the number of persons who will be regarded as "problems." If IQ is the only measure used and persons more than one standard deviation below the mean are "subnormal," then almost 30,000,000 persons would fall into the "problem" population.

How Does the Choice of Criterion Affect Differential Prevalence Rates?

Raising and lowering the norms for subnormality not only influences the number of persons regarded as "problems" but also influences the kinds of persons who are identified as "problems." In Riverside, we found that crude prevalence rates increased from 9.7 to 18.9 and 34.7 per 1,000 population when successively broader limits were used. Such increases seem modest. However, the population of Riverside is predominately middle-class Anglo and has a mean IQ well above the national norms for the test. Undoubtedly, the crude rates for the city are lower than they would be for a national sample. For this reason, rates based on significant segments of the population are more useful in comparing the impact of the criteria on the prevalence rates than are crude rates.

Table 13 shows what happens to prevalence rates by socioeconomic status within ethnic group as the criterion is raised. For middle- and high-status Anglos, raising the standards is inconsequential. Rates increase only 5 per 1,000 when we shift from the traditional to the AAMD criterion and are always under 10 per 1,000. Rates for low-status Anglos increase more sharply, rising from 16.8 to 25.3 as the limits are broadened. This pattern is similar to that found when we analyzed the impact of a one-dimensional compared to a two-dimensional definition of mental retardation. The addition of the adaptive behavior evaluation made little difference in middle- and high-status Anglo rates, just as the increase in criterion levels makes little difference in rates for middle- and high-status Anglos. It is possible that the issues both of the criterion and of developing Adaptive Behavior Scales have remained unresolved because they are of little practical importance to the middle-class, English-speaking majority. Perhaps little attention has been given to resolving the confusions and ambiguities growing out of multiple criteria because relatively few middle-class and/or Anglo children will be defined as mentally retarded and placed in special education classes regardless of which criterion is used.

The situation is quite different with rates for Blacks and Mexican-Americans. Overall rates for Blacks rise from less than 4.1, using the traditional criterion, to 53.1, with an AAMD criterion. Rates for Mexican-Americans double at each successive level, rising from 60.0 at the traditional criterion, to 127.4 at the educational criterion, to 238.4 at the AAMD criterion. Rates for low-status Mexican-Americans rise from 87.1 to 281.0.

Table 15 presents a more detailed picture of some of the other characteristics of persons in each criterion group, using the weighted frequencies from the tested subsample. There were an estimated 243 persons who would be eligible as clinical retardates, using the 16% cutoff level. Sixty-eight of them failed at the traditional criterion, 64 failed at the educational criterion but not the traditional criterion, and 111 failed only when the AAMD criterion was used.

Ethnic differences are quite distinct. The more physically disabled, traditional retardates include significantly more Anglos than either the educational or AAMD retardates. The latter contain significantly more Mexican-Americans and Blacks, the groups most affected by shifting the norms upward. The socioeconomic level of most persons who are clinically retarded is low, but the traditional retardates come from even more socioeconomically disadvantaged circumstances than those who fail only the educational or AAMD criterion. This relationship appears in spite of the fact that 37.3% of the traditional retardates are Anglos, and Anglos in general have a higher socioeconomic status than minority groups in Riverside. The traditional retardate is more likely to come from a deteriorated or dilapidated home located in a poor neighborhood than the other two groups; and the head of household in his family

Table 15: Background Characteristics of Persons Eligible as Clinical Retardates in the Field Survey for Each of the Three Criteria Levels

Characteristics	Failed Only Traditional Criterion (Nw = 68)	Failed Only Educational Criterion (Nw = 64)	Failed Only AAMD Criterion (Nw = 111)	Significance Level
Ethnic Group				
% Anglo	37.3	15.6	18.8	
% Mexican-American	59.8	70.3	67.7	<.01
% Black	2.9	14.1	13.5	
Socioeconomic Characteristics				
Mean Housing Decile	2.6	3.4	4.1	<.001
Mean SES Index of Head	12.3	18.7	19.9	<.01
% Occup. Unskilled Laborer	79.4	54.7	53.1	<.01
% Deteriorating or Dilapidated Housing	41.2	37.5	20.8	<.01
Educational Characteristics				
Mean Grades Completed by Head	6.7	7.6	10.1	<.001
Mean Grades Completed by Mother	7.1	5.2	10.1	<.001
% Head Had No Trouble Learning	41.2	71.9	82.0	<.001
Other Characteristics				
% Head Born in Mexico or South	63.2	32.8	36.9	<.001
% Lived in Riverside Over 10 Years	48.5	46.9	91.1	<.001
% Speak Spanish Most or All of the Time at Home	47.0	7.9	3.6	<.001

is more likely to work as an unskilled laborer. The average socioeconomic index score is only 12.3 for this group.

The environment of the traditional retardate is also significantly more disadvantaged educationally. The mother has completed an average of 6.7 years of schooling and the father 7.1 years of schooling, compared with an average of 10.1 years of schooling for parents of the AAMD retardates. The traditional retardate is more likely to live in a home in which the head of household was born in Mexico or in the southern states, is less likely to have lived in Riverside for 10 or more years, and is more likely to come from a home where Spanish is spoken most of the time or all of the time. The traditional retardates come from backgrounds less like the sociocultural mode of the community than either the educational or AAMD retardates.

Which Criterion Best Identifies Persons Who Need Assistance and Supervision?

Although the scope of the social "problem" of mental retardation is directly related to the criterion used to decide who is clinically retarded, the crux of the issue rests not with rates or numbers but with an analysis of the characteristics of the persons who will be defined as incompetent, using the three criteria. Even more significant than background characteristics are the social roles played by persons labeled as retarded, using the three different standards. Do most persons in the "borderline" category fail in their social roles? Do they belong to that class of mental deficients described in the California Legal Code as persons who are "incapable of managing themselves and their affairs independently, with ordinary prudence, of being taught to do so, and who require supervision, control, and care for their own welfare, or for the welfare of others, or for the welfare of the community [California Code Ann., 1952]." This legal definition, like most verbal descriptions of adaptive behavior, refers to adult behavior.

Statistical Comparisons of Social-Role Performance

The analysis of both the clinical case register and the field survey found that "borderline retardates" had fewer physical disabilities than those who failed the traditional criterion. In order to assess adult-role performance, we will concentrate on the social-role behavior of the estimated 175 adults who were identified as clinical retardates in the field survey.

In Table 16 the retardates who failed only the educational or AAMD criterion have been grouped together and called "borderline retardates" to permit more reliable statistical comparisons. The performance of the traditional retardate is compared with that of the borderline retardate on 26 different social-role items. Twenty-one of the comparisons are statistically significant at the .01 level or beyond. All differences, including those which do not reach statistical significance, show a higher percentage of the borderline retardates than the traditional retardates performing the role in question.

Educational and intellectual differences are large and consistent. While only 25.4% of the traditional retardates have completed eight

Table 16: Comparison of Behavioral Characteristics of Adults Scored as Retarded at the Three Criteria Levels Grouped in Mutually Exclusive Categories

Characteristics	Failed Traditional Criterion (Nw = 59)	Failed Educational or AAMD Criterion (Borderline Retardates) (Nw = 116)	Significance Level
Educational-Intellectual Roles			
% Completed 8 or More Grades	25.4	83.6	<.001
% Dropped School: Academic Reasons	35.6	0.0	<.001
% Trouble Learning in School	65.2	37.1	<.01
% Reads Newspapers	27.1	67.2	<.001
% Reads Magazines	6.8	72.4	<.001
% Reads Books	32.2	46.5	NS
% Reads and Talks about News	66.1	84.2	NS
Occupational Roles			
% Who Have Held a Job	54.2	82.6	<.001
% Semiskilled or Higher Occupation Status	14.3	64.9	<.001
% Financially Independent or Housewife or Student	62.7	80.2	<.001
Family Roles			
% Head of Household or Spouse of Head	69.5	78.4	NS
General Community Roles			
% Belongs to Social Clubs	11.9	33.3	<.01
% Votes in Elections	6.8	48.7	<.001
% Goes to Movies	35.6	89.7	<.001
% Works with Little Supervision	81.4	100.0	<.001
% Goes to Store Alone	67.8	96.3	<.001
% Travels Alone	69.5	96.3	<.001
Informal Community Roles			
% Writes Letters	50.8	92.6	<.001
% Attends Church	67.8	81.9	NS
% Visits Relatives Frequently	54.8	79.5	<.001
% Visits Neighbors Frequently	61.0	93.1	<.001
% Visits Friends Frequently	35.6	81.9	<.001
% Visits Co-workers Frequently	45.9	76.6	<.001
% Plays Parlor Games	30.5	71.3	<.001
% Goes Dancing	40.7	45.7	NS
% Participates in Sports	13.6	58.6	<.001

or more years of school, 83.6% of the borderline retardates had an eighth-grade education or better. None of the borderline retardates were reported to have dropped from school because of academic problems, but 35.6% of the clinical retardates were reported to have dropped out primarily because of academic problems. While 65% of the traditional retardates were reported to have had trouble learning in school, only 37% of the borderline persons were reported to have had academic difficulty. More borderline persons read newspapers, magazines, and books, and talk about the news; but only the first two differences are statistically significant.

Occupationally, borderline persons are doing distinctly better—82.6% have held a job at some time in their lives, while 54.2% of the traditional retardates have held a job. Of those who have worked, 64.9% of the borderline persons have had semiskilled or higher-level jobs, while only 14.3% of the traditional retardates have had more than an unskilled, laboring job. While 80.2% of the borderline group are either financially independent or are housewives or students, 62.7% of the traditional retardates are financially independent.

There is no difference in family roles between the two groups, but significantly more of the borderline persons play community roles. All can work without supervision, most travel alone and go to the store alone, and approximately half vote in elections. Even those informal social roles that did not distinguish the quasi-retarded and behaviorally maladjusted from the clinically retarded do distinguish those who fail the traditional criterion from those who fail only the educational or AAMD criterion.

Although statistical comparisons are interesting, the central concern of this discussion is to establish whether persons who are clinically "borderline retardates" are persons who, as adults, are "incapable of managing themselves and their affairs independently, with ordinary prudence." Table 16 makes it quite clear that most persons in this borderline category are managing their own affairs and do not appear to require "supervision, control, and care for their own welfare." Most have held jobs, and over half have had semiskilled jobs or better. Most are financially independent or else are playing the role of housewife or student. Most are married and are either the head of a household or the spouse of a head of household. They have had some difficulty in school, but most now read newspapers and magazines, although less than half read books. Most of them perform the usual roles in the community of shopping and traveling alone, working without supervision, and having frequent interaction with friends, relatives, neighbors, and co-workers. There is little in their role performance that appears either subnormal or particularly unusual. They do not fail the usual standards presented in the legal norms or verbal definitions that describe the mentally deficient.

Qualitative Comparisons of Social-Role Performance

This section presents vignettes of some of the persons who were identified in the field survey as clinically "eligible" to hold the status of mental retardate. This qualitative analysis of individual cases provides an opportunity to make a subjective assessment of the validity of the field identification procedures. It also reveals quite clearly the changing character of individuals who were screened as mentally retarded when the performance levels for normative expectations are increased from the lowest 3%, to the lowest 9%, to the lowest 16%. Personal names, composition of families, and family occupations have been completely changed to assure anonymity of the persons described in the vignettes. If the names selected to represent the persons described in the case studies bear any similarity to those of actual persons, the similarity is purely fortuitous.

Physically Disabled Clinical Retardates

In the social system epidemiology, we found that persons who had both physical disabilities and a low IQ test score, i.e., were deviant both from a medical-pathological and a statistical model of subnormality, were more likely to be labeled as mentally retarded by more than one formal organization in the community and to be perceived as abnormal by lay persons. For that reason, we have divided the case studies into two groups by their physical disability score. The first group of cases are persons with more than three failures on the Physical Disability Scales.

The Physically Disabled, Traditional Retardate (3% Criterion) is a person with an IQ below 70 and sufficient adaptive behavior failures to place him in the lowest 3% of the population for his age group. Although there were no preschool children in our sample in this category, there were several school-age children. The following two children are now in a state hospital for the retarded and illustrate school-age children in this category.

Janet, a ten-year-old Anglo girl, has an IQ of 18, an adaptive behavior score of 16, and a physical disability score of 5. None of the three other children in the family have any physical disabilities nor have they had trouble learning in school. Her youngest brother is in the program for gifted children in junior high school. Janet however, has had many problems. She experienced a lack of oxygen at birth and presently has epileptic seizures more than once a month. She has great difficulty walking, talking, dressing, and feeding herself. She failed all the Vineland and Gesell items at the ten-year level. She has never attended school except for the special education classes at the state hospital. Both parents are currently employed—her father is an auto mechanic and her mother is a secretary for an insurance firm.

Tony, a fouteen-year-old Mexican-American boy, has an IQ of 5, an adaptive behavior score of 16, and a physical disability score of 8. Institutionalized at an early age he has never attended school. He suffers from convulsions more than once a month and has great difficulty walking, seeing, feeding and dressing himself, and some difficulty sleeping and hearing. He failed all the Vineland and Gesell items in the Adaptive Behavior Scales. He is incapable of self-care. The mother does not believe he will ever attend school or that he will live long. The second youngest in a family of five children, Tony has never had any contact with his siblings. Spanish is spoken occasionally in his home. His widowed mother is a housewife, receiving social security and a veteran's pension. She never finished high school. His two older brothers, aged nineteen and twenty-one, did not finish high school and are currently working in a packinghouse. The sixteen-year-old sister is still in school. None of the other children have any physical disabilities.

Two cases were selected as typical of physically disabled adults who failed the intelligence test and Adaptive Behavior Scales at the 3% level. One is living in the state hospital, the other living in the community.

Paul is a twenty-six-year-old Anglo male who has an IQ of 45, an adaptive behavior score of 16, and a physical disability score of 4. Before entering the State Hospital for the retarded, he had been in a mental hospital in another state. Paul graduated from high school in Alabama, but his mother admits he "couldn't do high school work" and "they let him graduate." He has difficulty talking and sleeping. He has "fits" more than once a month and, before entering the hospital, had them two and three times a week. At times, Paul would become violent when he was at home. He never belonged to any social clubs or teams, could not go to the store and make purchases by himself, could not work without supervision, and did not travel to nearby towns by himself. Paul's father, a plumber, left school after the eleventh grade because of lack of interest. His mother, who is now a housewife, graduated from high school in Arkansas and worked for awhile as a salesclerk. Both parents were reared on farms. Paul is their only child. His mother, who also by chance appeared in the IQ subsample, has an IQ of 86, an adaptive behavior score of 6, and 1 physical disability.

The second case is an adult woman who spent her youth in a state hospital for the retarded but was living in an apartment by herself when contacted by the interviewer. She is apparently doing relatively well alone after spending several years in a family care home.

Mary is a thirty-year-old Anglo woman who failed each test at all three levels. Her IQ was 64, her adaptive behavior score was 12, and her physical disability score was 3. She was a patient in the state hospital until she was released on the family care program and has lived in an apartment by herself for the past two years. Mary receives Aid to the Totally Disabled and works a few hours a week housecleaning. She does not take a daily newspaper or any magazines, but has a radio and TV in working order. In her spare time, Mary plays the piano, listens to the radio, or watches TV. She never votes in elections, never participates in games nor goes to the movies. She attends church services more than once a week. She visits neighbors and friends, and turns to them for help when she is sick. Mary states that she had a great deal of trouble learning in school and that she never finished high school because "the other kids always picked on her." She had spinal meningitis when she was eighteen months old and still suffers from epileptic seizures about six times a month. She has no difficulty walking, talking, feeding and dressing herself, nor hearing or seeing.

All the Type 1 mental retardates who failed the traditional criterion show a clear symptomatology that fits the usual clinical picture of the mentally retarded. Regardless of ethnic background or social status, all the persons in this category have been defined as mentally retarded by their families and others in their environment as well as by the field survey. In this category, social system definitions and clinical definitions tend to converge.

The Physically Disabled "Borderline" Retardate is a person with an IQ between 70 and 85 and adaptive behavior in the lowest 16% of the population for his age. The following cases illustrate persons in this category.

Maria is a four-year-old Mexican-American girl with an IQ of 73, an adaptive behavior score of 8, and a physical disability score of 4. The second-oldest of four children, she lives with her mother, stepfather, grandmother, older brother, and two younger stepbrothers. Maria was born with a deformed foot and harelip. She has some difficulty hearing and cannot talk so that she is understood all the time. She has never had a serious operation or illness but fell off the bed when she was three months old. During pregnancy her mother "did not feel well and saw the doctor many times." Maria cries a lot but has no other problem behavior. She cannot dress herself when her clothes are laid out for her nor draw recognizable pictures with pencil or crayon. She has some trouble with coordination and cannot pour from a pitcher nor turn pages one at a time, although she can put on her own shoes and ride a tricycle.

Maria's father has lived in Riverside in the same house all of his life. His wife was born in Mexico and has not been in the United States very long. She had an IQ of 59, on the Spanish version of the Stanford-Binet, and an adaptive behavior score of 11, but no physical disabilities. English is never spoken in the home. The father, who had trouble learning in school, completed only five grades and is currently employed full time in construction work. The mother completed four grades in Mexico but left school for lack of interest. She is now a housewife and was employed in Mexico as a tortilla maker. Maria's six-year-old brother is repeating kindergarten this year and has attended speech therapy classes. He spends most of his time with his family "playing or fighting." Maria's two younger stepbrothers have no behavior problems or physical abnormalities.

William is a three-year-old Anglo boy with an IQ of 81, an adaptive behavior score of 6, and a physical disability score of 5. He lives with his divorced mother in a dilapidated house, which has been divided into seven apartments occupied by assorted alcoholics and unmarried women with their illegitimate children. William was born with the umbilical cord wrapped around his neck and, as a result, was placed in an incubator for three days after birth. He had pneumonia nine times in his first year of life and ran a fever of 106 degrees when he had the measles. This resulted in convulsions, which he still has a few times a year. His mother mentioned that her son has always been extremely fair-skinned and is only now beginning to have some color. He still is in diapers and is not speaking intelligibly. William's mother dropped out of school after the eleventh grade and is currently unemployed, receiving a monthly allotment from Aid to Needy Children. At one time she was a practical nurse in a nursing home. The family has moved approximately fifty times in the last ten years.

One woman has been selected to illustrate persons who would be eligible for a class for the educable mentally retarded if they were of school age. Her children have been taken from her by her ex-husband and the welfare agencies. She is unemployed and is dependent upon welfare. Her plight is very reminiscent of the mentally retarded described by Edgerton (Edgerton, 1967).

Martha is a forty-four-year-old Anglo woman with an IQ of 76, an adaptive behavior score of 8, and a physical disability score of 9. She is divorced from her husband and now lives alone. She has three children—two reside with her ex-husband in another state and a third child (illegitimate) is in a foster home. Martha left school after the tenth grade for health reasons, but indicated that she did have some trouble learning in school. At one time, Martha had spinal meningitis and was unconscious for one-and-a-half days. She still has epileptic seizures more than once a month. She has some difficulty walking, sleeping, and seeing. When sick, Martha turns to her mother, who helps "when I ask her." At one time, Martha spent three months in a state hospital for the mentally ill at her own request. Martha is currently unemployed and receives support from County Welfare. At one time, she did housework and was a live-in maid, but she lost her job when her employer learned that she had epileptic seizures. In her spare time, Martha reads detective stories, *True Story* magazines, and enjoys watching television. Martha does not belong to any clubs or organizations. She visits friends, but states that she is "afraid to visit neighbors."

Non-physically-disabled Clinical Retardates who fail at the traditional criterion are those with IQ test scores 69 and below who are in the lowest 3% in adaptive behavior. One case illustrates the school-age population, and three illustrate adults in this category.

Jimmy, a fourteen-year-old Anglo boy in the ninth grade had an IQ of 67, an adaptive behavior score of 11, and a physical disability score of 1. His father is employed as an electrician and his mother works on an assembly line making auto parts. She left school at the eleventh grade to get married, and his father joined the navy after completing the tenth grade. All his sisters are doing well in school, except the youngest who has received speech therapy.

Jimmy has some difficulty hearing and has interpersonal problems—especially with his sisters and teachers. According to his mother, he has great difficulty learning in school, but he has not received any special training nor been required to repeat a grade. He does not read books, newspapers, or magazines for his own enjoyment; does not make minor purchases at the store; is not a member of any group or social clubs of children his own age; never writes letters; has little interest in world affairs; tends to use physical violence rather than verbal expression to give vent to anger; and usually needs help with his homework. Jimmy spends most of his spare time helping with the yard and in the company of the neighborhood boys, with whom he goes water-skiing, camping, and plays baseball. His mother expects him to complete twelve years of school and do "professional work of some kind." His mother does not perceive him as retarded.

The characteristics of adults in this category are particularly revealing. Again, the life style of the Anglo woman described in the first case is reminiscent of the mentally retarded studied by Edgerton in his follow-up of former hospital patients (Edgerton, 1967). As a housekeeper and babysitter for two teachers, she has found protectors who are fellow church members and who make it possible for her to maintain an independent existence. Louise's employer was present throughout the interview.

Louise is a forty-five-year-old Anglo woman who had an IQ of 47, an adaptive behavior score of 10, and a physical disability score of 1. She has never been married and is now a live-in babysitter for an Anglo couple who have an 18-month-old child. Louise works 40 hours a week for this family and receives no additional financial support from a public or private agency. She completed seven grades in school, and has some trouble with arithmetic. Her one physical disability is a harelip, which has not been corrected. Her speech is very difficult to understand because of this deformity, and she speaks with her hand over her mouth much of the time. Louise frequently reads the newspaper, but never reads magazines or books. She is a member of the Baptist Church, attends church services regularly, and is involved in church work in her spare time. On the WAIS questions, she thought rubber comes from "cars and tires." When asked "Why does a train have an engine?" she replied "just on one end." When asked to name four men who have been President of the United States, she answered "all the time just studied that in history." "Strike when the iron is hot" to Louise means "don't touch the iron because it's hot."

Louise's employer, when asked if she knew of anyone who was retarded, named two female children but did not include Louise in her list.

The next two persons are of Mexican heritage. The most striking characteristic of these cases, and others like them, is the great disparity between the role performance one would expect on the basis of the clinical measures and the actual life pattern as revealed in interview data. They present a very different picture from Louise. All are adults who are filling normal adult roles as parents, housewives, and wage earners. Their social worlds center in family, neighbors, friends, and, perhaps, church. Bounded by limited educations and limited experience in American society, the printed word scarcely exists for them. Although they do not know the answers to questions on standard clinical measures, they are living out their lives within the social system of their community, unstigmatized and unhandicapped.

Thomas a thirty-four-year-old Mexican-American father of three, had an IQ of 45, an adaptive behavior score of 10, and no physical disabilities. Born in Mexico, he has never attended school and is presently working as a gardener. He doesn't read magazines or books, belong to any social organizations or write letters, but does watch television and is active in the Catholic Church. In his spare time, he prunes trees for extra money. His wife completed the seventh grade, and has worked as an orange picker. She also watches television, but doesn't read magazines or books. She and her husband visit relatives, neighbors, friends, and co-workers frequently. Both were reared in Mexico, although they have lived most of their lives in the United States. At home they speak English about half the time. They own a car, television, and radio, and subscribe to magazines but not to a newspaper. They listen to Spanish radio broadcasts daily. Their nine-year-old son scored 76 on the IQ test but is not in special education and, according to the mother, has no trouble learning in school.

Lupe, a thirty-nine-year-old Mexican-American mother of four, has an IQ of 55 on the Stanford-Binet, an adaptive behavior score of 11, and no physical disabilities. She did not continue beyond the seventh grade in Mexico because there were no teachers beyond that grade. Lupe has never held a job, never had a serious illness, and has never been in a hospital. She does not know how much education her husband has had. Although he goes out often she does not know where he goes and could give no information about his activities outside the home. The family seldom speaks English. They have a car and television, but do not subscribe to a newspaper or magazines and have no telephone. They watch Channel 34 Spanish broadcasts on television and listen to the Spanish programs on the radio. She and her husband go to the movies frequently and visit neighbors, friends, and relatives regularly. When given the WAIS items, she didn't know where rubber comes from, how many months there are in a year, or the capital of Italy, and could name only one President of the United States—Kennedy. Their eleven-year-old daughter is in a class for the educable mentally retarded in the public school.

Non-physically-disabled Persons in the "Borderline" Category are those with IQ test scores between 70 and 85 who are in the lowest 16% in adaptive behavior. One school-age case illustrates those children who have been placed in special education, and the other illustrates cases that have not been placed.

Barbara, an eight-year-old Mexican-American girl, has an IQ of 70, an adaptive behavior score of 7, and no physical disabilities. She has had some trouble learning and, after repeating first grade, is in a special education class for the mentally retarded. All of the items which she missed on the adaptive behavior measure were school-related, i.e., she failed the age-grade norm, was not able to count to 30 by ones, was not able to read or write sentences, could not tell time by the hour and minute, and so forth. However, she appears to perform adequately in all other social roles. Her mother reports that she gets along very well with her parents, school friends, and teachers, and rather well with brothers, sisters, and neighbors. She plays games with other children, is able to take care of her own dressing and physical needs, helps with regular household tasks, can talk on the telephone, and so on. She has had no serious illnesses, operations, or accidents. Her mother expects that she will be a seamstress. Barbara's father was reared in Mexico and completed the second grade. He dropped school to work and is now employed as a laborer in a steel mill. His wife, reared in New Mexico, never attended school and now works as a domestic. Their oldest daughter has seizures about once a year, but she is progressing normally in school and has no other clinical symptoms. The ten-year-old son is having trouble understanding in school and repeated the first grade.

The case of Daniel illustrates a situation in which a child is clinically qualified for the mental retardation label, but has not been identified by anyone at home or at school as a retardate. Although he has some trouble learning in school and has had remedial reading, he has never repeated a grade. His mother believes he is "lazy."

Daniel is a thirteen-year-old Anglo boy who had an IQ of 76, an adaptive behavior score of 7, and a physical disability score of 0. His father, who left high school after completing the ninth grade, later received special training and is now employed as a machinist. His mother graduated from high school and is employed as receptionist.

Daniel suffers from asthma, but has no history of serious accidents, illnesses, or operations and no indication of any physical disabilities. He has some trouble learning in school and received instruction in remedial reading. His mother believes he is "lazy" but sees a change since he has entered junior high school. Daniel has never repeated a grade, but he failed several of the academic items on the Adaptive Behavior Scales. He does not read books or enjoy picture magazines and doesn't belong to any social clubs of persons his own age nor does he make purchases at the store by himself of minor articles of clothing. He gets along rather well with his teachers and siblings and very well with his parents, school friends, and neighbors. He spends his spare time watching television, painting, or playing ball and swimming with his peers. His mother expects him to complete fourteen years of school and to become a commercial artist. She does not perceive Daniel as retarded. Daniel's brother is doing very well in school. He has no trouble learning, reads approximately fifty books a year, takes an active part in debates, and is president of his class.

The following two women, one Mexican-American and the other Black, would easily have qualified for a program for the educable mentally retarded. If judged by the criterion of IQ alone, they would even be eligible for a state institution. However, their adaptive behavior scores are barely failing.

Maria, a thirty-year-old Mexican-American mother of four, received an IQ of 69, an adaptive behavior score of 6, and has no physical disabilities. She was born in Riverside and completed the tenth grade in school. However the interview was conducted in Spanish, at Maria's request, and Spanish is spoken most of the time in the home. Maria has never done any kind of work except housework. Her husband was reared in rural Mexico and has never attended school. He now works in construction as a cement finisher. The family listens to Spanish radio broadcasts but does not participate in any other activities related to the Mexican culture nor do they attend church, although both are Roman Catholic. They do not take or read a newspaper or magazines. They are buying a five-room house in a Mexican-American residential area and have a car and a television. Maria reports that she reads stories to her young children occasionally and teaches them some songs and nursery rhymes. Both of the children who are in school are progressing normally, and the five-year-old son, who also appeared in the IQ subsample, scored a 94 on the Stanford-Binet.

Rebecca, a forty-nine-year-old Black mother of three, scored 68 on the Stanford-Binet, received a score of 6 on the Adaptive Behavior Scale, and has no physical disabilities. She was reared in rural Mississippi, the daughter of a farmer. The family moved to Riverside six years ago. She completed the fifth grade in school and used to work as a domestic. However, she and her family are now supported by Social Security payments from her deceased husband's account. She is very active in the Methodist Church, visits relatives, friends, and neighbors more than once a week, and is active in clubs and organizations in the Black community. Her oldest son is in the service, and the two sons remaining at home are both in high school. They have made normal progress through school and are engaged in a wide range of activities—singing in the church choir, playing ball, working on racing cars, attending dances, and working around the house. The mother would like the youngest son to become a doctor or a teacher and to complete at least four years of college. When Rebecca was administered the information and comprehension items from the WAIS, she passed both subtests at a high level.

Adults screened as borderline retardates lead much more restricted lives than most adults in Riverside and have a much smaller range of interests. However, in every case, they are filling usual, standard, adult roles, regardless of their difficulties with the intelligence test.

Suzanne, an eighteen-year-old Caucasian mother, scored 78 on the intelligence test and failed five adaptive behavior items. Although she graduated from high school in Riverside, she reported having some trouble learning in school. However, she never repeated a grade nor attended special classes. She has never held a job. On the WAIS items, she did not know where rubber comes from, the capital of Italy, nor what direction one would travel from Chicago to Panama. She believes a year has 6 months and that Brazil is in Colombia. She enjoys yardwork, sewing, sports, and likes to watch "soap operas" on television. Her favorite magazine is *Seventeen*. Her twenty-year-old husband also graduated from high school and is employed as a steel worker for a construction company. They do not belong to any formal organizations except the Baptist

Church, which they attend irregularly. They visit relatives and friends frequently and turn to their parents when they need help.

Josie, a thirty-one-year-old Mexican-American mother of six, with an IQ of 82, failed 5 adaptive behavior items. Although she graduated from a California high school, she had to repeat the second and third grades and says she had much trouble learning in school. She is presently a housewife, but has worked as a machine operator. She never reads books and does not belong to any formal organization, but likes to read *True Confessions* and *McCall's* magazines. Her husband completed the tenth grade in the Riverside schools. He had to repeat the first and second grades and had a great deal of difficulty with formal education. Today, he is a printer and active in the union. They own their home; have a car, television, and radio; subscribe to magazines and a newspaper; and have a telephone. They speak English and Spanish about equally in their home and enjoy listening to Spanish-language radio broadcasts. Their two oldest children, six and eight years of age, are both classified as slow learners in school and are receiving speech therapy.

A qualitative assessment of individuals identified as mentally retarded in the household screening reveals some general patterns. The physically disabled who fail the traditional criterion are quite distinctly subnormal, by both clinical and social definition, and they have usually been labeled as subnormal by their families and by others in their social worlds. Clinical definitions and social system definitions tend to converge.

On the other hand, nondisabled persons identified as "borderline" under the AAMD criterion, especially those from ethnic minorities, are frequently leading lives that are indistinguishable from those of other persons in their social groups, and they are not regarded as subnormal by other persons in their social world. However, they are mentally retarded in terms of the clinical measures of intelligence and adaptive behavior used in the study.

Persons identified under the educational criterion tend to fall between the two extremes. Some are retarded by both clinical and social definitions, while others labeled as retarded in the survey have not been labeled by the community. The more stringent the norms, the more divergent the clinical diagnosis and the social definition.

The presence of physical disabilities tends to increase agreement between clinical and social system definitions.

Anglo adults who fail the clinical measures are more likely to be perceived as retarded by others in their social worlds than are adults from minority groups. In general, it appears that clinical and social definitions are more likely to converge (1) when the 3%, traditional criterion is used as the clinical cutoff for defining subnormal, (2) when the person being studied has visible physical disabilities, and (3) when the person being studied is an Anglo.

Conclusion

Which criterion? The issue is less critical to middle- and upper-status Anglos because their rates of clinical retardation are not materially increased by raising the cutoff level. However, rates for low-status Anglos, Mexican-Americans, and Blacks are greatly inflated when the higher criteria are used.

Rates using the traditional criterion more closely approximate those of other major epidemiological studies of mental retardation than do rates using the educational or AAMD criterion. The traditional criterion also most closely approximates the actual rate of labeling in the community of Riverside as revealed in the clinical case register. Therefore, we must conclude that there is a significantly higher level of consensus among clinicians and researchers in the field of mental retardation on the traditional criterion than either of the other cutoff levels.

The number of persons defined as "problems" increases greatly as successively higher cutoff levels are used. If all "borderline" retardates were identified and labeled, the total number of persons defined as subnormal would become so large that it would be difficult for clinical definitions to guide responsible social action. We have seen in the clinical case register that few clinicians use the AAMD criterion.

Finally, we looked at the actual social-role performance of adults screened in the field survey as "borderline" retardates and compared it to the life style and roles of persons identified as clinical retardates at the traditional criterion level. We found that most of those adults who failed only the educational or AAMD criterion were filling the usual complement of marital, occupational, and community roles played by adults. Unlike those identified as clinically retarded under the traditional criterion, there was little in the role performance of the "borderline" retardate that would warrant calling them either subnormal or mentally deficient. Qualitative analysis of specific cases tended to confirm this conclusion, when there were no physical disabilities.

Therefore, we conclude that the traditional criterion comes closest to actual labeling practices in the community and best represents the findings of most epidemiologies. At this criterion level, persons are least likely to be labeled as retarded who, as adults, will be able to fill a normal complement of social roles.

Chapter 15

WHICH TAXONOMY?

In chapter 13, we concluded that the two-dimensional definition advocated by the AAMD nomenclature is defensible and that more adequate means for assessing adaptive behavior in the community are needed so that both IQ and adaptive behavior can be universally and systematically evaluated in clinical diagnosis. Those persons in the field survey who passed adaptive behavior, even though they failed the intelligence test, appear to be performing a normal complement of social roles and dealing intelligently with situations in their homes, neighborhoods, and communities. In chapter 14, we concluded that the traditional criterion is the criterion level on which there is the highest consensus among clinicians and the least risk of stigmatizing persons who, as adults, will be able to manage their own affairs and fill adult social roles. On the basis of these conclusions, we will, henceforth, regard only those persons who fail both adaptive behavior and IQ at the traditional 3% criterion as clinically retarded. All others are either quasi-retarded, "low normals," or "normals."

A One-Dimensional Taxonomy

Our scheme is a departure from the usual one-dimensional textbook definitions, which picture intelligence as normally distributed in the population and define mental retardates as persons whose IQ falls in the lowest 3% of the curve. Selecting any arbitrary cutoff point, whether it be an IQ of 70 or an IQ of 79, promotes a tendency to think of those persons who fall below that cutoff as a group who are organically and qualitatively different from persons having higher IQs. Such a conceptual scheme tends to lump all mental retardates together in a relatively undifferentiated cluster of persons who have one characteristic in common—they cannot pass an intelligence test. In this and similar schemes, mental retardates are treated as a relatively homogeneous group of persons, some of whom have more and some less of an attribute called "intelligence."

The AAMD nomenclature presents the idea of a two-dimensional definition of mental retardation but actually develops its classification scheme along only one dimension—the IQ. The five "levels" of mental retardation proposed in the nomenclature are names for statistical positions along a single dimension, IQ. They are a more elaborate exposition of the typical textbook definition but add nothing new conceptually to traditional constructs.

A Two-Group Taxonomy

Zigler has proposed a two-group taxonomy generated by introducing one additional dimension to that of IQ—organic pathology. His two-dimensional model, based on IQ and organic anomalies, generates two types of mental retardates: the organically damaged and the nonorganically damaged. The latter group he designates as familial-genetic retardates (Zigler, 1967). According to Zigler, the polygenic model of intelligence regards the genetic foundation of intelligence as dependent on a number of discrete genetic units which generate a distribution of intelligence that conforms to the normal curve. Statistically, the normal curve encompasses a range of six standard deviations. On the major intelligence tests, the mean IQ is 100 and the standard deviation is 15. Thus, the total range of expected IQ scores under a polygenic model of intelligence would be three standard deviations above and three standard deviations below 100, 55 to 145. Zigler's "familial-genetic" retardate is the nonorganically damaged person who falls genetically in the lowest portion of the normal curve of intelligence. Persons who are genetically retarded would be expected to have an IQ that falls within the lower limits of this range, i.e., an IQ that is not lower than 55. Their scores are regarded as just as integral a part of the normal distribution of intelligence as the scores of persons in the upper extremes of the normal curve.

According to Zigler, the "organics" are those who have physiological defects. Such persons tend to have IQs that fall below 50 and, hence, are outside the statistical distribution of the normal curve and are not a part of the polygenic distribution of intelligence. Their IQs form a separate distribution, which has a mean of approximately 35 and ranges from an IQ of 0 to an IQ of 70. "Their intellectual functioning reflects factors other than the normal polygenic expression—that is, these retardates have an identifiable physiological defect" (Zigler, 1967, p. 294). He cites data from Penrose, Roberts, and Lewis to support his view. By introducing the dimension of physical defect, Zigler generates his two groups, the "organics' and the "familial-genetics."

A Three-Group Taxonomy

The Riverside clinical epidemiology, in the field survey, developed a three-group taxonomy by introducing two additional evaluative dimensions to the usual one-dimensional textbook definition based solely on IQ. Like Zigler, the epidemiology introduced organic defect as the second dimension and, in addition, introduced adaptive behavior as the third dimension. The three dimensions produced three groups of persons among those who would be regarded as mentally retarded using only IQ: (1) Type 1 mental retardates are those with physical disabilities, roughly comparable to Zigler's "organics"; (2) Type 2 mental retardates are those without physical disabilities; and (3) the quasi-retarded are those with low IQs but adequate adaptive behavior. The latter two categories are mainly subsets of the nonorganic group, which Zigler called "familial-genetic" retardates.

Neither the Riverside clinical epidemiology nor the taxonomy of Zigler takes sociocultural factors into account. The omission is understandable, since both taxonomies are based on the clinical perspective, a supracultural model. Yet, we have seen throughout this volume that sociocultural background is significantly correlated with clinical measures, especially IQ and adaptive behavior. Can sociocultural factors be ignored? Should a taxonomy be developed which takes sociocultural factors into account?

A Latent Class Analysis of the Clinical and Sociocultural Characteristics of Labeled Retardates

A latent class analysis is a statistical model that generates typologies empirically by analyzing the interrelations of dichotomous attributes. The basis for classification into types requires that each latent class exhibit homogeneity with respect to the underlying dimensions that may be responsible for the interrelations, and that the intercorrelations between variables in the class be zero. Perfect homogeneity is not necessary if deviations from the class norm are random. In practice, this usually means that people within a class are much alike in their attributes and that exceptions are randomly distributed (Gibson, 1966; Lazarsfeld, 1959).

In order to describe the alignment of sociocultural and clinical factors in mental retardation, a latent class analysis was done on data collected in a follow-up study of the labeled retardates on the clinical case register. We did not secure a measure of adaptive behavior for labeled retardates at the time they were first nominated for the clinical register, because we did not interview the families of the nominees and there was not sufficient information in the clinical files on which to base a rating. However, in 1968, four years after the clinical case register was first collected, the clinical organizations that nominated persons to the register gave us permission, in all but 4.3% of the cases, to contact their nominees or the families of their nominees for an interview. Follow-up interviews were attempted with all labeled retardates or their families on the clinical case register who could be traced. Of the original cohort of 687 retardates labeled by clinical organizations, 9.8% had moved from town, 1% had died, 11.6% could not be located and/or contacted, and 12.1% refused to be interviewed. Interviews were completed with 421 of the labeled retardates or their families, 61.2% of the original register.

During this interview, the adaptive behavior scale appropriate for the age of the person was administered and an adaptive behavior score was computed. In addition, extensive information on the sociocultural characteristics of the person's family was also collected. Of those contacted, 177 were persons who had an IQ below 70 and who also failed 7 or more adaptive behavior items.

Ten sociocultural characteristics and three clinical characteristics—IQ, adaptive behavior, and physical disability—were dichotomized and used in the latent class analysis.[1] The sociocultural variables were selected from among those already shown to have epidemiologic significance: ethnic group; education of the head of household; education of the mother; occupation of the head of household classified by white-collar vs blue-collar; family income; occupation of the head of household classified by socioeconomic index score; whether the head of household was reared in a southern state; whether English is the only language spoken in the home; and whether the mother is married, divorced, or separated.

A Two-Group vs a Three-Group Taxonomy

The latent class analysis of persons who had been labeled as mentally retarded by clinical organizations in the community and who failed adaptive behavior and IQ at the traditional criterion was done to determine, empirically, the number of latent classes that best describe

[1] The variables in the latent class analysis were dichotomized as follows: IQ below 50 vs IQ 50–69; 7 adaptive behavior failures vs 8 or more failures; 0–2 physical disabilities vs 3 or more; Mexican-American vs non-Mexican-American; Black vs non-Black; education of the head of household 0–11 years vs 12 or more years; education of the mother 0–11 years vs 12 or more years; occupation of the head of household blue-collar vs white-collar; family income $0–$7,999 vs $8,000 or more; socioeconomic index score of the head of household 0–39 vs 40 or more; head of household reared in Mexico vs reared in the United States; head of household reared in a southern state, Texas, or Oklahoma vs head of household reared outside of those states; only English spoken in the home vs Spanish or some other language spoken in the home; mother married and living with spouse vs mother divorced, separated, or deceased.

the underlying structures responsible for the intercorrelation of these individuals' clinical and sociocultural characteristics.

According to Zigler's two-group taxonomy, which does not take sociocultural variables into account, we would expect two latent classes to emerge in the analysis. One class would consist of persons with very low IQs and many physical disabilities—the "organics." The second class would consist of persons he calls "familial-genetics." The latter would have somewhat higher IQs and fewer physical disabilities than the "organics."

Zigler recognizes that the normal-bodied group he calls "familial-genetic" retardates usually contains disproportionately large numbers of persons from lower social status and from ethnic minorities, the socioculturally nonmodal. There are two explanations that are commonly given for this phenomenon. Genetic theorists are prone to view the "familial-genetic" group as persons who are less well endowed intellectually, the lower end of the polygenic distribution of intelligence. They theorize that familial deficiencies in intelligence produce downward social mobility. Thus, the families of the genetically retarded gravitate to lower socioeconomic levels over several generations, and the preponderance of "familial-genetic" mental retardates in the lower social classes can be explained by this downward drift. While this hypothesis might have some validity for the Anglo population, it is hard to defend when applied to ethnic minorities, such as Blacks and Mexican-Americans, who have never held a high social status in American society from which they could "drift" downward and have been maintained in low-status positions by a variety of discriminatory practices.

Another school of thought, which Zigler calls the "defect theorists," holds that "all retardates suffer from a specific physiological or cognitive defect over and above their slower general rate of cognitive development" (Zigler, 1967, p. 294). They believe that failure to detect the exact organic nature of the defect in large numbers of mental retardates is due to the "relatively primitive nature of our diagnostic techniques." The overrepresentation of lower-status persons and persons from ethnic minorities in the "familial-genetic" group is explained as a result of the less adequate prenatal and postnatal care given to children living in socioeconomically disadvantaged circumstances. According to this view, less adequate medical care and diet produces a higher rate of organic damage, which in turn increases the rate of mental retardation.

Both "defect theories" and "genetic theories" assume a strict, supracultural clinical perspective so far as definition and diagnosis is concerned. Sociocultural factors enter into their schema only as possible "causal" agents or as incidental concomitants of lower genetic intellectual endowment. Neither of these viewpoints examines the possibility that some of the disproportions in rates of clinical retardation for socioculturally nonmodal groups could be related to the nature of the clinical perspective, its diagnostic procedures, and the nature of the population on which clinical measures were normed.

The Latent Class Solution

The latent class analysis program was set up to attempt all possible solutions from one through four classes and to retain the best-fitting solution.[2] The analysis formed three rather than two latent classes from the population of 177 clinical retardates. As shown in table 17, Class I contained 23% of the clinical retardates on the register, Class II contained 26%, and Class III, 51%.

Class I consists entirely of persons with three or more physical disabilities and eight or more adaptive behavior failures. Ninety percent of the Class I retardates have an IQ below 50. Their mean IQ was approximately 35, the hypothetical mean for Zigler's "organics." Clinically, they also resemble the Type 1 clinical retardates screened in the field survey, the physically disabled who are subnormal in both IQ and adaptive behavior.

Demographically, Class I contains retardates from each ethnic group in approximately the same proportion as they are found in the community. Only 65% of the heads of households and 62% of the mothers in the family had a high school education or more; the occupational and income level of the families of the "organics" was relatively low compared with the total community. Only 30% of the heads of households had white-collar jobs, only 27% had jobs that rated above an index score of 40 on the Duncan Socioeconomic Index, and only 37% had a family income over $8,000 per year. Six percent of the heads of households had been reared in Mexico, and 40% had been reared in the South or in Texas or Oklahoma. Most were from families that speak only English (75%), and there is a high rate of divorce and separation, 43% of the mothers.

In brief, Class I consists of organically damaged clinical retardates with low IQs, who come primarily from lower-middle-status families and represent all ethnic groups in about the same proportion as they

[2] This is to express appreciation to Mr. Curtis Miller, Socio-Behavioral Laboratory, Pacific State Hospital, who wrote the computer program for latent class analysis, which was used for the analysis presented in this chapter.

Table 17: Latent Class Structure among Those in the Follow-Up Study of the Clinical Case Register Who Are Retarded, Using a Two-dimensional Definition and the Traditional Criterion (IQ 0–69, 7 or More Adaptive Behavior Failures)

(N = 177)

Variables	Class I Organics	Class II Socioculturally Modal	Class III Socioculturally Nonmodal
Clinical Characteristics	%	%	%
IQ Below 50	90	52	20
Adaptive Behavior, 8 or More Failures	100	92	83
Physical Disabilities, 3 or More Failures	100	54	19
Sociocultural Characteristics	%	%	%
Anglo	74	99	27
Mexican-American	21	0	66
Black	5	1	7
Education of Head, 12 or More Years	65	97	32
Education of Mother, 12 or More Years	62	77	17
Occupation of Head, White-collar	30	84	0
Family Income $8,000 or More	37	89	43
SES Index of Head, 40 or Higher	27	87	0
Head Reared in Mexico or Foreign Country	6	2	13
Head Reared in South	40	5	16
Only English Spoken in Home	75	100	33
Mother Divorced, Separated	43	0	13
Percent of Total Population in Each Class	23%	26%	51%
Number of Persons in Each Class	41	46	90

appear in the community. For the most part, they are from English-speaking families, almost half of whom have a head of household who was reared in the South and migrated to California as an adult. The high rate of broken families is provocative. There is, of course, no way to determine from our data whether having an organically damaged, clinically retarded family member is a factor in this high rate of family dissolution or merely a corollary of the generally low socioeconomic level of the families in Class I. However, the rate of dissolution in Class I is over three times higher than that in Class III, a more socioeconomically disadvantaged group. This suggests that socioeconomic status alone cannot explain the high rate of divorce and separation.

Class II consists of more persons with higher IQs and fewer disabilities than Class I. About half the retardates in this category have less than three physical disability failures, and half have IQs above 50, thus falling into the lower ranges of the normal distribution of intelligence.

The demographic characteristics of the group are of particular interest because, educationally and socioeconomically, they are almost a mirror image of the Anglo population of the city. There were no Mexican-Americans and only 1% Blacks in Class II. The heads of households were better educated than those in Class I, 97% had a high school education or more, and 77% of the mothers had graduated from high school. Even more striking are differences in occupational level. Class II clinical retardates came from relatively high-status homes—84% of the heads of households had white-collar jobs, 89% had a yearly income of over $8,000 and 87% had occupations rated 40 or higher on the Duncan Socioeconomic Index. Few heads of households were reared in foreign countries (2%), and few were reared in the South (5%). The large majority were reared in the North or West. All of the families of retardates in this group spoke only English in the home. There were no divorced or separated mothers.

Thus, Class II retardates came mainly from middle- and high-status Anglo homes in which the parents were well educated and the family unit was stable. English was the only language spoken in the home, and most of the fathers were reared in the more economically advantaged regions of the United States, the North and West. Therefore, the subnormal performance of these individuals on intelligence tests and Adaptive Behavior Scales cannot be attributed to their coming from backgrounds that differ from the sociocultural mode of American society. Most retardates in this class had probably been exposed to the sociocultural materials needed to perform well on an intelligence test but had not acquired the necessary knowledge and skills needed to pass the test.

Class III consists mainly of persons with few or no physical disabilities and IQs between 50 and 69. Only 20% had an IQ below 50 and only 19% had three or more physical disabilities. In general, they had slightly better adaptive behavior scores than persons in the other classes but are, clinically, indistinguishable from Class II retardates.

The sociocultural characteristics of Class III retardates, however, were distinctly nonmodal. There was a heavy preponderance of Mexican-Americans (66%), about a third as many Anglos as would be expected (27%), and about the expected proportion of Blacks (7%). Only 32% of the heads of household and only 17% of the mothers had had a high school education. None of the heads of household had an occupation rated above 40 on the Duncan Socioeconomic Index or classified as a white-collar job, and 57% had a family income of less than $8,000 per year. Thirteen percent of the heads of household were reared in Mexico and 16% were reared in the South. Only 33% of the persons in this group came from families that spoke English all the time. Persons in Class III had probably had less exposure to the sociocultural materials needed to pass an intelligence test than persons in Class II.[3]

Internal Analysis of the Three Latent Classes

Is there any reason to distinguish persons in the three classes from each other in clinical practice? Is there any value in differentiating the socioculturally modal from the socioculturally nonmodal clinical retardate, i.e., persons in Class II from persons in Class III? Are persons in the two classes so similar that they can be treated as a homogeneous category and designated by a single title, such as "familial-genetic" retardate?

In order to answer these questions, the 123 persons in the latent class analysis who were sixteen years of age or over were regrouped so that all persons with three or more physical disabilities were classified as Class I and the remaining adults were left in either Class II or Class III, depending on the class to which they had been assigned by the latent class analysis. This regrouping clearly differentiated adults with major physical disabilities from those who were essentially normal-bodied, the "organics" from the "nonorganics." The analysis was restricted to adults so that a qualitative assessment of their adult social-role performance would be possible.

Regrouped in this fashion, Class I consisted of twenty-seven males and thirty-one females. Eighteen of the males and fifteen of the females (56.9% of the persons in this class) were institutionalized. Only two of the remaining persons in this class were married—both females. One of the married women, a Mexican-American, had returned to live with her parents and was working forty hours per week packing oranges. She was the only female in this class who had a job that was

[3] Labeled retardates in the follow-up study were the only group of persons who were clinically retarded by a two-dimensional definition using the traditional 3% criterion for whom we had complete clinical and sociocultural information on a large enough number of persons to do a latent class analysis. However, we did do a latent class analysis on persons screened as eligibles in the field survey, using the AAMD criterion in order to see if the three-group solution would also appear for the 120 eligibles screened in the field survey using this criterion. Three classes did appear for this group, and the classes had clinical and sociocultural characteristics almost identical to those found in the latent class analysis of labeled retardates on the clinical register reported in the text.

not part of a workshop program for the handicapped. The other female, a young Anglo, had been in special education classes from the fifth grade through high school, and was married and keeping house for her husband and daughter when interviewed. Only one of the noninstitutionalized males in this class was working at a regular job. He was a Mexican-American male, who was working forty hours a week at a trailer factory. On the basis of this subjective evaluation, there were probably two females and one male (5.2%) of the persons in Class I who, four years after the initial study, were leading lives in which they were filling what appeared to be the usual complement of marital and/or occupational roles for adults. The mean IQ for the adult Class I retardates was 39.6, not far from the mean of 35 hypothesized by Zigler for "organic" retardates.

Class II, the socioculturally modal group, contained fourteen normal-bodied adults, eleven males and three females. None of them had married or had had children. One male was institutionalized intermittently, and two males were in family care homes, but all were living in the community. The others were living with parents or relatives. Three males and one female were working regularly forty hours per week at a steady job. The males were all working as kitchen helpers, and the female was an elevator operator. These four persons appear to be relatively financially independent, 28.6% of the persons in this class. All others were only partially independent or were very dependent. Two of the other males worked part time, one as a kitchen helper and the other as a janitor. Four others worked in a workshop for the handicapped. Four persons in this class had never held a job and were totally dependent on their families for support. The mean IQ, 52.9, is significantly higher than that for Class I retardates.

Class III retardates, the socioculturally nonmodal, presented a wider range of performance. There were nineteen males, fourteen of whom were out of school and could be playing independent adult roles. Three of these adult males, all Anglos, were very dependent on their families and did not work. One Mexican-American male was in jail and another was in a foster home. However, the remaining nine adult males, eight Mexican-Americans and one Anglo, were all leading independent adult lives. The Anglo was married, had two children, and worked forty hours per week in a laundry. Two of the Mexican-American males were married and had children. One worked as a janitor and the other worked in construction. Another Mexican-American male supported his mother by working in a packing house and was head of her household. The other Mexican-American males still lived with their parents, and all were fully employed as truck drivers, laundry workers, or citrus packers. Thus, 64% of the adult males in Class III who were not still in school were leading independent adult lives.

Five of the thirty-two females in Class III were still in school, but twenty-seven were out of school and their performance as adults could be evaluated. Five of those out of school—three Mexican-Americans and two Anglos—lead very dependent, sheltered lives either with their families or in foster homes. They were perceived as subnormal by their families and carried no family responsibility. Two of them were in their 20s, one was in her 30s, and two were in their 40s.

There were six females—five Mexican-Americans and one Black—who, from their own or their parents' reports, appeared to be partially independent. Although they lived with their parents and were not holding a job outside the family, they did housework, cared for younger children, cooked, and filled other homemaker roles. They presented no problems to the family, and in most cases the family expected that they would eventually marry and leave home.

There were five young women—four Mexican-Americans and one Anglo—who were financially independent and had full-time jobs, but who still lived with their parents because they were not yet married. Two worked as kitchen helpers in the hospital, two worked as operators of sewing machines, and the fifth worked in a packing house. Another young Mexican-American woman was filling the role of mother in her parental family, rearing a large number of younger siblings because of her mother's illness.

The remaining women were either living alone and supporting themselves or were married and living with their husbands. One Mexican-American woman, separated from her husband, supported herself and her child as a fountain worker in a restaurant. One Anglo woman lived alone and supported herself by working as a domestic. The others, all Mexican-Americans, were married and taking care of their own families. Most of them had children. The mean IQ for Class III retardates was 57.4, significantly higher than either Class I or Class II.

These qualitative assessments give only a rudimentary picture of the lives of these adults, who were nominated as retardates and who failed both the intelligence test and adaptive behavior scales. However, it is clear from even this superficial picture that some of them were no longer playing the role of retardate and that many of them were filling the usual complement of social roles expected of persons of their age and sex when we contacted them four years after the original survey. We counted the number of men and women who were working full time and the number of women who were filling the role of housewife and mother. Thirty-two of the 123 labeled retardates over sixteen years of age in the latent class analysis (26%) fell into this category. However, they were disproportionately distributed over the three classes. Only 5.2% of the Class I retardates were leading relatively independent lives, while 28.6% of the Class II and 49% of the Class III labeled retardates fell into this category. There were no sex differences. However, there were large differences by ethnic group. Fully 45.3% of the Mexican-Americans who had been labeled as mentally retarded were leading independent adult lives, but this was true of only 11% of the 64 Anglos in the analysis. There were not enough Blacks on the register for a separate analysis of that group.

To summarize, 75% of the labeled adult retardates who had failed the 3% criterion on both IQ and adaptive behavior but were leading independent adult lives were Mexican-Americans and 78% of them were in Class III. All of the normal-bodied socioculturally nonmodal persons who failed the clinical measures were living in the community and half of them were leading independent adult lives. We conclude that clinical measures do not predict adult social-role performance for the socioculturally nonmodal as adequately as they predict for the socioculturally modal and the organically damaged. A supracultural clinical perspective that ignores the sociocultural background of the person being evaluated categorizes many socioculturally nonmodal persons as subnormal who, as adults, develop a life style indistinguishable from other persons in their group. Sociocultural factors need to be taken into account in diagnosis.

A Four-Group Taxonomy

As a result of the latent class analysis of the clinically retarded, we conclude that neither a two- nor a three-group taxonomy adequately describes the clinical and sociocultural characteristics of persons who have IQs below 70. There are at least four identifiable groups of persons who appear in the negative tail of the normal distribution of intelligence scores.

(1) The *quasi-retarded* are those who fail IQ but have normal adaptive behavior.

(2) The *organics* are those who have many physical disabilities and who fail both IQ and adaptive behavior. They come from all socioeconomic levels and all ethnic groups in approximately their expected proportion.

(3) The *socioculturally modal* are a group of relatively nondisabled persons who fail both IQ and adaptive behavior and come from homes that conform to the sociocultural configuration of the community.

Presumably, they have been exposed to the cultural materials needed to perform adequately on an intelligence test and on an adaptive behavior scale but have not acquired the knowledge and skills necessary to perform adequately.

(4) The *socioculturally nonmodal* are also relatively nondisabled persons who fail both IQ and adaptive behavior, but they come from homes that do not conform to the sociocultural mode for the community. Presumably, many of these individuals have not been exposed to the cultural materials and knowledge needed to perform acceptably on an intelligence test and adaptive behavior scales. A sizable percentage of them, as adults, are no longer perceived as retarded by persons in their social world, and they perform their social roles in a fashion indistinguishable from others in their sociocultural group.

Methods for distinguishing the quasi-retarded and the organics have been discussed. The problem remains, however, of distinguishing the socioculturally modal from the socioculturally nonmodal, and identifying those individuals within each group who have not acquired the knowledge and learned the skills needed to pass clinical measures because they could not learn them, from those who have not acquired those capabilities because they did not have the opporunity to learn them. Chapter 16 addresses this issue.

Chapter 16

SOCIOCULTURAL MODALITY

There are persons in all ethnic groups and from all socioeconomic levels who are organically damaged, cannot manage their own affairs, and need to be supervised and protected. These persons, Zigler's "organics," are readily identified. Their situation can be adequately conceptualized within the medical-pathological model. They present no particular dilemma to the clinical perspective.

However, the problem of differentiating the socioculturally modal from the socioculturally nonmodal person does pose a dilemma to the clinical perspective. How can we distinguish the person who fails adaptive behavior and IQ because he is not able to learn, from the person who fails both dimensions because he has had little opportunity to learn, but presumably could have learned if he had had the opportunity? Both groups have an average IQ between 50 and 69, both groups have few physical disabilities, and both have many adaptive behavior failures. They cannot be distinguished clinically when a "culture-blind" diagnosis is used. In this chapter, we will pursue the issue of the relationship between sociocultural modality and performance on the two basic measures that were used in the clinical epidemiology–IQ and adaptive behavior–in order to develop a pluralistic model of mental retardation that is sensitive to sociocultural modality and converges with social system definitions.

The Sociocultural Component of IQ

The Inferential Model Used in Interpreting the IQ

The IQ is ordinarily treated as a measure of an individual's intellectual capacity, his mental ability. Obviously, intellectual capacity cannot be measured directly, because that would require assessment of the genetic component of performance, the genotype. An individual's genotype can only be expressed through behavior learned in a social and cultural setting, his phenotype. The intelligence test measures what a person has learned, his phenotype. On the basis of his performance, inferences are made about the nature of his genotype. The clinical perspective is based on the assumption that it is possible to make valid inferences about the genotype from a properly normed and administered intelligence test. Those who make diagnoses from the clinical perspective are constantly making inferences about genotypes on the basis of the performance of phenotypes. The logic behind these inferences is relatively simple, but the assumptions are rarely, if ever, met in actual practice. The reasoning is as follows.

(1) If two persons have an equal opportunity to learn certain types of cognitive, linguistic, and mathematical skills and to acquire certain types of information; (2) if they are equally motivated to learn these skills and to acquire this information; (3) if they are equally motivated to exert themselves in a test situation and equally familiar with the demands of the test situation; (4) if they are equally free of emotional disturbance and anxieties that might interfere with their performance; (5) if they are equally free of biological dysfunctions and organic difficulties that might interfere with their performance, *then* any difference between their performance on a test that measures the extent to which they have learned these cognitive, linguistic, and mathematical skills and acquired certain types of knowledge is probably the result of differences in their genetic intellectual endowment. Simply stated, if learning opportunities and all other factors are equal, those persons who learn the most and who perform the best probably have greater mental capacity than those who learn the least and perform most poorly. Of course, the major difficulty in applying this logic in clinical situations in which inferences are made about human behavior is that all other factors are never equal.

The extent of these inequalities is clearly shown when we analyze the interrelationship between sociocultural background variables and IQ. There were 100 Mexican-Americans, 47 Blacks, and 556 Anglos from seven months through forty-nine years of age for whom IQs were secured in the field survey and for whom we also had information on eighteen of the sociocultural characteristics of their families. Most of them were tested by research staff psychometrists, though some IQs were secured through the public schools. The eighteen sociocultural characteristics were dichotomized so that one category corresponded to the modal sociocultural configuration of the community and the other category was nonmodal.[1] IQ was used as the dependent variable in a step-

[1] The eighteen independent variables analyzed were dichotomized as follows: segregated vs desegregated neighborhoods; head of household reared in Mexico vs reared in the United States; head of household reared in rural (under 10,000 population) vs reared in urban area (over 10,000 population); spouse of head of household reared in Mexico vs reared in the United States; spouse of head of household reared in rural vs reared in urban area; family moved 0–2 times in the last 10 years vs family moved 3 or more times; religion of head of household Catholic vs non-Catholic; number of persons in the family less than 6 vs 6 or more; education of mother 0–8 years vs 9

wise multiple regression in which the eighteen sociocultural characteristics were used as independent variables. The multiple regression coefficient for this large heterogeneous sample was .50 ($p < .001$), indicating that 25% of the variance in the IQs of the 703 culturally and ethnically heterogeneous individuals in this group could be accounted for by sociocultural differences.

In a similar analysis, 1,513 elementary school children in the public schools of Riverside were studied, using thirteen sociocultural characteristics of their families as independent variables and Full Scale IQ as the dependent variable. During the school year 1966–67, 598 Mexican-American, 339 Black, and 576 Anglo elementary school children in the Riverside Unified School District were tested using the Wechsler Intelligence Scale for Children. In addition to training received in regular university courses in test administration, the team of psychometrists who tested these children were given supplementary training to assure that their testing and scoring procedures were standard. They were closely supervised throughout the testing. The Mexican-American and Black children in the sample included the total school population of the three segregated minority elementary schools which then existed in the district. The Anglo children were randomly selected from eleven predominately Anglo elementary schools in the district. The multiple correlation coefficient was .57, indicating that 32% of the variance in the IQs of this socioculturally heterogeneous group of children could be accounted for by differences in family background factors. The more socioculturally modal the background, the higher the IQ. When sociocultural factors are so highly correlated with IQ, and the sociocultural characteristics of the three groups are not constant, no inferences can be made about the comparative innate mental ability of these children on the basis of the scores. The assumptions on which such inferences are based are not met. We cannot assume that any difference in the performance on an intelligence test reflects differences in the genotype of Anglo, Mexican-American, and Black children.

Ethnic groups in American society are not socioculturally homogeneous. Not only do sociocultural characteristics account for a large

---

or more years; owning or buying home vs renting home; English spoken in home all or most of the time vs half of the time, seldom, or never; nuclear family structure vs extended family structure; male head of household vs female head of household; head of household citizen of the United States vs noncitizen; head of household married and living with spouse vs divorced, separated, or never married; occupation of the head of household white-collar vs blue-collar; Duncan Socioeconomic Index Score of occupation of the head of household 0–29 vs 30 or higher; and 1.4 persons or less per room vs 1.5 or more persons per room.

amount of the variance in IQ in multi-ethnic groups, but they also account for a large amount of the variance in IQ within each ethnic group. A series of stepwise multiple regressions were run for Mexican-Americans and Blacks, using IQ as the dependent variable and sociocultural variables as independent variables. The analysis served two purposes: to determine the amount of variance in the IQs of persons in each ethnic group that can be accounted for by sociocultural modality, and to determine which sociocultural characteristics are most significantly correlated with IQ. We will first discuss data on persons studied in the field survey of the clinical epidemiology and then we will discuss data collected from the group of elementary school children who were administered the WISC.

Sociocultural Modality and IQ for Mexican-Americans and Blacks in the Field Survey

As reported earlier, there were 100 Mexican-Americans and 47 Blacks in the field survey for whom we have IQs and for whom we also have information on a large number of sociocultural background variables.

Eighteen sociocultural variables were treated as independent variables in the analysis of the 100 Mexican-Americans. All of these variables describe a characteristic of the family or of family members and are not characteristics of the person himself. Each variable was dichotomized as in the analysis descibed earlier. One side of the dichotomy was socioculturally modal and the other socioculturally nonmodal.

The first set of correlations in table 18 presents the findings for the Mexican-Americans. Together, the eighteen sociocultural variables were correlated .61 with IQ and account for 37.2% of the variance in the measured intelligence of this group of Mexican-Americans ($p<.001$). The five sociocultural characteristics that were most significant in the stepwise multiple regression are listed in order. Living in a household in which the head of household has a white-collar job is the best single predictor, .37. A family with five or fewer members contributes the most additional information, followed by a socioeconomic index score for the head of household's occupation of 30 or above. Living in a family in which the head of household was reared in an urban environment and was reared in the United States were next in importance. These five variables, combined, generate a multiple correlation of .54 and account for 29.2% of the variance in IQ.

Some other variables in the analysis were significantly correlated with IQ but did not add much new information beyond that provided by these five. For example, living in a nonsegregated neighborhood is correlated .21 with IQ; an urban childhood for spouse of the head of

Table 18: Sociocultural Component of IQ for Mexican-Americans and Blacks

Field Survey						Full Scale WISC: Children 6–14 Years					
Mexican-Americans (N = 100)			Blacks (N = 47)			Mexican-Americans (N = 598)			Blacks (N = 339)		
Sociocultural Variable[a]	R	% Variance	Sociocultural Variable[a]	R	% Variance	Sociocultural Variable[a]	R	% Variance	Sociocultural Variable[a]	R	% Variance
Head White-			Mother Reared	.27[b]	7.3	Less than 1.4	.24[c]	5.8	1–5 in Family	.21[c]	4.4
collar	.37[c]	13.7	in North			per Room					
1–5 in Family	.43[c]	18.5	Head White-	.33[b]	10.9	Mother Expects	.32[c]	10.2	Mother Expects	.30[c]	9.0
SES Index	.47[c]	22.1	collar			Some College			Some College		
Head 30+			Head Male	.35	12.3	Head 9+ Years	.34[c]	11.6	Head Married	.35[c]	12.2
Head Reared	.49[c]	24.0				Education					
Urban Area			Nuclear	.38	14.4	English All or	.36[c]	13.0	SES Index	.39[c]	15.2
Head Reared	.54[c]	29.2	Family			Most of the Time			Head 30+		
in U.S.			Own Home	.41	16.8	Own Home	.37[c]	13.7	Own Home	.41[c]	16.8
Total – 18	.61[c]	37.2	Total – 17	.52	27.0	All 17	.39[c]	15.2	All 16	.44[c]	19.4
Variables			Variables			Variables			Variables		

[a] All sociocultural variables are stated in the direction of sociocultural modality.
[b] Significant at the .05 level of significance.
[c] Significant at the .01 level of significance.

household is correlated .23; and non-Catholic religion for the head is correlated .24.

All but one of the five primary variables relate to characteristics of the head of household. His occupational level and childhood environment are of central importance. For Mexican-Americans, having a higher IQ is positively correlated with living in a small family in which the head of household has a white-collar job rated 30 or above on the Duncan Socioeconomic Index and who was reared in the United States in an urban environment.

There were only 47 Blacks in the field survey for whom we had information on all variables in the analysis. Such a small number of cases makes it difficult to achieve statistical significance, and findings are less reliable. However, the pattern of relationships is still worth noting. The multiple correlation between IQ and sociocultural characteristics was .52. The variables studied were identical to those in the analysis of Mexican-Americans except that the item on use of English was omitted and three items were scored differently. The two items on the region in which the head of the household and spouse were reared were dichotomized so that persons reared in the South, including Texas and Oklahoma, were compared with persons reared elsewhere. The item on religion was dichotomized to compare Baptists and Methodists with persons of all other religious preferences.

For Blacks, the region in which the mother of the family spent her childhood was the most important predictor, followed by whether the occupation of the head is blue-collar or white-collar. Sex of the head of household, family structure, and whether the family owns or is renting its home follow in that order. Blacks with higher IQs tended to come from intact nuclear families that owned or were buying their homes. They had a male head of household who had a white-collar job, and a mother who was reared outside the South.

A similar regression run on the 556 Anglos in the sample yielded a correlation coefficient of .31 when all sociocultural variables were used, indicating that sociocultural factors accounted for only 9.6% of the variance in IQ. As noted in chapter 3, the Anglo population of Riverside consists mainly of middle- and upper-middle-class adults (79%) with white-collar jobs (64%) and at least a high school education (80%). The estimated mean IQ for the entire Anglo sample in the field survey was 112.4. The mean IQ of Anglo children in the WISC testing reported earlier was 106.9, and the median IQ for Anglo children, based on the school testing program, ranged from 106 to 108 for various age groups.

The high-status and sociocultural homogeneity of the Anglo population and the fact that the mean IQ for the Anglo population of Riverside was so high makes intraethnic comparisons for Anglos less useful. Because the full range of social statuses and IQs are not represented in the Anglo population, sociocultural modality and IQ are not analyzed further for this ethnic group.

Sociocultural Modality and Children's Full Scale WISC IQs

Because the amount of IQ data on Mexican-Americans and Blacks was limited in the field survey, we turned to information provided by the parallel research study that we were conducting in Riverside on elementary school children, using the WISC. The purpose of this replication was to validate the findings from the field survey and to provide data for a more complete analysis than was possible with the small number of cases yielded by the field survey. Insofar as possible, the same sociocultural variables found to be significant in the field survey were used as independent variables to predict the Full Scale WISC IQ of these elementary school children, using a stepwise multiple regression. Information on sociocultural variables was secured in interviews with each child's parents.

All but two of the variables used in the earlier analysis were used to predict the IQs of Mexican-American children. Segregated vs desegregated neighborhood was deleted because all of the children in the elementary school sample lived in segregated neighborhoods. Where the mother was reared was also omitted for lack of information. A new variable, which was not available in the epidemiology, was included—the number of years of schooling the mother expected the child to complete. This variable was dichotomized high school graduation or less vs thirteen or more years of education. Education of the head of household was substituted for education of the mother.

As shown in table 18, all seventeen variables were correlated .39 with Full Scale IQ and accounted for 15.2% of the variance. This correlation is not as high as that secured in the analysis of field survey data that included adults as well as children. It could be that the IQs of adults are more influenced by sociocultural factors than those of children.

Overcrowding is the primary predictor (r = .24). Children who come from homes that have 1.4 or fewer persons per room have higher IQs than those from homes with an average of 1.5 or more persons per room. The number of years of schooling the mother expects the child to complete ranks second, raising the multiple correlation coefficient from .24 to .32 for Full Scale IQ. Education of the head of household, use of English in the home, and whether the family owns or is renting their home all contribute to the prediction.

In brief, Mexican-American elementary school children with higher IQs come from less crowded homes, have mothers who expect them to complete some education beyond high school, have fathers who had a ninth-grade education or more, and live in a family that is buying its home and speaks English all or most of the time. Thus, the more socioculturally modal the family, the higher the IQ of the child.

The variables found significant in the field survey and those found significant for elementary school children are very similar. Both analyses found that some measure of family size was significantly related to IQ. Occupation of the head of household does not appear in the children's analysis but education of the head does. Education of the head of household is correlated .32 with the socioeconomic index score of the head of household and .23 with white-collar vs blue-collar job. Therefore, education is accounting for approximately the same sociocultural components as occupation of the head. Speaking English in the home is correlated −.24 with having the head of household reared in Mexico. Consequently, these two variables have much in common. We conclude that there is a basic similarity between the variables found significant for Mexican-Americans in the field survey and those found significant in the analysis of elementary school children. Findings from the two analyses substantiate each other. Sociocultural modality is related to the WISC IQs of Mexican-American adults and children.

The sociocultural component of IQ is slightly greater for the 339 Black children than for the Mexican-American children. Exactly the same sociocultural variables were included in the analysis of Black children as those that were used in the field survey analysis except that segregated vs desegregated neighborhood was again omitted. Together, the sixteen sociocultural variables produced a multiple regression of .44 with Full Scale IQ. This means that 19.4% of the variance in Full Scale IQ can be accounted for by sociocultural factors.

The primary variables for Black children are similar to those found for Mexican-American children. Instead of overcrowding, the size of family emerges as the most important single variable for Blacks ($r = .21$). Here again, the two are measuring approximately the same characteristic of the family environment. Just as with Mexican-American children, the mother's educational expectations for the child appear as the second most significant variable after its common variance with size of family is taken into account. Marital status of the head of household, socioeconomic index score of the occupation of the head of household, and whether the family is buying or renting its home appear in that order.

In brief, the Black children with higher IQs come from families that have characteristics similar to the modal sociocultural configuration of the community. They come from families with less than six members. They have mothers who expect them to get some college education and fathers who have an occupation rated 30 or higher on the Duncan Socioeconomic Index. They have parents who are married and living together in a home which they either own or are buying. These variables are similar to those found significant in the field survey. Some measure of the father's occupation appears on both lists as well as some measure of family intactness. Sex of the head of household and marital status of the head are parallel variables because most families in which the head of household is separated or divorced have a female as head of household. Living in a family that is buying its home is a positive predictor in both the field survey analysis and the analysis of the elementary school children.

To summarize, sociocultural factors were able to explain from 15% to 30% of the variance in the IQs of Mexican-Americans, while sociocultural factors explained from 19% to 27% of the variance in Black IQs. It is clear that, even within ethnic group, the assumptions of the inferential model on which the interpretation of the IQ is based are not met. There is cultural heterogeneity within each minority ethnic group. The differential behavior that results has an impact on performance on an intelligence test. The more socioculturally modal the background of the individual, the higher his IQ.

Developing an Index of Sociocultural Modality

The findings from both multiple regressions were used to assign each Mexican-American and Black child in the WISC sample to one of five groups according to the extent of sociocultural modality in his family background. Children were first grouped using the five most significant sociocultural variables based on the field survey and then were grouped according to the five most significant sociocultural variables in the sample of children given the WISC. See table 18 for the variables used in each of these indices.

Each child was given one point for each family background characteristic that was like the sociocultural mode for the community on the five primary sociocultural variables predicting high IQ for his group. When grouped by the variables significant for the sample given the

WISC, a Mexican-American child received one point for each of the following: a family with 1.4 or fewer persons per room; a mother who expected him to go to school beyond high school; a head of household who had a ninth-grade or higher education; a family that speaks English all or most of the time at home; and a family that owns or is buying a home. If his family was like the sociocultural mode on four characteristics, he was given a score of 4, and so forth.

When the variables significant in the field survey were used as the basis for determining sociocultural modality, each Mexican-American child received one point for each of the following: living in a family in which the head of household has a white-collar job; living in a family with five or fewer members; living in a family in which the head of household has an occupation rated 30 or above on the Duncan Socioeconomic Index; living in a family in which the head of household was reared in a place with a population of 10,000 or more; and living in a family in which the head of household was reared in the United States.

The same procedure was followed for Black children, using the five sociocultural variables most predictive of Full Scale WISC IQ. A child received one point if he lived in a family with five or fewer members; if he had a mother who expected him to attend school beyond high school graduation; if he lived in a family in which the head of household was married and living with his spouse; if his family had a head of household whose occupation rated 30 or above on the Duncan Socioeconomic Scale; and if he lived in a family that owned or was buying its home.

When Black children were classified according to the sociocultural modality of their family background, using variables found to be significant in the field survey, each received one point for each of the following characteristics: having a mother reared in the North; living in a family in which the head of household has a white-collar job; living in a family which has a male head of household; living in a nuclear family consisting of a mother and father and their biological children; living in a family that owns or is buying its home.

The mean Full Scale IQ for children in each sociocultural modality group was calculated. The number of children in each group, the mean IQ, and the standard deviation for each group are presented in table 19.

Sociocultural Modality Groups for Mexican-American Children

There were only 25 Mexican-American children who came from backgrounds that included all five of the modal sociocultural characteristics found most predictive of high IQ in the sample of children given the WISC, 4.2% of the children tested. When we scored Anglo

Table 19: Mean IQs for Sociocultural Modality Groups Based on Variables Found Significant in Two Samples

		Sociocultural Modality					
		High 5	4	3	2	Low 1–0	Total
Mexican-American Children							
Children's Sample Variables	Number	25	174	126	146	127	598
	Mean	104.4	95.5	89.0	88.1	84.5	90.4
	Standard Deviation	10.4	12.1	11.8	11.6	11.3	12.7
Field Survey Variables	Number	21	75	139	94	74	403
	Mean	100.0	94.6	89.1	90.5	87.4	90.7
	Standard Deviation	12.3	13.1	11.5	12.9	11.6	12.6
Black Children							
Children's Sample Variables	Number	17	68	106	101	47	339
	Mean	99.5	95.5	92.8	87.1	82.7	90.5
	Standard Deviation	12.1	11.3	11.0	10.5	11.4	12.0
Field Survey Variables	Number	37	87	60	66	44	294
	Mean	95.3	90.4	93.5	89.6	85.8	90.8
	Standard Deviation	13.1	12.4	12.5	10.9	9.9	12.2

children using the same variables and scoring procedures used for Mexican-American children, 68.7% came from family backgrounds that scored five points. This large difference in the percentage of Mexican-American and Anglo children from backgrounds that promote high performance on an intelligence test emphasizes how very few of the Mexican-American children in Riverside come from sociocultural backgrounds that are even roughly comparable to those of Anglo children in the same schools. However, for the group of 25 children who were most like the sociocultural mode, the mean Full Scale IQ was slightly above the norms for the test, 104.4. Their mean Verbal IQ was 100.6, and their mean Performance IQ was 108.2. Mexican-American children with cultural backgrounds most similar to those of the community as a whole had a mean IQ not significantly different from that of the Anglo children on whom the tests were normed.

The 174 children with four modal sociocultural characteristics had a mean Full Scale IQ of 95.5, a Verbal IQ of 91.8, and a Performance IQ of 105. All scores were approximately nine points lower than the group most like the community mode. This is more than half a standard deviation difference and indicates how highly sociocultural factors are correlated with IQ.

The 126 Mexican-American children with three modal characteristics had a mean Full Scale IQ of 89.0; the 146 with two modal characteristics had a mean Full Scale IQ of 88.1; and the 127 with no or only one modal characteristic had a mean Full Scale IQ of 84.5. The group least like the modal sociocultural configuration was one standard deviation below the Full Scale norm for the population. In other words, about half the 127 children least like the sociocultural mode for the community would qualify as borderline retardates under the AAMD criterion if only an intelligence test were given.

When the sociocultural characteristics found to be most highly correlated with IQ in the field survey served as the basis for the index, there were 403 Mexican-American children for whom we had all the necessary background information needed to classify their family backgrounds by sociocultural modality. This subset of 403 children had a mean IQ of 90.7, while the total set had a mean IQ of 90.4. Therefore, it appears that the set and subset have essentially equivalent IQs.

Even though the sociocultural modality index based on the field survey variables was generated from a completely different sample of 100 Mexican-Americans of all ages, it still differentiated the elementary school children almost as well as the index generated on the children themselves. The 21 children from the most socioculturally modal homes had a mean Full Scale WISC IQ of 100.0, exactly the norm for the test. Those in the group with the lowest sociocultural modality had a mean IQ of 87.4 ($p < .001$).

Sociocultural Modality Groups for Black Children

The situation is just as dramatic for Black children. There were only 17 in the group which had all five modal characteristics as determined in the multiple regression on the elementary school children themselves, 5% of the total. We scored Anglo children using the same variables and procedures used for Black children and found that 39.6% of them had all five of the modal background characteristics, and 35.2% had four modal characteristics. As with Mexican-American children, there were many more Anglo than Black children in Riverside who came from homes that were similar to those of the sociocultural mode on these five characteristics. The dissimilarity of sociocultural characteristics occured in spite of the fact that the Black population of Riverside is socioeconomically more advantaged than the Black population in many other communities in the United States. Discrepancies would probably be much greater elsewhere.

The 17 Black children who did come from families that resembled the modal configuration on all five characteristics had an average IQ of 99.5, exactly at the national norms for the test. Thus, Black children who came from backgrounds even roughly comparable to those of persons in the modal society did just as well on the WISC as the Anglo children on whom the norms were based.

The mean Full Scale IQ of the 168 children with four modal characteristics dropped five points below the national norms to 95.5. The 106 children with three modal characteristics had a mean Full Scale IQ of 92.8, while those with only two characteristics had a mean of 87.1. The 47 children who had none or only one of the five modal characteristics had a mean IQ of 82.7. The average child in this group would also qualify as retarded, using the AAMD criterion. Here, again, we find over one standard deviation difference in IQ between the children from homes most like the sociocultural mode and those least like the modal configuration. The Verbal and Performance IQs of Black children in different sociocultural modality groups did not differ in any systematic way from the Full Scale IQ.

There were 294 Black children for whom we had all the family background information needed to classify them into sociocultural modality groups, using the variables found to be significant on the 47 Blacks of all ages tested in the field survey. Although the selection of the items in the index was based on a multiple regression on a small, completely different sample of Blacks of all ages, it still differentiated Black children over a ten-point range in IQ. The most socioculturally modal group on this index had a mean IQ of 95.3, which dropped to 85.8 for those with family backgrounds least like the sociocultural mode ($p<.001$). The deviation of the mean of the most modal group from 100 is not statistically significant and can be explained by chance variation.

A similar correlational analysis could be done on Anglo children in a population containing a sufficiently large number of Anglos from socioculturally nonmodal backgrounds. This was not possible in Riverside. Only 5 Anglo children in the 576 who were administered the WISC came from family backgrounds that scored 2 or below on the Mexican-American sociocultural modality index and only 31 scored two or below on the Black sociocultural modality index.

This analysis leads to two conclusions. Sociocultural modality explains a relatively large percentage of the variance in IQ. There is no way to hold sociocultural factors strictly constant across the three ethnic groups. Therefore, direct comparisons between IQs achieved by Anglos, Mexican-Americans, and Blacks are not legitimate. Second, when the variation in IQs is studied within ethnic group, sociocultural modality accounts for 20% to 30% of the variance. Therefore, it is not possible to treat Mexican-Americans or Blacks as homogeneous social categories or to hold sociocultural factors strictly constant by controlling only for ethnic group. A more differentiated, pluralistic approach is desirable in interpreting the meaning of a given IQ.

Pluralistic Norms for Interpreting an IQ

One way in which sociocultural factors could be taken into account in interpreting the meaning of an IQ is to compare an individual's performance only with other persons who come from comparable sociocultural backgrounds and who, presumably, have had similar opportunities to acquire the knowledge and skills needed to answer the questions on an intelligence test. In this way, the evaluation procedure would come closer to meeting the assumptions of the inferential model on which the test is based than do present procedures.

For example, a Mexican-American child who has only one sociocultural characteristic that is modal would fall into the group we have called 0–1 in table 19. For him, an IQ of plus or minus 11.3 points from 84.5 is within the normal range for his sociocultural modality group using standard statistical definitions. That is, an IQ of 73.2 to 95.8 is statistically normal for a child from his sociocultural background. An IQ between 61.9 and 73.2 would be "low normal" but not subnormal, if the 3% criterion were used. At the other end of the scale, an IQ between 95.3 and 106.6 would indicate "high normal" ability. An IQ above 106.6 would indicate very superior performance on an intelligence test for a child from such a nonmodal sociocultural background. Only an IQ below 61.9, the lowest 3% for his group, would be diagnosed as evidence of intellectual subnormality and be interpreted as a symptom of mental retardation.

The same would apply for Black children. We would expect the average IQ for a Black child from the 0–1 group to be 82.7. If his IQ falls between 71.3 and 94.1, he is in the normal range for his group. If he has a score between 94.1 and 105.5, he is high normal. If he scores above 105.5, he is in the superior range. Likewise, a score between 59.9 and 71.3 would be low normal, and only a person with a score below 59.9 would be diagnosed as subnormal.

A pluralistic approach would evaluate the intelligence of a person only in relation to others from similar sociocultural backgrounds. If the person scores more than one standard deviation above the mean for his sociocultural group, then he would be diagnosed as high normal in ability, even if his actual IQ were 100, average by the standard test norms. Conversely, if he is a Mexican-American child and manages to achieve a 75 on an intelligence test when he comes from an overcrowded, Spanish-speaking home in which the father has less than an eighth-grade education and was reared in a rural area, and his mother does not expect him to finish high school, he would be diagnosed as normal in ability. He would be within one standard deviation of the mean for his sociocultural modality group and, hence, in the normal range for children who have had little exposure to the cultural materials needed to take the WISC. The fact that he had not acquired the knowledge and skills needed to produce a high score on the test would be interpreted as a lack of opportunity rather than a lack of ability to learn. The same pluralistic procedure could be used in evaluating the meaning of an IQ for specific Black children except that Black sociocultural modality groupings would be the framework for interpretation.

The Sociocultural Component of Adaptive Behavior

Adaptive behavior was conceptualized as an age-graded dimension on which the individual gradually increases the number and complexity of the social roles that he plays. The Adaptive Behavior Scales attempt to assess the individual's success in coping with the increasing societal demands of various social roles in comparison with other persons of his age and sex.

The kind of roles which persons play and the level and complexity of their role sets differ markedly from one sociocultural group to another. We would expect that the adaptive behavior scores of persons from different ethnic groups would have a high sociocultural component and that persons within an ethnic group would also show considerable heterogeneity.

To study the sociocultural component of IQ, we generated a sociocultural modality index on the population studied in the field survey and then tested its efficacy by using it to classify individuals from a different sample, i.e., children attending public elementary schools. We followed a similar procedure in the analysis of adaptive behavior. We divided the screened sample into two mutually exclusive subsamples each representative of the entire screened sample. We generated a sociocultural modality index on one subsample and then tested the efficacy of the index by using it to classify persons in the second sample.

Table 20 presents the findings when the adaptive behavior scores of the 207 Mexican-Americans and the 162 Blacks in representative subsample one were used as the dependent variable in a stepwise multiple regression in which the same sociocultural variables were used as

Table 20: Sociocultural Component of Adaptive Behavior Scores for Mexican-Americans and Blacks

	Mexican-Americans (N = 207)			Blacks (N = 162)	
Sociocultural Variable[a]	R	% Variance	Sociocultural Variable[a]	R	% Variance
Head Reared in U.S.	.36[b]	13.0	Head Votes Frequently	.25[b]	6.3
Moved 2 or Fewer Times in 10 Years	.42[b]	17.6	1–5 Persons in Family	.32[b]	10.2
Own Home	.45[b]	20.3	SES Index Head Occupation 30+	.35[b]	12.3
Live Outside Segregated Minority Areas	.48[b]	23.0	Own Home	.37[b]	13.7
Mother Reared Urban Area	.49[b]	24.0	Education of Mother 9+ Years	.38[b]	14.4
All 18 Variables	.54[b]	29.2	All 17 Variables	.42[b]	17.6

[a] All sociocultural variables are stated in the direction of sociocultural modality. Correlations were done on persons in representative subsample one.

[b] Significant at the .01 level of significance.

independent variables as those employed in the analysis of the sociocultural component of IQ.

The multiple correlation coefficient for all eighteen sociocultural variables for Mexican-Americans was .54, explaining 29.2% of the variance in adaptive behavior. That for Blacks was .42, explaining 17.6% of the variance in adaptive behavior scores. These correlations are of approximately the same magnitude as the correlations between sociocultural factors and IQ. All are significant beyond the .01 level.

As in the analysis of IQ, Mexican-Americans who live in households in which the head of household was reared in the United States, in which the mother was reared in an urban area, and in which the family owns or is buying its home have fewer adaptive behavior failures. Living outside the segregated minority residential area and being less geographically mobile are new variables, which did not appear among the first five in the analysis of the sociocultural component of IQ.

For Blacks, the list of relevant sociocultural variables is almost identical to those most predictive of high IQ. Head of household voting frequently or occasionally is the single new predictive variable among the first five.

The 452 Mexican-Americans and 312 Blacks in representative subsample two were scored for sociocultural modality using the five variables found most significant in the stepwise multiple regressions for their group in representitive subsample one. For Mexican-Americans, the average number of failures on adaptive behavior increased from 2.9 for the group which was most socioculturally modal, to 5.2 for the most nonmodal group ($p<.001$). For Blacks, the average number of failures increased from 1.4 to 4.3 over the five categories. ($p<.001$). As in the case of IQ, the sociocultural component of adaptive behavior is sizable and there is meaningful differentiation within each ethnic group along a sociocultural continuum.

Pluralistic Norms for Interpreting Adaptive Behavior Scores

Our analysis indicates that a pluralistic system for taking sociocultural differences within the Mexican-American and Black groups into account in evaluating the meaning of a particular adaptive behavior score has possibilities. Unfortunately, there were not enough Mexican-Americans and Blacks screened in the field survey in each of the three age groups to provide sufficient data for further exploration and elaboration of such a pluralistic procedure in this study.

For this reason, it was necessary to treat each ethnic group as if it were a socioculturally homogeneous group. Distributions of adaptive behavior scores for each of the three major age groups (preschool, school-age, and adult) within each ethnic group were used to determine the cutoff score for the lowest 3% of the population in each group. This is exactly the same procedure as that used in the clinical epidemiology for establishing community-wide cutoffs.

When the three ethnic groups were normed separately, there was no change in the traditional 3% cutoff score for Anglos or Blacks. The cutoff score for the lowest 3% in adaptive behavior was still 7 or more failures for preschool children, 9 or more failures for school-age children, and 8 or more failures for adults. However, there were major changes in the cutoff scores for Mexican-Americans. Preschool children required one additional failure to be in the lowest 3%; school-age children required 2 additional failures, and adults, 6 additional failures. Thus, the adaptive behavior cutoffs for the traditional criterion for Mexican-Americans, based on Mexican-American norms, are 8 or more failures for preschool children, 11 or more failures for school-age children, and 14 or more failures for adults.

Rates for Clinical Retardation Based on Pluralistic Norms

What happens to prevalence rates for clinical retardation in the Riverside field survey when pluralistic norms and evaluation procedures are systematically applied? We reanalyzed the field survey data, using a two-dimensional definition, the 3% criterion, and pluralistic norms. Table 21 presents the rates per 1,000 for each ethnic group for all possible combinations of procedures.

The prevalence rate per 1,000 for Blacks was 44.9 when a one-dimensional definition was used based only on the individual's IQ and the standard test norms. There was a large drop in prevalence rate for Blacks when a two-dimensional definition, using the standard norms for IQ and the community-wide norms for adaptive behavior, was applied, 44.9 to 4.1 per 1,000. Because the pluralistic norms for Blacks on the Adaptive Behavior Scales are the same as the community-wide norms, there is no drop in rate of clinical retardation when a partial pluralistic two-dimensional definition is used, i.e., standard norms for IQ and pluralistic norms for adaptive behavior. By chance, all the Blacks in the failing group in our sample had IQs that were low enough so that they failed the pluralistic norms for IQ as well as the standard norms. Hence, there was no decrease in rate when pluralistic IQ norms were applied as well as pluralistic adaptive behavior norms. The Black rate for clinical retardation was essentially identical to the Anglo rate when pluralistic procedures were used.

Table 21: Rates per 1,000 of Clinical Retardation by Ethnic Group, Using Successively More Pluralistic Evaluative Procedures and the Traditional 3% Criterion

Screening Procedure Used at the Traditional Criterion (lowest 3%)	Black	Mexican-American	Anglo	Total Population Rate
One-dimensional Definition (IQ Only, Using Standard Test Norms)	44.9	149.0	4.4	21.4
Two-dimensional Definition (Standard Norms for IQ and Adaptive Behavior)	4.1	60.0	4.4	9.7
Partial Pluralistic Two-dimensional Definition (Standard Norms for IQ and Pluralistic Norms for Adaptive Behavior)	4.1	30.4	4.4	6.8
Pluralistic Two-dimensional Definition (Pluralistic Norms for IQ and Adaptive Behavior)	4.1	15.3	4.4	5.4

Mexican-American rates were greatly reduced when pluralistic norms were applied. The rate for clinical retardation using a one-dimensional definition based only on IQ and standard test norms was 149.9 per 1,000 for Mexican-Americans, approximately 15% of the population. When a two-dimensional definition was used and adaptive behavior as well as IQ was evaluated, the rate dropped to 60 per 1,000, even though the standard norms were still used. When pluralistic adaptive behavior norms were applied and the standard IQ norms were maintained, the rate dropped to 30.4. When pluralistic norms were used to interpret both adaptive behavior and IQ, the rate was 15.3 per 1,000. This was still slightly higher than either Anglo or Black rates, but the difference between 4.1 per 1,000 (.41%) and 15.3 per 1,000 (1.53%) is relatively minimal.

Nothing happens to Anglo rates when pluralistic norms are applied. They are 4.4 per 1,000 regardless of whether adaptive behavior is evaluated or not. Since the standard norms are Anglo norms, there is no change in norms for either the Adaptive Behavior Scales or the intelligence test when pluralistic procedures were used. Anglos are those for whom diagnostic procedures were designed, and there is little in our epidemiological findings that would suggest the need for significant modification in screening procedures for them. However, an epidemiological study in a community containing large numbers of low-status, disadvantaged Anglos would probably reveal the value of pluralistic norms based on Anglo sociocultural modality groups. Such norms would come closer to meeting the assumptions of the inferential model on which the intelligence test is based and to providing a framework for taking sociocultural factors into account in interpreting the meaning of the clinical scores of disadvantaged Anglos. A larger sample and further development of measures of adaptive behavior appropriate for use in the community would make similar procedures possible in evaluating adaptive behavior.

Chapter 17

SOCIOCULTURAL PLURALISM: CONVERGENCE OF THE CLINICAL AND SOCIAL SYSTEM PERSPECTIVES

What is true mental retardation? Who is really mentally retarded? What is the real prevalence rate for mental retardation? All of these are nonsense questions, which cannot be answered. Individuals have no name and belong to no class until they are assigned to one. The definer determines the terms of his definition and sets the boundaries for his classes. He constructs the model and prescribes the operation he will use to organize the world according to his categories. His model circumscribes not only what he will perceive but the kinds of questions he will be able to ask about the empirical world.

Tactics in the Pursuit of Meaning

One of the distinguishing attributes of the human intellect is its ability to simplify its environment by the process of selecting from the varied characteristics of assorted individuals those characteristics which they have in common and using these common characteristics as the basis for developing a mental construct while ignoring differences between individuals. The process of abstraction makes it possible to treat all objects in a common class as if they were identical. Ignoring differences simplifies the environment and allows for economy of action and decision-making, but it also tends to reduce sensitivity to the characteristics on which individuals placed in the same category continue to differ. The definer frequently begins to act as if persons classified into a particular category by his mental construct are identical in all respects, not just in those respects by which they have been classified.

Two elements of the process of abstraction need special emphasis. First, the choice of the characteristics by which objects or persons in the real world shall be grouped is entirely at the discretion of the person doing the abstracting. There is nothing predetermined about the basis for classification. The taxonomy will depend on the purpose of the definer.

Second, when a classification system has been evolved, names are usually applied to the various classes and mental constructs. Language is essential. It fixes labels on the categories created by abstraction and makes it possible to contemplate and manipulate them intellectually. Thus stabilized and objectified by language, mental constructs tend to be treated as "given" and to be regarded as the "natural" or the "right" way to organize the empirical world. When this happens, the stabilization of mental constructs through labeling may block the development of potentially more useful or more creative ways of conceptualizing human experience.

Mental retardation is such an abstraction. It exists as a category of thought, a way of classifying people. Traditionally, two models have been used in making such classifications: the pathological model of medical practitioners, and the statistical model of psychologists and other behavioral scientists. Although these two models are operationally and conceptually very different and do not always allocate people to comparable categories, they are both based on a set of assumptions about the nature of mental retardation, which we have called the "clinical perspective." They regard mental retardation as individual pathology characterized by symptoms that manifest themselves in comparable forms in all sociocultural segments of American society. They assume that these symptoms can be diagnosed using standardized instruments and that persons can be classified on the basis of these procedures into the "mentally retarded" and the "normal" without regard to the sociocultural milieu in which they are living or the manner in which they are perceived by persons in their own social groups.

The clinical perspective starts at the top of the abstraction ladder with the mental construct "mental retardation" and moves downward from the ideal to the empirical world to classify individuals by operationalizing the critical concepts that make up the construct. Philosophically, this orientation is known as the operationist approach. A set of operations are developed for evaluating the objects of experience along those dimensions which have been selected as the basis for classification. Each concept has a set of operations for its measurement. The operations used in manipulating the concept scientifically *are* the scientific meaning of the concept. The clinical epidemiology was based on the assumptions and procedures of the clinical perspective.

The social system perspective starts in the empirical social world at the bottom of the abstraction ladder and moves upward to the mental construct. In this approach, the meaning of the concept "mental retardation" rests in understanding the use to which the concept is put, i.e., the plan of action engendered by the concept. Observing the concept "mental retardation" in action as it is used to sort out and categorize persons as "retarded" or "normal" in the empirical social world reveals the contours of its meaning. Meaning rests in outcomes rather than origins. From the social system perspective, the meaning of mental retardation rests in how the concept is used to sort out, classify, and label people. When we comprehend this sorting and labeling process and the outcomes of the process in terms of who is and who is not labeled, then we will comprehend the meaning of mental retardation in an American community.

In the social system epidemiology, we began in the empirical world of Riverside and attempted to locate all those persons who were holding the status and playing the role of mental retardate in any of the social systems of the community. The characteristics of persons who were holding the status of mental retardate in any of these social systems were studied and inferences were drawn about the content of the norms, the focus of the norms, and the level of the norms being applied by various social systems in defining mental retardation. Beginning at the level of experience and analyzing the characteristics which persons labeled as mentally retarded by different types of social systems had in common and those characteristics on which they differed, we moved, inductively, from the empirical world up the abstraction ladder to the mental construct of the meaning of mental retardation in the city of Riverside.

What is mental retardation? Who is retarded? What is the prevalence rate for mental retardation? The answers to these questions depend on the definer's perspective, his assumptions, and the tactics he uses in the pursuit of meaning. There is no single answer. There are no "true" responses. The human intellect can organize the empirical world into myriad categories and sort people according to an infinite number of characteristics. The definer selects the system that best serves his purposes.

As social scientists, we could have let the matter rest with the description of the meaning of mental retardation in the community from a clinical and from a social system perspective. Instead, we chose to move one step beyond exposition to an analysis of the implications of each perspective. We have studied divergences between the outcomes when clinical and social system perspectives are applied and have discussed those procedures which maximize convergence of the two perspectives. The point where clinical and social system definitions converge is the point of maximum consensual validation.

Convergence of Clinical and Social System Perspectives: Sociocultural Pluralism

Clinical and social system perspectives tend to converge when clinical procedures are made sensitive to sociocultural differences. The pluralistic clinical procedures developed in this study regard the performance of an individual on standardized measures such as an intelligence test or Adaptive Behavior Scales simply as a manifestation of his phenotype. The phenotype is a product of continuous interaction between the individual's genetic endowment and his developmental experience in a particular sociocultural environment. Inferences about the contribution of the genotype to the performance of the phenotype on clinical measures can only be made when the interaction of the genotype with the sociocultural environment is taken into account. If the phenotypical performance of two or more persons is to be compared and inferences are to be made about the relative nature of their genotypes, then a minimum of two factors must be held constant: the physiological condition of the sensory, motor, and other biological systems of the individuals being compared, and the sociocultural environments in which they were socialized.

If we agree that all three factors are significant in the performance of the phenotype, then, in simplest terms, poor performance on an intelligence test or Adaptive Behavior Scale may result from any one or any combination of these three factors. The person may achieve a statistically subnormal performance because he is organically impaired and/or because his polygenically inherited learning potential is low and/or because he has been reared in a sociocultural environment that does not teach him the kinds of knowledge and skills or develop in him the motivational patterns required to perform well on the kinds of tasks and in the kinds of situations that are typical of psychometric testing. Given the Anglo-oriented content and the nature of the performances evaluated in the clinical measures commonly used by clinicians, those normal-bodied persons who do least well tend to be persons from socioculturally nonmodal backgrounds.

Thus, three types of low performers on intelligence tests and Adaptive Behavior Scales were identified: the physiologically damaged; the socioculturally modal who have presumably had the opportunity to learn the materials in the intelligence tests but have not learned them; and the socioculturally nonmodal who have presumably not had as much opportunity to learn the skills and acquire the knowledge needed to pass an intelligence test as have persons from socioculturally modal backgrounds. The primary task of a pluralistic clinical perspective is to differentiate between these three groups and thus bring about greater convergence between clinical and social system definitions.

The use of pluralistic interpretations is foreign to the clinical perspective, especially to the pathological model. This model has evolved in the field of medicine as a conceptual tool for comprehending and controlling disease processes. Based on functional analyses of pathological processes in living organisms, the pathological model is not geared to take sociocultural factors into account except as they produce biological changes in the organism. Such a perspective is quite appropriate when dealing with physiological conditions. The pathological-medical model has been a very powerful conceptual tool when used to study disease processes and organic dysfunctions. It is appropriate for conceptualizing the clinical retardates whom we have called Type 1 retardates in the field survey, whom Zigler has called the "organics," and who appeared as Class I retardates in the latent class analysis. Their condition can be described through functional analysis. Their pathologies can be identified as organically based. It is reasonable to assume that stable patterns of comparable biological symptoms will manifest themselves in similar form in many societies and in a variety of cultures.

On the other hand, the socioculturally modal and nonmodal, both classified as Type 2 retardates in the field survey and as "familial-genetics" by Zigler, cannot be differentiated by standard clinical procedures. As biological factors become more obscure, the pathological model becomes less useful as a conceptual tool. Both the socioculturally modal and the nonmodal are normal-bodied. The standard statistical model cannot distinguish them. Both groups have low IQs that fall within the range described by the normal distribution. Both groups have subnormal adaptive behavior as measured by community-wide norms. We have examined the possibilities of using a pluralistic statistical model rather than a medical-pathological model or a standard statistical model to conceptualize cases in which persons are not physically disabled and show no evidence of biological damage. The key clinical problem in such cases is to distinguish between the socioculturally modal and the socioculturally nonmodal.

A pluralistic clinical perspective makes this distinction by taking sociocultural differences into account during evaluation by evaluating each individual in relation to others from comparable sociocultural backgrounds, who presumably have had similar opportunities to acquire the knowledge and skills measured in intelligence tests and Adaptive Behavior Scales. Pluralistic evaluation defines a person as clinically retarded only if he scores in the lowest 3% of his own sociocultural group on both IQ and adaptive behavior. If he scores above the lowest 3% in his own sociocultural group on IQ and/or adaptive behavior, he is evaluated as quasi-retarded, low normal, or normal, but not clinically retarded. In such cases, the discrepancy between his score and the community-wide norms for adaptive behavior or IQ is interpreted as a measure of the distance he will have to go if he is to acquire the knowledge and skills needed to achieve in the mainstream of American society, but *not* as evidence of intellectual deficit or genetic inferiority.

A Pluralistic Evaluation Procedure

Pluralistic evaluation is most concerned with normal-bodied persons who are usually diagnosed solely by means of an intelligence test. A pluralistic clinical perspective would require abandoning the supracultural stance of the customary clinical perspective when evaluating persons who are not biologically damaged. On the basis of the findings in this epidemiology, we have examined the possibility of taking sociocultural differences into account by using a pluralistic clinical perspective to interpret the meaning of any set of clinical scores. Such a diagnosis would have three characteristics not presently a part of clinical evaluations. It would use the traditional criterion of the lowest 3% to define subnormality. It would use two dimensions, IQ and adaptive behavior, to evaluate mental retardation, and both measures would have to be failed before making an evaluation of clinical retardation. It would use pluralistic norms to interpret the meaning of a specific IQ or adaptive behavior score. Such norms would evaluate the individual's performance in relation to others from similar sociocultural backgrounds.

In this procedure each person would be assigned to the sociocultural modality group that comes closest to describing his background. His IQ and adaptive behavior would be classified as subnormal, low normal, normal, high normal, or superior according to the location of his scores in the distribution of scores earned by persons who had had similar opportunities to acquire the knowledge and skills required to do well on these measures.

An Experimental Application of Pluralistic, Socioculturally Sensitive Procedures

During the academic year 1969–70, the Pupil Personnel Departments of the Riverside and Alvord Unified School Districts reevaluated all 268 children in their classes for the educable mentally retarded, using a social system perspective and pluralistic evaluative procedures.[1] The

[1] We wish to thank key persons from the Riverside Unified School District for their support and advice in our research efforts. We would especially like to thank Albert

students ranged from seven through nineteen years of age. Fifty-five percent were males, 54% were Anglos, 23% were Mexican-Americans, and 23% were Blacks. Most of the children were from lower socioeconomic statuses. Seventy-seven percent of them were from homes in which the head of household had a blue-collar job. The mean socioeconomic index score of the heads of households was 24.1. Thus, five years after the original social system epidemiology, children from lower socioeconomic levels and ethnic minority groups continued to be overrepresented in classes for the mentally retarded, although the percentage of Mexican-American children had been somewhat reduced by a conscious, informal effort on the part of psychologists in the two districts to take sociocultural factors into account in evaluating Mexican-American children.

In the reevaluation, a school psychologist retested each child, using the WISC. Interviewers, employed by the research project, interviewed the parents of each child. Interviewer and parent were matched for ethnic group, and a Spanish version of the interview was used when the parent preferred being interviewed in Spanish. Information on the adaptive behavior of each child and the sociocultural characteristics of his family was secured. Each child was placed in the sociocultural modality group appropriate for his family background as rated on the five-question index developed on the sample of children reported in chapter 16.

In making the pluralistic evaluation, the standard WISC norms were used for all Anglo children. The community-wide adaptive behavior norms were used for all Anglo and Black children. The pluralistic IQ norms derived from the sample of children given the WISC as described in chapter 16, were used for Mexican-American and Black children. Pluralistic norms were used for evaluating the adaptive behavior of Mexican-American children. The traditional 3% cutoff and a two-dimensional definition were used.

Labeled Retardates with IQs 69 and Below

Figure 4 shows, schematically, how the 268 children in special education classes in these two public school districts performed, using pluralis-

---

Marley, of the Riverside Unified School District, and Robert W. Hooker and J. Martin Kaeppel, of the Alvord School District, and their staffs for their assistance in the reevaluation of the labeled mental retardates in their school districts. Without their interest and the support of their staffs the experimental application of pluralistic procedures would not have been possible. We also wish to thank Rosa McGrath and Lillian Redmond, who served as interviewers in the reevaluation study.

Figure 4: Reclassification Resulting from the Application of Socioculturally Pluralistic Procedures in Reevaluating Labeled Retardates in the Public Schools

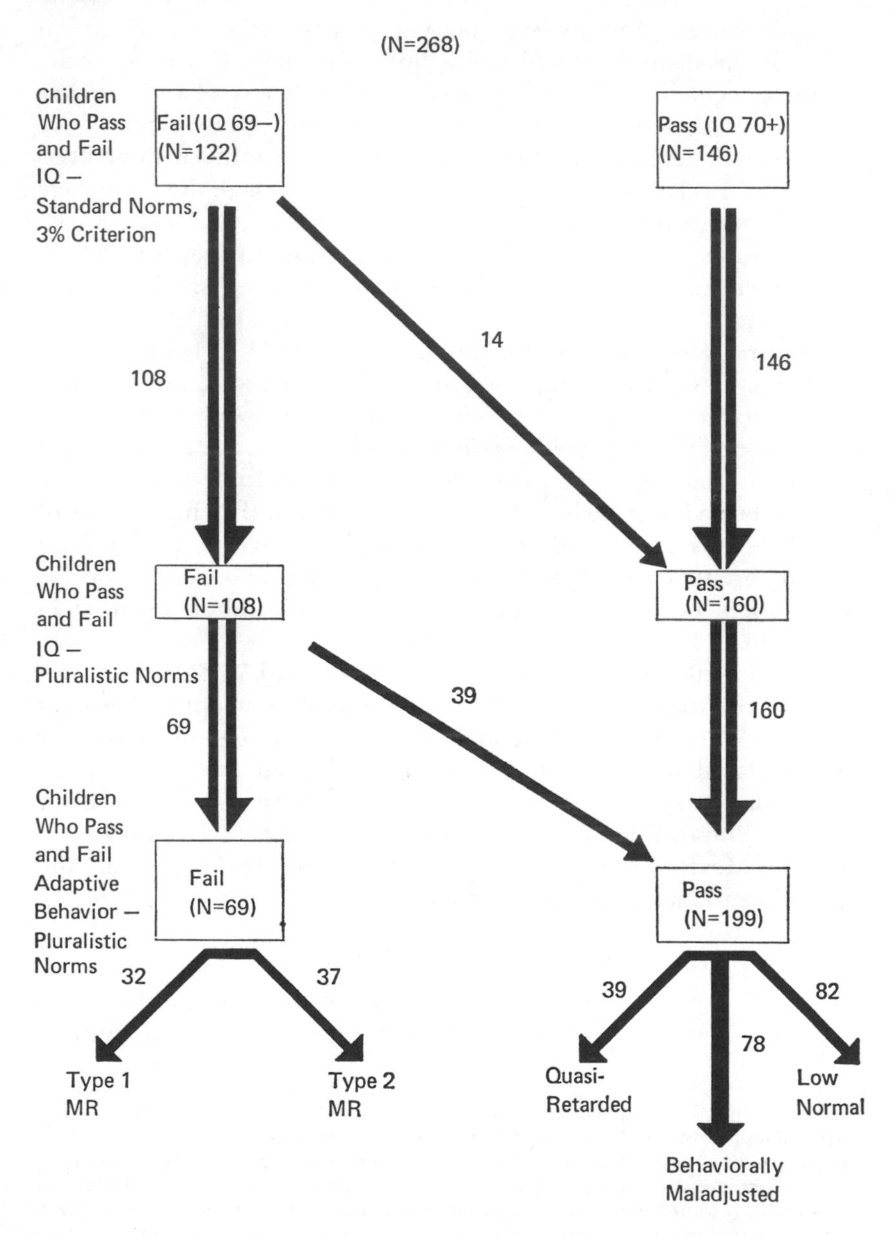

tic norms. There were 122 children who had an IQ of 69 and below. When pluralistic IQ norms were used, there were 14 children in this group from socioculturally nonmodal homes whose IQs fell in the normal range for their sociocultural modality group even though they were below the standard norms for the test. These children's IQs ranged between 62 and 69. They passed the IQ dimension and are shown in figure 4 by an arrow drawn to the "Pass" column from the "Fail" (IQ 69–) column.

Thirty-nine of the 108 children who failed pluralistic IQ norms, passed the pluralistic norms for adaptive behavior. They, too, are shown by an arrow drawn to the "Pass" column. These children are the quasi-retarded. This leaves 69 children who failed both the pluralistic norms for adaptive behavior and IQ who were "clinically retarded." Thirty-two of these children failed the Physical Disability Scale and were classified as Type 1 mental retardates.

Labeled Retardates with IQs 70 and Above

The "Pass" column in figure 4 shows that there were 146 children who had an IQ of 70 or higher. When the 3% criterion is used, these 146 children were classified as in the low normal range for IQ. There were 14 children in this high IQ group who had an IQ above 84, and 5 of these children had IQs in the 90s. These 19 children with IQs above 84 are in the "normal" range, even by standard IQ norms, while the remaining 132 are "low normals."

The 14 children from socioculturally nonmodal backgrounds who had IQs below 69 but rated as "normals" when pluralistic IQ norms were used were added to the 146 with IQs of 70 or above. Thus, there were 160 labeled retardates who passed the pluralistic norms for IQ. Seventy-eight of them failed the pluralistic norms for adaptive behavior and were classified in the behaviorally maladjusted category. Eighty-two of them passed the Adaptive Behavior Scales and were classified as low normals. Thus, the application of a two-dimensional screening procedure, which takes sociocultural factors into account, classified 11.9% of the 268 labeled children as Type 1 mental retardates, 13.8% as Type 2 mental retardates, 14.6% as quasi-retardates, 29.1% as behaviorally maladjusted, and 30.6% as normals. Table 22 compares some of the characteristics of children in the five groups.

Clinical Characteristics

Because IQ and adaptive behavior were used to classify children into the various types shown in table 22, no statistical tests were made of the differences in IQ and adaptive behavior. However, the patterns of

Table 22: Characteristics of Labeled Retarded When Classified Using Pluralistic Procedures

	Type 1 Retardates (N = 32)	Type 2 Retardates (N = 37)	All Mental Retardates (N = 69)	Behaviorally Maladjusted (N = 78)	Quasi-retarded (N = 39)	Normal (N = 82)	Significance Level
Clinical Characteristics							
Mean IQ	59.9	59.5	59.6	76.4	59.7	75.9	a
Mean Adaptive Behavior	12.8	11.8	12.3	11.8	6.4	6.5	a
Mean Physical Disability	3.3	.5	1.8	1.7	1.2	.9	$<.001$[b]
Sociocultural Characteristics							
Ethnic Group							
% Anglo	84.3	70.2	76.8	61.5	41.0	32.9	
% Mexican-American	6.2	16.2	11.6	17.9	20.5	40.2	$<.001$
% Black	9.3	13.5	11.6	20.5	38.4	26.8	
% Speak English All the Time	84.4	86.5	85.5	80.8	76.9	57.3	$<.001$
% White-collar—Head	31.3	30.6	31.0	15.1	16.7	11.8	$<.05$
Mean SES Index—Head	28.7	28.5	23.6	24.6	22.1	21.2	NS

[a] Not appropriate.

[b] In calculating the overall significance of difference, all the mentally retarded (Type 1 + 2) were combined for purpose of comparison.

scores are interesting. The mean IQs of both types of mental retardates and of quasi-retardates were just below 60 and are about identical. The quasi-retardates did not have an average IQ higher than the children classified as mentally retarded. The mean IQs of the behaviorally maladjusted and the normals were in the middle 70s. These two groups have almost identical IQs, as measured by the test. Both the mental retardates and the behaviorally maladjusted had an average of about 12 adaptive behavior failures, while the quasi-retardates and normals had about 6.5 failures. Therefore, within the group of children who failed the Adaptive Behavior Scales, i.e., the mentally retarded and the behaviorally maladjusted, there were no differencs in adaptive behavior. There were also no differences in adaptive behavior between those classified as quasi-retarded and "normal."

Although physical disability scores were used to differentiate Type 1 from Type 2 mental retardates, they were not used to distinguish mental retardates from the quasi-retarded, behaviorally maladjusted, or normal. Therefore, a statistical test in which the average physical disability score of the two types of mental retardates (1.81) is compared to the mean physical disability scores of the other three classes is appropriate. The F ratio was significant ($p<.001$). When all mental retardates were combined, they had significantly more physical disabilities than the normals ($p<.001$) and the quasi-retarded ($p<.05$). The behaviorally maladjusted had about the same number of physical disabilities as all mental retardates and significantly more disabilities than the normals ($p<.001$). Physical disabilities tended to distinguish both the behaviorally maladjusted and the mentally retarded from the quasi-retarded and the normals.

Sociocultural Characteristics

Age was not a differentiating factor, nor was sex. However, sociocultural differences were pronounced. When pluralistic norms were applied, the ethnic characteristics of the group of children still categorized as mentally retarded closely approximated the ethnic distribution of the two school districts. About 77% were Anglo, 12% Mexican-American, and 12% Black. Disproportionately large numbers of children reclassified as quasi-retarded and normal rather than mentally retarded were Mexican-American and Black. The ethnic distribution of those children reclassified as behaviorally maladjusted fell between the two extremes ($p<.001$). Children who were reclassified as quasi-retarded or normals were significantly less likely to come from families that speak English all the time ($p<.001$). All three groups of reclassified children were more likely to come from homes in which the head of household had a blue-collar occupation. The average socioeconomic index score of the head of household was also lower for the three reclassified groups, but differences were not quite statistically significant. In brief, reclassification of labeled retardates, using pluralistic norms, essentially eliminated ethnic disproportions among those who continued to be labeled as mentally retarded and identified a sizable number of labeled retardates who were from socioculturally nonmodal backgrounds as quasi-retarded, behaviorally maladjusted, or normal when judged only in relation to other children from similar sociocultural backgrounds.

Convergence of Social System and Clinical Definitions

The experimental application of pluralistic norms eliminated the disproportionately large number of children from ethnic minorities who were labeled as retarded and produced an ethnic and sociocultural distribution that approximated community percentages. Did pluralistic evaluation bring about a convergence of social system and clinical definitions of mental retardation?

When parents were interviewed in the reevaluation of the 268 labeled mental retardates, they were asked to rate their child on 25 bipolar behavior dimensions, using a semantic differential rating based on seven categories. Five of these 25 ratings were directed at measuring the parent's perception of the child's intellectual competence: slow–quick; bright–dull; capable–not capable; difficulty learning–learns easily; and retarded–accelerated. The average parental ratings given the children in each of the pluralistic categories is shown in table 23.

All but one of the five parental ratings significantly differentiated the children in the five categories. The children who were classified as mental retardates or behaviorally maladjusted, using the pluralistic norms, were rated as significantly duller, more retarded, less capable, and having more difficulty learning than the children who were classified as normals. They were rated as significantly duller and having more difficulty learning than the quasi-retarded. There were no significant differences between the "normals" and the quasi-retarded except on the accelerated–retarded dimension. The normals were rated significantly more accelerated. Thus, the normals and the quasi-retarded tended to be perceived similarly by parents, and both were consistently given better ratings on these five dimensions than children in the other three categories.

The behaviorally maladjusted, those who failed the Adaptive Behavior Scales but had passing IQs, were rated by their parents more like persons in the mentally retarded categories, especially the nondisabled

Table 23: Convergence of Clinical and Social System Definitions With Pluralistic Interpretations of Clinical Measures

Parent Rating	Type 1 Physically Disabled MR N = 32	Type 2 Nondisabled MR N = 37	Behaviorally Maladjusted N = 78	Quasi-retarded N = 39	"Normal" N = 82	Significance Level
Retarded	4.9	3.8	3.7	3.3	2.5	<.001
Difficulty Learning	5.4	4.7	4.8	4.2	4.1	<.05
Not Capable	3.5	2.9	2.9	2.6	2.1	<.001
Dull	3.3	3.2	3.5	2.6	2.7	<.01
Slow	5.9	5.8	5.7	5.2	5.3	NS

NOTE: A high score indicates ratings in the direction of the pole named in the table. Ratings were Accelerated–Retarded; No Difficulty Learning–Difficulty Learning; Capable–Not Capable; Bright–Dull; Quick–Slow.

mental retardates. There are no statistically significant differences between the nondisabled mentally retarded and the behaviorally maladjusted on any of the ratings, and there is only one significant difference (accelerated–retarded) between ratings given the physically disabled mentally retarded and the behaviorally maladjusted.

We conclude that parents see labeled mental retardates who are reclassified as normals and quasi-retardates, using the pluralistic norms, as more competent than the children who remain categorized as mentally retarded. The behaviorally maladjusted child, who is failing on adaptive behavior but has a higher IQ than the mental retardate, is rated about as incompetent as the mentally retarded child. Parents did not differentiate as clearly between the children with poor adaptive behavior who had higher and lower IQs as they differentiated between the quasi-retarded and normals. We conclude that a pluralistic typology does result in closer conformity to the social system evaluations of the family than a clinical perspective, which ignores sociocultural differences and treats all children with low IQs as one homogeneous group—the mentally retarded.

The following quotation from an interview with the mother of a fourteen-year-old, quasi-retarded, Black boy illustrates some of the frustration felt by parents who believe their child has been incorrectly labeled and placed. Similar complaints were recorded in many of the interviews with mothers of quasi-retarded and normal children.

> Donald mows the lawn, keeps his room clean, takes out the trash, and likes to cook and bake. He helps me around the kitchen and fixes food for the other children. He's a very dependable person for babysitting. He likes music and dancing and is well coordinated. He's good at mechanical things—takes bikes apart and remodels them. He's interested in tailoring and he's good at it. He does his own pants to remodel them to make bell-bottoms and puts hems in his sister's skirts. He'll sew buckles on the little children's shoes, anything to help other people. If we're out, I don't worry about the children's welfare. Donald will look after them.
>
> We were not told about the special education. The people from the school said that Donald needed help in reading and if he was put in special class he would be able to get better help, that is, the class would be smaller. A man from the school got us to sign for Don to go into special education. Don is being retarded in special education. He doesn't like being labeled as retarded. It's affecting him. He begs us to have him removed from that class. . . . There are boys from Juvenile Hall in that class who are real delinquents. They are trouble makers plus the mentally retarded kids who are in that class. We have to make Don go to school because that class does not offer a challenge to him. What they do is very repetitious, the same thing over and over. They all do the same thing in class. That's ridiculous because all children don't like the same thing. . . . If they don't do something for Don, he'll be a dropout.

Don does not like it at that school. He's very unhappy there. We have to make him go. The only reason he consents to go is because we have been promised that he will be taken out of that EMR class. The teachers have asked us to let them put another one of our kids in EMR. We said an emphatic "no," because now we know what it's all about.

Implications and Limitations of the Riverside Epidemiology

If there are four distinct types of persons who fail intelligence tests, as the findings of the Riverside epidemiology seem to indicate, this situation has two major implications for persons operating from a clinical perspective. First, socioculturally sensitive diagnostic measures and procedures are needed to reliably differentiate the four types. Second, programs need to be designed which address the specific difficulties each type of person has in participating in American society. These programs should replace the undifferentiated existing programs, which treat all persons with low IQs as a homogeneous group.

Developing Socioculturally Sensitive Diagnostic Measures and Procedures

Adaptive Behavior Scales developed for the field survey were designed for screening in a survey interview and were not intended for rigorous evaluation. Because of the limitations imposed by the length of the interview, the scales were short and had a very low ceiling. There was no validation of the respondent's report by independent assessments from other sources. In spite of these obvious deficiencies, the measures still worked toward the convergence of social system and clinical definitions of subnormality.

A more thorough evaluation of adaptive behavior would require the development of a scale, (1) that covers a broader range of social-role performance in greater depth than the scales used in the screening interview; (2) that is longer and more reliable than the scales used in the survey screening; (3) that has a higher ceiling; (4) that has been checked for validity by securing independent reports on the individual's performance from more than one source; and (5) that has been normed on a larger, more representative population.

The standardized scales currently in use, e.g., the Vineland Social Maturity Scale, the Gesell Developmental Scales, the Parson's Adaptive Behavior Scales, have been designed primarily for screening institutional populations and/or young children. More comprehensive measures of adaptive behavior are needed, which cover a wide range of social roles and behaviors in the community and are applicable to school-age persons and adults living outside of institutions.

The Adaptive Behavior Scales used in this epidemiology are limited in their applicability because they were normed on the population of Riverside. Although the size of the norming sample was relatively large for Anglos (5,677 persons), the Anglo population of Riverside tends to be primarily middle- and upper-middle-class, with a relatively small representation of persons from low socioeconomic status. The norming samples for Mexican-Americans (659 persons) and Blacks (474 persons) were relatively small. No pluralistic norms based on sociocultural modality groups were calculated because of the small number of cases. Any measures of adaptive behavior intended for general use should be normed on larger, more representative samples of the major sociocultural groups that comprise American society.

Pluralistic Intelligence Test Norms for the major sociocultural segments of Riverside are not applicable beyond that community. The sociocultural modality groups generated on the basis of findings from the multiple regression analyses were small. Only 25 Mexican-American and 17 Black children fell into the group that was socioculturally modal on all five variables used in the index. Because the Anglo population of Riverside has few low-status persons, there were too few socioculturally nonmodal Anglos for a study of the relationship between sociocultural modality and IQ and adaptive behavior in that group. Consequently, it is not possible to determine from the Riverside sample whether a more heterogeneous population including sizable numbers of nonmodal Anglos—Anglos such as might be found in the rural South or Appalachia—would produce a higher correlation between sociocultural background variables and IQ.

Although the findings of the Riverside epidemiology point a direction that brings closer a convergence of clinical and social system definitions, the measures and procedures used in the epidemiology are not sufficiently refined and the samples on which the measures were normed are not sufficiently general for use in their present form. More refined instruments based on more representative samples are needed.

Implications for Programs

If pluralistic procedures were developed that could differentiate those with low IQs into five categories—the physically disabled retardate, the nondisabled retardate, the quasi-retardate, the behaviorally maladjusted, and the low normals—then it follows that programs, especially educational programs, could be developed to meet the specific needs of each group. Present programs for trainable mental retardates and educable mental retardates are designed to meet the needs of persons who are presumed to be constitutionally subnormal and to have a very low potential for learning. Today, the three other groups we have identified among the labeled retarded, i.e., the quasi-retarded, the behaviorally maladjusted, and the low normals, are classified as mental retardates and are placed in these programs designed for persons assumed to have limited intellectual capacity, programs that have low academic expectations and that focus on developing nonacademic skills.

The quasi-retardate, who is coping intelligently with problems outside the psychometric situation, cannot be regarded as comprehensively incompetent. Having demonstrated by his adaptive behavior that he does cope intelligently with nonacademic situations, programs could be developed for the quasi-retardate, based on the assumption that he has problem-solving ability that is not evaluated in the intelligence test situation. Programs could be addressed to his specific verbal and cognitive difficulties on the assumption that he has the potential for learning, given appropriate educational experiences.

The socioculturally nonmodal do not do well on either intelligence tests or Adaptive Behavior Scales. Coming from a background that is socioculturally different from the modal culture, they need educational programs that will build upon and enhance the cultural heritage from which they come and assist them in acquiring the skills needed to succeed in the mainstream of American society. Classes for the mentally retarded are not designed to meet these needs.

Conclusion

Throughout this volume, we have found that there are points at which clinical and social system definitions of mental retardation tend to converge and other points at which they diverge sharply. We have concluded that the convergence of clinical and social system definitions is enhanced by the use of a pluralistic, social system perspective on mental retardation, which takes sociocultural factors into account in evaluating the meaning of a particular IQ or adaptive behavior score.

If such instruments and pluralistic procedures were available, the clinician would have more information on which to make an assessment. Knowing the person's location on the standard norms for IQ and adaptive behavior, he would be able to predict the amount of difficulty that person is likely to have in achieving in the American public schools. Knowing the person's location on the distribution of IQs of persons from similar sociocultural backgrounds, he would be able to assess how much of the person's seeming "subnormality" is related to sociocultural factors. Knowing something about the person's coping behavior in nonacademic situations, he would be in a better position to decide whether the person is comprehensively incompetent or whether his incompetence is primarily school-specific. With this larger fund of information and a broader normative framework, there could be a greater convergence of clinical and social system definitions of subnormality.

Appendix A

METHODOLOGICAL NOTES

A clinical epidemiology is based upon the assumptions and definitions of the clinical perspective. The purpose of a clinical epidemiology is to describe the distribution of a pathology in the population studied, and to calculate prevalence and/or incidence rates for both the total population and subpopulations within the total population.

Field Survey Pilot Study

A pilot study was conducted in Pomona, California (65,000 population), one year preceding the field work in Riverside. Two samples were used in the pretest. The first sample was composed of 498 individuals, 49 years of age and younger, living in 213 households which fell into an area-probability sample of 1% of the census blocks in the pretest community. The second sample consisted of 127 individuals from the families of 30 children selected randomly from the roster of students in public school special-education classes.[1] The special-education sample was chosen to increase the total number of retardates screened and to determine whether refusal rates would be higher for families with labeled mental retardates. Interviewers did not know whether they were interviewing a family selected in the area-probability sample or one from the special-education sample. An adult member of each family was interviewed. The overall response rate was 89.2% for the area-probability sample and 96% for the special-education sample. We concluded that families with labeled retardates were no more likely to refuse an interview than families from the general population and that parent responses to interview questions were not altered to hide the presence of a mental retardate.

The behavior screening for the pilot study was a single "social-developmental" measure containing both the items later incorporated into the Adaptive Behavior scales and the items later organized into separate Physical Disability scales (Mercer, Butler, and Dingman, 1964). The

[1] We are indebted to the following persons who were associated with the Pomona Unified School District, for their advice and assistance: the late Superintendent, Dr. Aubrey H. Simons; Miss Arlene Pederson, District Psychologist; Mrs. Veda Vroman, Director of Pupil Personnel Services; and Dr. George Sitkei, Research Statistican.

pretest indicated that adaptive behavior, physical disability, and measures of intelligence are distinguishable dimensions, especially for older children and adults. Therefore, a three-dimensional rather than a two-dimensional typology was used in the final study conducted in Riverside.

Pretest evaluation procedures were organized as a series of multilevel screens. At each level, individuals not eligible as clinical retardates were identified and eliminated from further screening. Those failing all levels were defined as social-developmental failures. Because of weaknesses revealed in the pretest, the screening procedures were extensively modified for the Riverside survey.

(1) The social-developmental scale was separated into two different measures: adaptive behavior and physical disability.

(2) The multilevel screening design was abandoned, and the final scales consisted of a series of equally weighted questions.

(3) Sex biases revealed in the pilot-study analysis were reduced by eliminating some questions and by modifying the occupational questions to allow for the culturally approved roles of housewife and student as alternatives to paid employment.

The pilot study also produced information on the most effective field procedures. Some investigators have advised approaching a community with little publicity, quietly negotiating interviews individually with each respondent, and leaving town as quickly as possible. Because of the scope of our study, we did not feel that an unobtrusive approach was possible. Therefore, we experimented with the opposite approach: a well-placed news story describing the study as a health survey focused on chronic illness, primarily mental retardation, with a picture of one of our interviewers conducting an interview. Each interviewer was given a copy of the story to use when explaining the study to each respondent. The newspaper publicity proved an effective way to allay fears, to legitimate the study, and to secure entrée to households. So far as we were able to determine, local newspaper coverage increased cooperation and did not generate any opposition to our endeavors. A similar approach was used in Riverside.

To determine whether an introductory letter would improve our response rate, we randomly assigned households in the pretest probability sample to two groups: one group received an introductory letter by mail before the arrival of the interviewer, and the other group received no advance warning. We found that 92.4% of the households receiving introductory letters were willing to be interviewed, compared with 86.2% of those not receiving a letter. The interviewers reported that the introductory letters helped them to gain entrée and made it easier to develop rapport. Therefore, we decided to send out introductory letters to sample households in Riverside even though it meant additional expense in prelisting housing units, securing the names of householders, and addressing and mailing letters.

In the pilot study, we were able to test 68% of the preschool children in the area-probability sample and 83.3% of those in the special-education sample who were selected for testing. However, only 43.2% of the adults selected for testing were actually tested: 46.9% of the area-probability sample and 33.3% of the special-education sample. We surmised that this low response might be due to two characteristics of the pilot study. Because of insufficient time during the fieldwork for the two psychometrists to complete the testing, there was a three months lag between date of interview and date of test for many respondents. In addition, we neglected to forewarn respondents in the pretest that a second interview might be required if a member of the family were selected for testing. As a result of this experience, we organized Riverside fieldworkers into two groups, interviewers and psychometrists. Persons to be tested were contacted within two weeks after the initial interview. We rewrote the introductory letter to emphasize that some households would be visited twice. The "thank-you" letter also emphasized the possibility of a return visit. Finally, we added a closing question to the Riverside interview, which asked each respondent whether he would be willing to have another person from the study return to interview an individual member of the family, if one happened to be chosen for the subsample. These changes in field procedures greatly improved respondent cooperation with the intelligence testing in Riverside.

The sampling plan for Riverside called for a multistage area-probability sample based on clusters of six housing units chosen randomly from each sample census block. Such clusters could introduce a biasing factor if the families of mental retardates tend to reside on particular blocks. When the within-block variance in social-developmental scores was compared with the between-block variance, there was no evidence in the pilot study that mental retardates cluster on particular blocks and we decided to proceed with the sampling plan as projected and select six housing units per block.

Riverside Field Survey

We defined the population at risk as persons under fifty years of age with a family residence at the time of the study within the political boundaries of Riverside as they existed at the time of the 1960 census.

There were some mental retardates who were in institutions, private boarding homes, foster homes, and other types of living arrangements away from their families. We counted them as part of the study population if their parents or legal guardians lived in Riverside. Mental retardates who were living in foster homes in Riverside, but whose families lived elsewhere, were not included in the study. Persons in military service, prison, college, and other types of group settings were counted as residents of Riverside if they were members of a family living in Riverside and were not members of a household located elsewhere. The population at risk was identical for both the clinical epidemiology and the social system epidemiology.

Sample Design for The Screened Sample

In the 1960 census, Riverside had a population of 84,300 persons living in 28,600 housing units. The first stage of the field survey was a screening interview in which the adaptive behavior and physical disabilities of each member of each sample household were evaluated on the basis of information obtained from an adult respondent.

The basic sampling unit was the housing unit, as defined by the United States Census.[2] Certain types of group living quarters were not considered housing units, i.e., convents, dormitories, prisons, hospitals, convalescent homes, and so forth. Persons living in temporary quarters such as motels, hotels, and jails were also excluded. We estimated that a sample of 3,000 housing units would yield approximately 7,000 persons under fifty years of age.

Our sampling frame was stratified along two dimensions, geographic area and socioeconomic level. Stratification by Riverside's seventeen census tracts assured that each geographic area was represented in the final sample in proportion to the number of persons living in that area in the 1960 census. The United States Census reports the average dollar value of owner-occupied housing units and the average contract rent for renter-occupied housing units on each census block. We combined these two values to form an index of the average value of housing for each census block and divided the blocks according to housing values so that 10% of the population of the city fell into each group. Decile 1 contained the blocks with the 10% of the population in the least ex-

[2] A housing unit is a house, an apartment or other group of rooms, or a single room which is occupied or intended to be occupied as separate living quarters, that is, the occupants do not live and eat with any other persons in the structure and there is either (a) direct access from the outside or through a common hall, or (b) a kitchen or cooking equipment for exclusive use of the occupants. Trailers, tents, boats, and railroad cars are included if they are occupied as housing units, but excluded if they are vacant, used only for sleeping space or vacations, or used only for business.

pensive dwellings, decile 2 contained the next lowest 10%, and so forth.[3] All the census blocks in the city were sorted into their proper category in the 170-cell grid formed by the cross tabulation of census tract and housing-value decile. Five hundred blocks were selected, on a probability basis by population, so that their populations would be distributed in the same proportions across the 170 cells of the grid as the population in the sampling frame.

University students canvassed each of the five hundred blocks and listed every structure, noting whether it was used as a housing unit or for other purposes. They also listed all vacant structures as well as all structures under construction. Apartments in the same building were listed separately. Subdivided, single-family units were investigated thoroughly. Special care was taken to explore any trailers, tents, garages, alleys, courts, and passageways. It is precisely in these kinds of locations that many adult mental retardates live out their lives, and it was essential that every dwelling, however unlikely, be listed for sampling (Edgerton, 1967).

We selected fifty blocks at random and assigned a second student to make an independent listing of the structures on these blocks. There was 95% agreement on blocks in housing-value deciles four through ten, and 85% agreement on blocks in deciles one through three. To correct for possible omissions in the prelisting, three questions concerning additional dwelling units were added at the end of each interview. Only six additional housing units were discovered in this fashion. We concluded that the prelisting was accurate.

A sampling ratio was calculated for each block by dividing the num-

[3] Housing Value per Block = (Average Value of Owner-Occupied Housing Units on the Block) x (Number of Owner-Occupied Housing Units) + [(Average Monthly Rent x 100) x (Number of Rental Housing Units)] ÷ (Total Number of Housing Units on the Block). The index is based on the assumption that the monthly rental of a housing unit represents approximately 1% of its value. The range of housing values for each decile, as of the 1960 census, were as follows: Decile 1, $6,300 and below; Decile 2, $6,338–$8,192; Decile 3, $8,197–$9,500; Decile 4, $9,507–$10,711; Decile 5, $10,723–$11,975; Decile 6, $12,000–$13,282; Decile 7, $13,286–$14,380; Decile 8, $14,390–$15,836; Decile 9, $16,000–$18,999; Decile 10, $19,000 and over.

Some of the 1,113 census blocks in Riverside were not occupied in 1960 and consequently had no average housing value. However, these blocks could not be ignored because Riverside, like most California cities, had been growing rapidly. A block vacant in 1960 could easily be filled with tract homes by the time of fieldwork. These blocks had to be included in the sampling frame and given some probability of being selected for the sample. This end was achieved by combining vacant blocks with adjacent blocks containing occupied housing units in 1960. These "contrived" blocks were constructed so that each would contain a minimum of six housing units. As a result of combining vacant blocks with occupied blocks to form "contrived" blocks, the total number of blocks in the city was reduced to 864. There were 65 contrived blocks and 799 census blocks in the final sampling frame.

ber of housing units on the block in 1960 by six. Using this ratio, housing units to be interviewed were chosen randomly from the list of dwelling units on each block. Instead of the 3,000 housing units which we had anticipated, the selection produced 3,192. The increase of 192 units reflected community growth after the census and occurred mainly in areas where relatively expensive tract homes had been constructed. Consequently, the actual sample has more persons in upper socioeconomic deciles than appeared in the sampling frame.

Fieldwork

Using electric-utility billing lists, we were able to determine the name of the householder at each address within two weeks prior to fieldwork, and prepared individually addressed introductory letters for 95% of the housing units in the sample. The remaining 5% were vacancies. Our pretest experience indicated that an interviewer could complete 60 interviews with Anglo and Black families in six weeks, but could complete only 40 interviews with Mexican-American families because of the larger number of persons to be screened per family. Projecting from the ethnic distribution of Riverside, we estimated 2 Black, 4 Spanish-speaking, and 35 Anglo interviewers could complete most of the interviewing in two months, matching interviewers and respondents for ethnic group (Hyman, 1955).

All interviewers employed for the field survey were college graduates and 36 were teachers: 14 elementary teachers, 17 junior high teachers, 3 senior high school teachers, and 2 junior college teachers. Sex distribution was approximately equal. Spanish-speaking interviewers were assigned to all households in which the head of the household had a Spanish surname. Black interviewers were assigned to interview in housing units located in predominantly nonwhite blocks according to the 1960 census. Anglo interviewers were randomly assigned the remainder of the households with each interviewer receiving approximately equal numbers of units on all socioeconomic levels.

Each interviewer had 44 hours of formal training before and during the fieldwork, not including their individual consultations with supervisors. The training consisted of a concentrated four-day workshop prior to fieldwork, followed by a series of half-day meetings interspersed throughout the fieldwork. There were weekly team meetings with the project director. Collegiate-level readings in the theory and technique of interviewing were required. Interviewers received university extension credit for their course work and practicum. Each interviewer conducted two supervised interviews before starting to work in the field. The supervisors reinterviewed 163 randomly selected respondents and asked about the composition of the household, the number of years the family had lived in Riverside, and the occupation, birthplace, and education of the head of the household. These questions were selected because they are matters of fact, are critical variables in the study, and would be difficult for an interviewer to falsify. Although eleven of the reinterviews were not with the same respondent as the initial interview, there were no significant discrepancies. In addition, approximately 350 families selected in the subsample for intelligence testing were recontacted by psychometrists. There were no cases in which a psychometrist appeared at a household to interview a nonexistent person and only two cases in which there were age discrepancies. We concluded that there had been no undetected falsification of interview reports.[4]

In each occupied housing unit, one adult family member served as respondent and provided information about all other members of the household to whom he was related. A qualified respondent was any member of the household eighteen or more years of age and/or married who was mentally competent to answer.[5] In general, information about an adult was supplied by the person himself, his spouse, a parent, or an adult son or daughter residing in the household. Information about children was supplied by a parent, unless some other adult was usually responsible for their care. No person was asked to supply information about a person unrelated to himself. Thus, servants, lodgers, or unrelated individuals living in the same household were individually interviewed. The average interview lasted an hour and fifteen minutes. Each screening interview consisted of three parts: a section asking questions about each individual member of the household, another asking about characteristics of the family, and a third covering attitudes of the respondent.

Most respondents were female. Approximately 26% of the sample of

[4] During the first two weeks of the fieldwork, we discovered that one of the teacher-interviewers was turning in completed interview schedules for families which he had not interviewed. This falsification was initially suspected because of discrepancies in the reported number of hours he logged in the field, his reported mileage, and the number of completed interviews. A check by telephone of the three households in which he claimed to have completed interviews revealed that he had not interviewed any of the respondents. When confronted directly with the evidence, he admitted that he had falsified the schedules and that he had been painting his house during the hours he reported himself in the field. Unfortunately, it was not possible to retrieve the wages he collected for the training session nor those collected during the two weeks he spent painting his house.

[5] This definition of a qualified respondent corresponds to that used by the National Health Survey, Vital and Health Statistics, U.S. Department of Health, Education, and Welfare, National Center for Health Statistics, Series 1, Number 2, May 1964.

6,998 persons under fifty responded for themselves. A husband or wife responded for a spouse in 21.0% of the cases, and a biological parent answered questions about a child in 47.4% of the cases. A foster, adopted, or step-parent answered questions about a child in 4% of the cases, and in 2% of the cases some other relative responded for the individual.

Spanish-speaking interviewers conducted all interviews in Mexican-American homes and used Spanish in the interview, if this was preferred by the respondent. Sixty-five interviews, 2.4% of the total, were conducted in Spanish, and 21 interviews, .8%, were conducted in a combination of English and Spanish. The first contact with each household was made by a stranger. However, we did use prior acquaintance as an asset in retrieving refused interviews. There were 51 completed interviews, 1.9% of the total, in which the interviewer was slightly acquainted with the respondent, and 12 cases, .4%, in which interviewer and respondent were well acquainted. The majority of completed interviews, 97.6%, were conducted by interviewers who were unacquainted with the respondent before the field contact. There were only 41 "unable to contact" housing units. In 15 cases, we learned from neighbors that the occupants were out of town and would not return during the fieldwork period. Several others were in the hospital, and one family moved before they were contacted.

There were 299 cases in which the respondent refused to be interviewed the first time he was contacted. For each refusal, the interviewer completed a "refusal report form" on which he recorded the estimated age of the respondent, his sex, his ethnic group, his reason for refusal, and the condition, type, and size of the housing unit. When possible, he secured information on family composition. By switching the sex of the interviewer, sending a member of another ethnic group, or sending an acquaintance, it was possible to retrieve 65 interviews which had initially been refused, 2.2% of the sample. There remained 234 housing units, 7.9% of the sample, which were refusals and were never interviewed. An intensive study was made of the characteristics of these households (Mercer and Butler, 1967). The city directory, the voter registration rolls, and the public utility rolls were used as sources of additional information. There were no differences between those who refused and those who participated, except for age. Older respondents refused to be interviewed significantly more frequently than younger respondents. For this reason, an age correction factor is used whenever aggregates are reported.[6]

[6] The usual procedure for estimating the characteristics of nonrespondent households in survey research is to assign the mean value of the interviewed households on a block to the households on that block not interviewed. This method was used to estimate the ages of persons in the noninterviewed households. These estimates were

The final distribution of completed interviews deviated only slightly from the expected percentage in each of the 170 cells in the sampling frame. There was no significant bias in response rate either by census tract or housing decile.

Analysis of Adaptive Behavior and Physical Disability Scales

An item analysis was done of the Adaptive Behavior and Physical Disability scales to determine item difficulty and the relationship between responses to individual items and the total score on each scale. Item difficulty was measured by the percentage of persons who passed an item. Some scales had items passed by less than half the persons screened. On the other hand, every scale had at least one item which was passed by everyone or almost everyone.

Using a log likelihood ratio test (*Annals of Human Genetics,* 1957), those questions which best differentiated the 85% to 90% having the highest scores from the 10% to 15% having the lowest scores were retained in the scales, and the other items were dropped. The school-age and adult scales were more discriminating than the preschool scales. The final adaptive behavior score for each person screened was calculated by totaling the number of *failing* responses. Distributions for the total sample were skewed, as anticipated. A raw score of seven or more failures placed a preschool child in the lowest 3.0% of the total sample, a score of nine or more failures placed a school-age child in the lowest 3.0%, and a score of eight or more failures placed an adult in the lowest 3.4%.

Cutting points for the educational criterion were somewhat lower than the theoretical 9%. A score of 6 or more failures placed a preschool child in the lowest 6.5%, a score of 7 or more failures placed a school-age person in the lowest 8.0%, and a score of 6 or more failures placed an adult in the lowest 8.1% of the total sample.

In establishing the cutoff scores for the AAMD criterion, the lowest 16%, we had a choice of taking either the lowest 21.4% or 11.9% of the preschool group, the lowest 19.1% or 12.4% of the school-age group, and the lowest 19.5% or 12.4% of the adults. We selected the lower percentage as the cutoff. Approximating the three criterion levels was more difficult for the Physical Disability scales because they were shorter and the items were less difficult.

---

then compared with the actual ages of persons in the refusing households as reported by the interviewer on his refusal report form. We found a systematic error which overestimated the number of persons under 16 years of age by 3.88%, overestimated the number of persons 16 through 49 years of age by 3.43%, and underestimated persons 50 years of age and over by 2.67%. These percentages are the correction factors that are used when aggregates are estimated for age groups.

The Validity of the Adaptive Behavior Scales

Two methods were used to test the validity of the Adaptive Behavior measures: their ability to differentiate known groups and their correlation with ratings by "experts" (Selltiz, et al., 1965).

We tested the ability of the Adaptive Behavior scales to identify persons in the household survey who had been labeled as mentally retarded and, presumably, had failed in adaptive behavior. There were two groups of labeled retardates in the survey: thirteen persons of school age who were currently enrolled in special education classes and eleven adults who had been in special education when they were in school.

All thirteen school-age children had nine or more failures in adaptive behavior, placing them in the lower 2.5% of their age peers. Twelve of the thirteen were in the lowest 1.5%. The average number of failures on the Adaptive Behavior scales was 12.5 for the 6-through-10-year-olds and 13.2 for the 11-through-15-year-olds compared to an average of 2.0 and 3.4 failures on the scale for other children their age. All eleven persons over 16 years of age failed the AAMD criterion. Nine scored in the lowest 5%, and five scored in the lowest 1.5%. Their average number of failures on the Adaptive Behavior scales was 10.6, compared with an average of 2.2 for the general adult population.

There is some circularity in this method of identifying known mental retardates from the household survey itself because the external criterion is not completely independent of the scores on the Adaptive Behavior scales. Fortunately, there were 37 persons nominated by "clinical" informants as mentally retarded who, by chance, also appeared in the screening sample. This approximates the situation in which an "expert" makes an independent judgment about the performance of the individuals in question. Twenty-four of the 37 nominated persons failed the scales at the AAMD criterion, an overall agreement of 64.9%. The average agreement varied with age. Neither of the preschool children who were nominated failed the Adaptive Behavior scales, but 15 of the 24 school-age children failed, 62.5% agreement. Agreement on adult cases was even higher, 81.8% of the 11 cases. The average number of adaptive behavior items failed by nominated school-age children and adults (7.4 and 9.7 items, respectively) was much higher than the average for the sample as a whole (2.7 and 2.2 failures, respectively). We combined the school-age and adult populations and compared the characteristics of those nominees who passed the Adaptive Behavior scales with those who failed. There were no significant differences by sex, IQ, or socioeconomic level. However, those who failed the Adaptive Behavior scales were significantly more likely to be nominated by more than one informant ($p<.001$), to have more physical disabilities ($p<.01$), and to be Anglo ($p < .05$). The Adaptive Behavior scales show least agreement with the assessment of "experts" when screening Mexican-American, school-age children who have been nominated by only one agency, usually the school.

Tested Subsample

Five psychometrists were employed to administer approximately 450 tests to the subsample selected for testing. A sixth psychometrist, who spoke Spanish, was employed to administer the Spanish Stanford-Binet to adults who did not speak English or preferred to speak Spanish. Scores from the school testing program were used for public school children. All Catholic elementary school children were administered group intelligence tests by the project staff. Those scoring 85 or below were then individually evaluated.

The sampling frame for the tested subsample was stratified along three dimensions: score on the composite index including both physical disability and adaptive behavior items, age, and housing-value decile. The 10% of persons with the most failures on the composite measure were sampled at the rate of 75% for preschool children, 100% for school-age children, and 33% for adults. Those who scored in the top 90% were sampled at lower rates: 10% of the preschool and school-age children and 10% of the adults with scores between 11% and 25% on the composite scale. Adults with scores in the top 75% were sampled at the rate of 2%.

Testing conditions in the home, although not always optimal, were better than anticipated (Watts, Sitkei, and Meyers, 1969). In the opinion of the psychometrists, 66.7% of the tests were very reliable, 29.6% were somewhat reliable, and only 3.7% were unreliable.

There were 483 persons selected for individual testing: 196 between seven months and five years of age, 60 between six and fifteen years, and 227 over fifteen years of age. Of those selected, 423 were tested, an overall response rate of 87.6% One hundred percent of the children between seven months of age and two years selected for the subsample were tested, 93.7% of the children three to five years of age, 91.7% of the school-age children, and 80.2% of the adults. The 44 nontested adults were compared with the 182 who were tested. There were no differences between the two groups on any of the variables examined: age, sex, socioeconomic decile, ethnic group, amount of education completed, or score on the combined Adaptive Behavior-Physical Disability Scale. We used information available through the regular school testing program to supplement the tests administered by the research staff. This supplement produced a total of 296 IQ test scores for school-age children. Each case in the subsample was assigned a weight according to the number of cases in the screened sample it represented.

Validity of the Intelligence Testing

The estimated mean IQ of the population based on reconstructed distributions from the tested subsample was 112.4, ranging from 105.6 for school-age children to 116.8 for adults. Because persons in the Riverside sample scored much higher than national norms, we checked the validity of the results from the tested subsample with two different public school testing programs—one using the WISC and one using the Lorge-Thorndike.

The mean Full Scale WISC IQ of Anglo children in the school testing program was 106.9 compared to a mean of 109.5 estimated from the epidemiology. The mean Full Scale WISC IQ for Mexican-American children was 91.1, compared with 85.8 in the epidemiology, and the mean for Black children was 91.5, compared with 91.6 in the epidemiology. The median IQ for Anglo children on the Lorge-Thorndike was 107. The median IQ of Mexican-American and Black children combined on the Lorge-Thorndike was 90, compared with a median of 88 in the epidemiology for the two groups combined. We concluded that the survey sample estimates were accurate. The higher average IQ test score probably reflects the relatively higher social status of families in Riverside. For this reason, rates of clinical retardation are more meaningful when reported for subgroups of the Riverside population than for the city as a whole.

Methods Used in the Social System Epidemiology

The census month for the social system epidemiology was one year after the census month for the field survey. The actual collection of data, however, required a span of two years beginning one year prior to the field survey and continuing for one year thereafter. Two hundred and forty-one organizations and governmental agencies were contacted, representing every facet of community life. Each organization was asked to nominate for the study all mentally retarded persons known to that organization and to share any demographic and clinical information about the nominee that the agency had in its files. All organizations in Riverside who were asked to contribute to the case register agreed to participate. Many agencies required absolute assurance that we would not contact any of the persons whom they had nominated without their explicit permission. This understanding precluded the possibility of individual clinical evaluation by members of the project staff.

The term "mental retardate" was deliberately left undefined. Persons participating in each organization were asked to nominate those persons who were regarded as mental retardates by their organization. Procedures for securing nominations were adapted to the institutional structure and record-keeping system of each agency. A few social systems, such as the public schools, preferred to have members of their own staff work in their own files. In these cases, the research project reimbursed members of the regular agency staff for time spent on weekends and during vacations collecting needed information from agency records. In most cases, however, agencies preferred to have research assistants from the project do the actual clerical work involved in the search of the records.

The public schools of Riverside provided information on all persons who had ever been diagnosed as mentally retarded by the city school system. The list of labeled retardates provided by the city schools extended from 1948 until the time of the study, 914 individuals. There were 429 nominees still living in the community at the time of the survey.

All agencies of the California State Department of Mental Hygiene providing services for mental retardates were contacted. The state hospital serving Riverside had 63 patients whose families lived in Riverside. Four additional Riverside residents were located in other hospitals in the state system, 28 were found on hospital waiting lists, and another 13 were located who had been discharged from the hospital to their families in the community. The files of the Riverside Mental Hygiene clinic revealed 11 additional persons who had been diagnosed as mentally retarded by the clinic but had never been patients in a state hospital.

Files of the State Department of Vocational Rehabilitation were analyzed, and 14 labeled mental retardates were located in these records. The local chapter of the Retarded Children's Association, which operates a school and workshop for the mentally retarded, provided information on 72 mental retardates. The files of the Crippled Children's Clinic operated by the County Health Department provided names of 77 retardates who were living in the community at the time of the census. The 49 persons receiving Aid to the Totally Disabled from the County Welfare Department by reason of mental retardation were included. Five additional cases were contributed by case workers nominating persons on their regular case load. The State School for the Deaf, located in Riverside, provided 11 nominations based on psychological evaluations made by the school psychologist. Sixty-five cases were located through nominations by psychiatrists, pediatricians, physicians, and psychologists in private practice.

Contacts with non-clinical organizations were usually made with the director of the agency or with the pastor of a church. These persons usually served as informants and provided whatever information was available. In a few large non-clinical organizations, such as the Catholic Church, information was supplied by a special group devoted to serving the mentally retarded.

Seven basic variables were matched to determine whether a nominee had been nominated before: name, birthdate, sex, address, mother's name, father's name, and ethnic group. Other information was also used in difficult cases. If five variables matched, the case was treated as a duplicate.

The geographic boundaries for the case register were coterminous with those for the field survey. If the nominee was reported as living at a Riverside address and was on the active case load of any organization during the census month, he was accepted as a resident, 47% of all cases nominated. If a telephone was listed in the name of the family, 16% of the cases, or the family was being billed for utilities at the home address during the month, 35% of all cases, they were counted as residents. For those cases which could not be definitely located by these indirect methods, telephone calls, visits to friends and neighbors, visits to the home address, registered letters, and other tracing devices were used, 2% of all cases. Only persons certified by these methods to be living in Riverside during the census month were included in the final comprehensive register. Patients in the Department of Mental Hygiene hospitals were counted as residents of Riverside if they had a home address within the geographic limits defined for the study.

Appendix B

ITEMS USED FOR MEASURING THE ADAPTIVE BEHAVIOR OF PERSONS OF VARIOUS AGES

[The questions in the Adaptive Behavior and Physical Disability Scales were designed for field screening in a survey research project. Although they proved adequate for that purpose, they are not sufficiently reliable or adequately normed for use in a clinical setting. They are research instruments and should *not* be used to make decisions about individuals. We are now in the process of collecting standardization data for a series of measures from a representative sample of 2,100 California public school children, 5 through 11 years of age: 700 Black, 700 Mexican-American and 700 Anglo. Pluralistic norms will be developed from the data. The normed measures will be incorporated into a System of Multicultural Pluralistic Assessment (SOMPA) which will provide information for a comprehensive assessment of a child's performance from the mother, or principal socialization agent, and from the child. The mother will respond in an interview to the Adaptive Behavior Inventory for Children (ABIC); the Sociocultural Modality Index, a measure of socialization milieu; and a Health History and Impairment Inventory. For the child the system will include pluralistic norms for the 1973 revision of the Wechsler Intelligence Scale for Children, 5 through 11, and a Physical Dexterity Battery of items covering gross and fine motor dexterity, as well as visual-motor coordination and development. This investigation is supported by Public Health Service Grant MH 20646 from the National Institute of Mental Health, Department of Health, Education and Welfare.]

	Age in Months
Does———babble and imitate sounds as a start toward talking and letting you know what he/she wants? (Do not include crying, or sounds made only to indicate annoyance or discomfort.) Pass=Yes Fail=No	7–9
Does———pull him/herself up to a standing position without anyone's help? (He/she may hold onto some object to help him/her stand up, but not onto a person.) Pass=Yes Fail=No	7–9

	Age in Months
Does———creep and crawl on the floor without getting into trouble so that it isn't necessary to do more than "keep an eye on him" while you do other things? Pass=Yes Fail=No	7–9, 10–12
Does———when held in standing position bounce up and down? Pass=Yes Fail=No	7–9
Does———take solid food well? Pass=Yes Fail=No	7–9, 10–12
Does———sit up by him/herself for a minute or more? Pass=Yes Fail=No	7–9
Does———cry a lot? Pass=No Fail=Yes	7–9, 16–18, 19–21, 22–24, 30–35, 36–47, 48–59, 60–71
Does———transfer objects from one hand to the other? Pass=Yes Fail=No	7–9, 10–12
Does———usually drink from a cup or glass with little or no spilling if someone helps him/her hold it? (Alternate: Can———be spoonfed liquids with little or no messing?) Pass=Yes Fail=No	7–9
Does———open mouth when he/she sees food? Pass=Yes Fail=No	7–9
Does———recognize a stranger? Pass=Yes Fail=No	7–9
Does———stare at a rattle in his/her hand? Pass=Yes Fail=No	7–9
Does———coo, squeal, and make many different sounds? Pass=Yes Fail=No	7–9
Does———grasp a toy when held before him/her? Pass=Yes Fail=No	7–9
Does——pat his/her bottle when eating? Pass=Yes Fail=No	7–9
Does———wave "bye-bye" or play "pat-a-cake"? Pass=Yes Fail=No	10–12
Does———usually follow simple instructions when they are given without gestures; for example, when asked to do so, will he/she point to things, wave bye-bye? Pass=Yes Fail=No	10–12, 13–15
Does———say "Dada" or "Mama"? Pass=Yes Fail=No	10–12

	Age in Months
Does———pull self to feet at a rail? Pass=Yes Fail=No	10–12
Does———recognize his/her own name? Pass=Yes Fail=No	10–12
How often does———have temper tantrums? Pass=Less than 1 a week Fail=1 or more a week	10–12, 13–15, 16–18, 19–21, 22–24, 30–35, 36–47, 48–59, 60–71
Does———sit by him/herself? Pass=Yes Fail=No	10–12
Does———stand by him/herself without anyone's help for at least a minute? Pass=Yes Fail=No	10–12
Does———drink from a cup? Pass=Yes Fail=No	10–12, 13–15
Has———stopped drooling? (A bib may be needed while feeding.) Pass=Yes Fail=No	10–12
Does———regularly indicate the wish to be talked to, played with, moved about? (May include familiar and unfamiliar people.) Pass=Yes Fail=No	10–12
Does———pick up small things with just his/her finger and thumb? Pass=Yes Fail=No	10–12
Does———give up a toy when asked? Pass=Yes Fail=No	13–15
Does———cooperate when he/she is being dressed? Pass=Yes Fail=No	13–15, 16–18
Does———say words besides "Dada" and "Mama"? Pass=Yes Fail=No	13–15, 16–18
Does———walk around? Is he/she usually careful enough about his/her movements so that you can let him/her go about the room with only occasional watching and reminders? Pass=Yes Fail=No	13–15
Does———walk when only one hand is held? Pass=Yes Fail=No	13–15
Does———repeat acts people laugh at? Pass=Yes Fail=No	13–15, 16–18
In his/her play, does———frequently spend 15 minutes or more doing such things as scribbling, stringing beads, or building with blocks? Pass=Yes Fail=No	13–15

	Age in Months
In his/her play, does——often arrange toys or other objects into some pattern, take things out of one box and put them into another, etc.? Pass=Yes Fail=No	13–15, 16–18
Does——creep? Pass=Yes Fail=No	13–15
Does——usually chew solid and semi-solid foods? (If solid foods are withheld because chewing is unmastered, do not score pass.) Pass=Yes Fail=No	13–15
Does——usually take off his/her own socks, booties, stockings or unlaced shoes, not just in play, but part of undressing? Pass=Yes Fail=No	13–15, 16–18
Does——feed him/herself crackers? Pass=Yes Fail =No	13–15, 16–18
Does——recognize some pictures? Pass=Yes Fail=No	16–18, 19–21
Does——usually drink from a cup or glass without help and without spilling or messing? Pass=Yes Fail=No	16–18, 19–21
When——wants something he/she cannot reach by him/herself, does he/she use a stick, climb upon a chair, or open a door to get at what he/she wants? Pass=Yes Fail=No	16–18
When you ask him/her to, will——usually move something from one place to another or bring you some object you ask for? Pass=Yes Fail=No	16–18
Does——offer toys to others? Pass=Yes Fail=No	16–18, 19–21
Does——try to throw a ball when playing with it? Pass=Yess Fail=No	16–18
Does——walk alone? Pass=Yes Fail=No	16–18, 19–21
After——'s food is cut up, does he/she usually feed him/herself with a spoon; that is, can he/she manage with little or no spilling or messing and without help? Pass=Yes Fail=No	19–21
When you take——out does he/she usually walk with you—that is, does he/she no longer use a baby carriage? Pass=Yes Fail=No	19–21
Does——ask for food or drink? Pass=Yes Fail=No	19–21, 22–24

	Age in Months
Does———tell you when he/she is wet? Pass=Yes Fail=No	19–21, 22–24
Does———hand you his/her empty dish when finished? Pass=Yes Fail=No	19–21, 22–24
Do you usually let———freely move about the house or yard if you are within call? Pass=Yes Fail=No	19–21
Does———feed him/herself most of the time? Pass=Yes Fail=No	19–21, 22–24
Does———pull you when he/she wants to show you something? Pass=Yes Fail=No	19–21
Can you count on———to avoid putting in his/her mouth or eating things which might be harmful (if examples necessary–clay, dirt, crayons, marbles, etc.). Pass=Yes Fail=No	19–21, 22–24
Has———'s speech developed to the point where he/she uses short sentences or meaningful phrases? How many words do you think he/she says? (25 expected–if doesn't know, would it be as many as 25?) Pass=Yes Fail=No	22–24, 25–29
Does———usually unwrap or peel candy, gum, bananas, before eating them? When———eats fruit, does he/she leave the pits? Pass=Yes Fail=No	22–24
Does———make 2- or 3-word sentences? Pass=Yes Fail=No	22–24, 25–29
Does———say the name of some person other than "Mama" and "Dada"? Pass=Yes Fail=No	22–24, 25–29
Does———ask to go to the toilet? Pass=Yes Fail=No	22–24, 25–29
Are there half-a-dozen or so common objects which ———names without difficulty when he/she sees the object or a picture of it? Even if his/her pronunciation is not exact does he/she say these words clearly enough so that people outside the family understand him/her? Pass=Yes Fail=No	22–24
Does———walk down steps with someone holding one hand? Pass=Yes Fail=No	22–24, 25–29
Does———pull a toy by a string? Pass=Yes Fail=No	22–24, 25–29
Can———tell you his/her own name? Pass=Yes Fail =No	25–29, 30–35

	Age in Months
Does———usually let you know when he/she has to go to the toilet so that you don't have to worry about catching him/her in time? (He/she may let you know by words or by some regular sign.) Pass=Yes Fail=No	25–29
Does———tell about things that have just happened to him/her? Pass=Yes Fail=No	25–29, 30–35
When———is thirsty does he/she usually get his/her own drink from the tap without spilling? Does——— stay away from dirty or unknown liquids? Pass=Yes Fail=No	25–29, 30–35
Does———frequently decide for him/herself that he/she'll spend his/her time on such activities as building blocks, looking at books alone, coloring with a crayon or dressing dolls and do so without getting into mischief although he/she is not watched? Pass=Yes Fail=No	25–29
When———'s food is cut up, does he/she usually use a fork with little spilling? Pass=Yes Fail=No	25–29
Does———put on simple pieces of clothing for him/herself? Pass=Yes Fail=No	25–29, 30–35
When buttons are opened, does———usually take off his/her own coat, dress, or sweater, without tearing things and without help? Pass=Yes Fail=No	25–29
Does———play quite a bit or is he/she content to be still most of the time? Pass=Plays quite a bit Fail=Is still most of the time	25–29, 60–71
Does———run fairly well? Pass=Yes Fail=No	25–29
Is———careful to avoid things which might be harmful or dangerous to him/her? For example: Does——— keep away from matches, broken glass, hot radiators? Is———careful in handling things which are heavy or breakable? Is———careful not to approach strangers and unknown animals? Pass=Yes Fail=No	30–35
Does———hold a crayon with his/her fingers rather than with a fist? Pass=Yes Fail=No	30–35, 36–47
Does———usually put on a dress, coat, sweater and overcoat without help except with buttons? Pass=Yes Fail=No	30–35

	Age in Months
Does———use "I," "me," and "you" when he/she talks? Pass=Yes Fail=No	30–35, 36–47
Does———repeat things others say? Pass=Yes Fail=No	30–35, 36–47
After———'s hands are washed, does he/she usually dry them satisfactorily, using a towel? (Wiping hands on clothes not credited.) Pass=Yes Fail=No	30–35
Does———regularly carry on a conversation and get across what he/she wants to say? Does———tell you simple little stories or tell you about something he/she has done? In talking with you, does———'s conversation include nouns, pronouns, verbs, adjectives, and adverbs? Pass=Yes Fail=No	30–35
Does———help put toys away? Pass=Yes Fail=No	30–35, 36–47
Does———understand simple directions? Pass=Yes Fail=No	30–35, 36–47
Does———satisfactorily use a child's scissors to cut as one of his/her playthings without damaging things and with only occasional supervision? (Alternate: Does———paint with water colors without much messing?) Pass=Yes Fail=No	30–35
Does———no longer use baby talk, can be understood all the time? Pass=Yes Fail=No	36–47, 48–59
Can———give his/her full name? Pass=Yes Fail=No	36–47, 48–59
Does———button clothing without help? Pass=Yes Fail=No	36–47
Can you count on———to help you with some household tasks when you ask him/her to do so? For instance, will he/she run an errand in the house, help set or clear the table, dust, or feed the dog or cat if you have one? Pass=Yes Fail=No	36–47
Does———usually walk downstairs by him/herself using only one foot per step? That is, does he/she not place both feet on a step, before going on to the next step? Pass=Yes Fail=No	36–47
When———'s hands are dirty, does he/she usually wash them satisfactorily without help? This would mean that without too many reminders, he/she runs the	36–47

	Age in Months
water for him/herself and uses soap, washing without messing and dries them with a towel. Pass=Yes Fail=No	
Does———make three-word sentences? Pass=Yes Fail=No	36–47, 48–59
Does———do "stunts" to express him/herself or to entertain adults or other children—for example, does he/she sing, or dance or recite or do some sort of gymnastic well enough to consider the performance fairly good and not just cute or show-off? Pass=Yes Fail=No	36–47
Does———regularly play group games with other children—games in which he/she has to cooperate with the others like in Ring-a-Rosy, London Bridge, Tea Parties? Pass=Yes Fail=No	36–47
Does———put on his/her own shoes? Pass=Yes Fail =No	48–59, 60–71
Does———know a few rhymes? Pass=Yes Fail=No	48–71
When———'s clothes are all laid out for him/her, does he/she routinely dress him/herself without help except for tying and back buttons? Pass=Yes Fail=No	48–59
Does———regularly play games in which there is a winner and a loser and stick to the rules of the game? This would include such games as Tag, Hide-and-Seek, Rope Jumping, Statue, Marbles, Hopscotch, and spinning tops? Pass=Yes Fail=No	48–59, 60–71
Does———frequently draw recognizable objects with a pencil, crayons, or paint or use clay or Play-Doh to make something recognizable and without messing things up in the process? Pass=Yes Fail=No	48–59
Does———usually wash and dry his/her face satisfactorily without too many reminders or much messing? (Ears may be omitted.) Pass=Yes Fail=No	48–59
Does———ride a tricycle? Pass=Yes Fail=No	48–59, 60–71
Does———usually take care of him/herself at the toilet? This would include flushing and cleaning him/herself without reminders and handling his/her clothes ex-	48–59

	Age in Months
cept perhaps for some help with back buttons. Is daytime toilet training complete? Is nighttime training complete or limited to rare accidents? Pass=Yes Fail=No	
Can———pour from a pitcher? Pass=Yes Fail=No	48–59, 60–71
Can———turn pages one at a time? Pass=Yes Fail=No	48–59
Can———count up to five? Pass=Yes Fail=No	48–59
Can———name the capital letters? Pass=Yes Fail=No	48–59
Does———print or write his/her name or a few 3- or 4-letter words so that they are legible? (For credit—does he/she do this without having to copy, that is, from dictation or just on his/her own?) (Spelling errors are permissible.) Pass=Yes Fail=No	60–71
Does———run errands in which he/she is trusted with money? Pass=Yes Fail=No	60–71
Does———regularly play some of the more complicated table games which require taking turns, appreciating the goals, observing the rules, judgment, and some friendly rivalry? The kind of games we're thinking of are Tiddly-Winks, simple card games, dominoes, checkers, spinning games, and so on. Pass=Yes Fail=No	60–71
Does———lace his/her own shoes? Pass=Yes Fail=No	60–71
Can———go on errands outside home, without crossing streets? Pass=Yes Fail=No	60–71
Does———go beyond the street on which you live alone or with other children? Pass=Yes Fail=No	60–71
Does———regularly engage in play which requires both skill and the use of caution—because of possible dangers—for example, does he/she use skates, stilts, a skooter, or bicycle on his/her own outside the house or does he/she climb trees, skip rope or go on a playground swing by him/herself? Pass=Yes Fail=No	60–71

	Age in Years
Has———ever repeated any grades? Pass=No Fail=Yes or never attended school	6, 7, 8, 9, 10, 11, 12, 13, 14, 15, 16–19, 20–29, 30–39, 40–49
Does———have trouble learning in school? Pass=No Fail=Yes or never attended school	6, 7, 8, 9, 10, 11, 12, 13, 14, 15, 16–19, 20–29, 30–39, 40–49
What is———'s grade in school? Pass=At or above age grade norm[a] Fail=Below age grade norm	6, 7, 8, 9, 10, 11, 12, 13, 15
Can———name the capital letters? Pass=Yes Fail=No	6
Does———recognize several numbers on clock, calendar, or telephone dial? Pass=Yes Fail=No	6, 7
Does———run errands in which he/she is trusted with money? Pass=Yes Fail=No	6
Does———lace his/her shoes? Pass=Yes Fail=No	6
Does———legibly write a dozen or more 3- or 4-letter words in which he/she spells fairly well? (for credit—does he/she do this without having to copy—from dictation or on his own?) (Grammar unimportant.) Pass=Yes Fail=No	8
Does———know four colors? Pass=Yes Fail=No	6, 7
Can———name a penny, a nickel, and a dime? Pass=Yes Fail=No	6, 7
Does———have any difficulty getting along with his/her sisters? Pass=No Fail=Yes	6, 8, 9, 10, 11, 12, 13, 14, 15
Can———tell how many fingers on each hand? Pass=Yes Fail=No	6
Does———name one or more colors? Pass=Yes Fail=No	6
Does———usually use a knife to spread butter or jam? When he/she uses a knife does he/she manage not to mess so that there isn't more clean-up to do than when butter or jam are spread for him/her? Pass=Yes Fail=No	6

	Age in Years
If you draw a bath for———, does he/she usually bathe and dry him/herself satisfactorily so that he/she needs no help except in washing his/her ears, back, and hair? Pass=Yes Fail=No	6
Does———skip, using feet alternately? Pass=Yes Fail=No	6, 7
Can———sing a few songs? Pass=Yes Fail=No	6
Does———ever engage in any spare time activity? Pass=Yes Fail=No	6, 14, 16–19, 20–29, 40–49
Does———have any difficulty getting along with his/her teachers? Pass=No Fail=Yes	6, 9, 11, 12, 14, 15
Does———have any difficulty getting along with his/her school friends? Pass=No Fail=Yes	6, 8, 10, 11, 14
Does———have any difficulty getting along with the neighbors? Pass=No Fail=Yes	6, 7, 8, 10, 11, 12, 14, 15
Has———had any trouble with the police? Pass=No or noncriminal acts only Fail=Yes, criminal acts	6, 7, 8, 12, 14, 15
Can———go on errands outside home without crossing streets? Pass=Yes Fail=No	6
Does———tell time to the nearest quarter hour and use this information to keep track of where he/she should be or of what he/she should be doing? If he/she cannot tell time does he/she ask others for these purposes? Pass=Yes Fail=No	7
Does———count by ones to thirty or more? Pass=Yes Fail=No	7, 8
Does———usually cut up food served without help? (Help may be given with fowl, meat on bones, and tough meat.) Pass=Yes Fail=No	7
Can———write numbers from 1 to 20? Pass=Yes Fail=No	7
Does———routinely and satisfactorily comb his/her hair as part of dressing and when necessary at other times? Pass=Yes Fail=No	7, 8
Does———print both names? Pass=Yes Fail=No	7, 8
Does———tie shoe laces? Pass=Yes Fail=No	7

	Age in Years
Does——play girl and/or boy type games with other children his/her own age or a bit older? Pass=Yes Fail=No	7, 8
Has——given up believing in Santa Claus, fairies, goblins, bogymen, gremlins? Pass=Yes Fail=No	7
Does——have any difficulty getting along with his/her father? Pass=No Fail=Yes	7, 9, 10, 13, 15
With whom does——spend most of his/her spare time? Pass=Family and/or others Fail=No one	7, 8, 9, 12
Has——ever been upset by parental conflict in the family? Pass=No Fail=Yes	7, 8, 10, 13
When bedtime comes, does——routinely get ready for bed on his/her own—regularly brush his/her teeth, wash, go to the toilet, undress and turn out the light? (Keeping him/her company and tucking him/her in is OK.) Pass=Yes Fail=No	7
Does——have any difficulty getting along with his/her mother? Pass=No Fail=Yes	7, 11, 13, 14, 15
Does——read stories, comic strips, news items, etc., on his/her own initiative at about the fourth grade level? Pass=Yes Fail=No	8, 9
Does——enjoy reading to him/herself? Pass=Yes Fail=No	8, 9
Does——read and write sentences? Pass=Yes Fail=No	8, 9
Does——tell time by hour and minutes? Pass=Yes Fail=No	8, 9
Are there tools or utensils which——uses to fix or make something simple? For example, a hammer, saw, screw driver, rake, shovel, needle, other sewing or cooking utensils for practical purposes? Pass=Yes Fail=No	8
Is——greatly interested in comic books? Pass=Yes Fail=No	8, 9
Does——count by two to twenty? Pass=Yes Fail=No	8, 9
Does——have any difficulty getting along with his/her brothers? Pass=No Fail=Yes	8, 9, 10, 11, 12, 13, 14, 15

	Age in Years
Does———have a regular task around the house which is his/hers and which he/she carries out regularly with few reminders and little supervision? Pass=Yes Fail=No	8, 9
Has———ever run away from home? Pass=No Fail =Yes	8, 9, 12, 13, 15
Can———use the table of contents and index of a book? Pass=Yes Fail=No	9, 10
Does———show judgment in his/her choice of things to buy out of his/her allowance or from other money he/she has, handle money and what he/she buys with it carefully, and make correct change from a dollar or more? Does he/she make appropriate decisions when sent to make purchases? Pass=Yes Fail=No	9, 10
Does———know the multiplication tables through four? Pass=Yes Fail=No	9, 10
Can———take down a simple phone message? Pass=Yes Fail=No	9, 10
Does———usually take a bath without any help in drawing the bath, washing and drying him/herself? Pass=Yes Fail=No	9
Does———write or print all letters correctly? Pass=Yes Fail=No	9, 10
Does———usually take care of him/herself satisfactorily at table so that he/she needs little or no help or attention? Pass=Yes Fail=No	9
Does———use a dictionary? Pass=Yes Fail=No	10, 11
Does———spend a good deal of time reading by him/herself? Pass=Yes Fail=No	10, 11
Does———write with good proportions? Pass=Yes Fail=No	10, 11
Does———occasionally write short letters, including addressing and mailing them? Pass=Yes Fail=No	10
Does———look up telephone numbers and make telephone calls? Pass=Yes Fail=No	10, 11
Does———make things—boys hammer and saw, girls knit and sew? Pass=Yes Fail=No	10, 11

	Age in Years
Does———take care of him/herself sufficiently so that he/she routinely crosses the street either alone or with other children going beyond the street on which you live? Pass=Yes Fail=No	10
Does———answer ads in newspapers and magazines or make purchases by mail? Pass=Yes Fail=No	10, 11
Does———seek work in home or neighborhood to earn some money? For example, do housework tasks, gardening, babysitting, and newspaper route? Pass=Yes Fail=No	10, 11
Does———often read books, newspapers, or magazines for his/her own enjoyment? Pass=Yes Fail=No	11, 12, 13, 14, 15
Does———know most of the states and their capitals? Pass=Yes Fail=No	11, 12
Does———enjoy doing oral problems in arithmetic? Pass=Yes Fail=No	11, 12
Does———take care of him/herself or someone else an hour or longer at a time? Pass=Yes Fail=No	11, 12
Does———like to follow the funnies in the newspaper? Pass=Yes Fail=No	11
Does———seek to do simple, creative work? For example, cooking, simple repair work, construction work, gardening, painting, or writing? Pass=Yes Fail=No	11
Does———enjoy competition in class and on the playground? Pass=Yes Fail=No	12, 13
Is———an active member of an athletic team, social club, or any group his/her own age? Pass=Yes Fail=No	12, 13, 14, 15
Does———play competitive games or team sports that require following rules and keeping score, such as card games, checkers, baseball, basketball, football? Pass=Yes Fail=No	12, 13, 14, 16–19, 20–29, 40–49
Does———prefer active outdoor type of games? Pass=Yes Fail=No	12
Does———seem especially interested in clubs of one kind or another? Pass=Yes Fail=No	11, 12

	Age in Years
Does———usually go to the store by him/herself to buy minor articles of clothing, such as shoes, belts, socks or undergarments? Pass=Yes Fail=No	12, 13, 14, 16–19, 20–29, 30–39, 40–49
Is———afraid of being left alone? Pass=No Fail=Yes	12, 13
Does———seem interested in current picture magazines? Pass=Yes Fail=No	12, 13
Does———like to carry on debates or discussions of a political or civic nature? Pass=Yes Fail=No	13, 14
Does———go to the movies every week or two? Pass=Yes Fail=No	12, 13
Does———do work either at home or on a job in which he/she needs little or no supervision? Pass=Yes Fail=No	13, 14, 16–19, 20–29, 30–39, 40–49
Does———admire or idolize an older brother, sister, friend, or neighbor? Pass=Yes Fail=No	13
Does———show great interest in clothes (boys) or enjoy dressing up (girls)? Pass=Yes Fail=No	13
Does———openly express interest in the opposite sex? Pass=Yes Fail=No	13
Does———show a high degree of consideration for friends and for younger children? Pass=Yes Fail=No	13, 14
Does———usually not need help with homework? Pass=Yes Fail=No	14, 15
Is———interested in world affairs, clips newspaper items, reads editorials? Pass=Yes Fail=No	14, 15
Does———like athletic and adventure stories (boys), or teenage stories about people their own age (girls)? Pass=Yes Fail=No	14
Does———sometimes write letters to friends or relatives, giving or asking for important information? Pass=Yes Fail=No	14, 15, 16–19, 20–29, 30–39, 40–49
Does———usually give vent to rage by words rather than by physical violence or crying? Pass=Yes Fail=No	14, 15

	Age in Years
Is———concerned about appearance—drawn to a mirror as to a magnet? Pass=Yes Fail=No	14, 15
Does———usually listen and respond well? Pass=Yes Fail=No	15
Does———make an attempt to keep his/her room a little neater? Pass=Yes Fail=No	15
Does———take care of his/her fingernails? Pass=Yes Fail=No	15
Does———show an interest in people with different backgrounds? Pass=Yes Fail=No	15
Does not———include too much in his/her activities or planning? Pass=Yes Fail=No	15
How many books does———read in a year? Pass=One or more a year Fail=None	16–19, 20–29, 30–39, 40–49
How often does———read the newspaper? Pass=Frequently Fail=Seldom or never	16–19, 20–29, 30–39, 40–49
Is———dependent on others for any financial support? Pass=No or housewife Fail=Yes or no occupational role or not housewife	16–19, 20–29, 30–39, 40–49
Are there any magazines that———usually reads? Which ones? Pass=Yes, not comics Fail=None or comics only	16–19, 20–29, 30–39, 40–49
Does———participate in any organizations? Pass=Yes Fail=No	16–19, 20–29, 30–39, 40–49
Does———ever travel to nearby towns by him/herself? Pass=Yes Fail=No	16–19, 20–29, 30–39, 40–49
Does———read and talk about local news and sports? Pass=Yes Fail=No	16–19, 20–29, 30–39, 40–49
Does———participate in sports? Pass=Yes Fail=No	16–19, 20–29, 30–39, 40–49
Is———working now? Pass=Yes; or no, housewife or retired or in school Fail=No, unemployed, or never worked.	16–19, 20–29, 30–39, 40–49
Does———participate in religious activities? Pass=Yes Fail=No	16–19, 20–29, 30–39, 40–49
Has———ever worked? Pass=Yes, or no, still in school Fail=No	16–19, 20–29, 30–39
Did———drop school because of academic or discipline problems? Pass=No Fail=Yes or never attended school	16–19, 20–29, 30–39, 40–49

	Age in Years
Does———visit neighbors? Pass=Yes Fail=No	16–19, 20–29, 30–39, 40–49
Has———completed eight or more grades in school? Pass=Yes Fail=No or never attended school	16–19, 20–29, 30–39, 40–49
Has———ever received special education for the mentally retarded? Pass=No Fail=Yes	16–19, 30–39
Does———go to the movies? Pass=Yes Fail=No	16–19, 20–29, 30–39, 40–49
What is———'s usual occupation? Pass=4 thru 10th decile Fail=0 thru 3rd decile (Duncan Scales)[b]	16–19, 20–29, 30–39, 40–49
Does———ever watch TV programs other than children's programs or cartoons? Pass=Yes Fail=No	16–19, 40–49
Does———visit relatives? Pass=Yes Fail=No	16–19, 20–29, 30–39, 40–49
If old enough, does———vote? Pass=Yes or too young Fail=Never	16–19, 20–29, 30–39, 40–49
Does———visit friends? Pass=Yes Fail=No	20–29, 30–39, 40–49
Does———visit co-workers? Pass=Yes Fail=No	20–29, 30–39, 40–49

[a] Age grade norms are determined according to the following schedule: A child is considered at the norm if 5 or 6 years of age in Kindergarten; 6–7 in grade 1; 7–8 in grade 2; 8–9 in grade 3; 9–10 in 4th; 10–11 in 5th; 11–12 in 6th; 12–13 in 7th; 13–14 in 8th; 14–15 in 9th; 15–16 in 10th; 16–17 in 11th. If at or above the norm the child "passes" the item. If below norm, in an ungraded class, in a school for retarded, or not in school, the child "fails" the item.

[b] Persons in the lowest three deciles as rated by the Duncan Socio-economic Index are those who have an occupation that ranked in the lowest 30% of the male, experienced civilian labor force population on that Index. The Index is based upon the education and income of persons in various occupations adjusted for the age composition of the occupations and based on the 1950 Census. Following is a summary list of the occupations ranking in the three lowest deciles:

Hucksters and peddlers
Loom fixers
Paperhangers
Shoemakers and repairers
Blasters and powermen
Dyers
Fruit, nut, and vegetable graders and packers
Mine operatives and laborers
Coal miners
Bootblacks
Charwomen and cleaners
Janitors and sextons
Motormen in mines, factories, logging camps, etc.
Sawyers
Textile spinners
Taxicab drivers and chauffeurs
Textile weavers
Farm laborers
Private household workers
Laundresses
Service workers in hospital and institutions
Elevator operators
Porters

Fishermen and oystermen
Gardeners
Lumbermen, raftsmen, wood choppers
Garage laborers, carwashers, greasers
Longshoremen and stevedores
Teamsters

Laborers in all industries, for example: Construction, transportation, iron and steel, food preservation and preparation, textile, all manufacturing.

For further details, see Reiss, Albert J., Jr., *Occupations and Social Status,* The Free Press of Glencoe, Inc., 1961, Glencoe, Illinois.

Appendix C

ITEMS USED FOR MEASURING THE PHYSICAL DISABILITY OF PERSONS OF VARIOUS AGES

	Age in Months	*Age in Years*
Was———placed in incubator or oxygen tent after birth because he/she had problems of any kind? Pass=No Fail=Yes	7–12, 13–18, 19–24, 25–29, 30–35, 36–47, 48–59, 60–72	
Has———been in a hospital for any illness since birth? Pass=No Fail=Yes	7–12, 13–18, 19–24, 25–29, 30–35, 36–47, 48–59, 60–72	
Did———have any birth injuires or defects? Pass=No Fail=Yes	7–12, 13–18, 19–24, 25–29, 30–35, 36–47, 48–59, 60–72	
Was———'s mother sick or did she have any complications during pregnancy? Pass=No Fail=Yes	7–12, 13–18, 19–24, 25–29, 30–35, 36–47, 48–59, 60–72	
Was———'s birth either premature or overterm? Pass=Fullterm + or − 3 weeks Fail=Premature or overterm more than 3 weeks	7–12, 13–18, 19–24, 25–29, 30–35, 36–47, 48–59, 60–72	
Does———vomit regularly after eating? Pass=No Fail=Yes	7–12, 13–18, 19–24, 25–29, 30–35, 36–47, 48–59, 60–72	
Has———'s mother had two or more stillbirths or miscarriages? Pass=No Fail=Yes	7–12, 13–18, 19–24, 25–29, 30–35, 36–47, 48–59, 60–72	
Did———weigh under five pounds or over nine pounds at birth? Pass=No Fail=Yes	7–12, 13–18, 19–24, 25–29, 30–35, 36–47, 48–59, 60–72	

	Age in Months	*Age in Years*
Did———have yellow jaundice when brought home from the hospital? Pass=No Fail=Yes	7–12, 13–18, 19–24, 25–29, 30–35, 36–47, 48–59, 60–72	
Has———ever had an epileptic seizure, fit, or convulsion? Pass=No Fail=Yes	7–12, 19–24, 25–29, 36–47, 48–59, 60–72	6–10, 11–15, 16–19, 20–29, 30–39, 40–49
Does———have any trouble sleeping? Pass=No Fail=Yes	7–12, 19–24, 25–29, 30–35, 36–47, 48–59	6–10, 11–15, 16–19, 20–29, 30–39, 40–49
Was———an Rh baby? Pass=No Fail=Yes	13–18, 19–24, 25–29, 30–35, 48–59, 60–72	
Has———had any serious illnesses affecting the central nervous system such as meningitis, polio, encephalitis, sleeping sickness, or complications with scarlet fever or measles? Pass=No Fail=Yes	7–12, 13–18, 25–29, 30–35, 36–47, 60–72	6–10, 11–15, 16–19, 20–29, 30–39, 40–49
Has———ever had a serious operation involving prolonged unconsciousness or injury to his/her brain or spinal cord? Pass=No Fail=Yes	13–18, 25–29, 30–35	6–10, 11–15, 16–19, 20–29, 30–39, 40–49
Does———have any trouble talking? Pass=No Fail=Yes	25–29, 30–35, 36–47, 48–59, 60–72	6–10, 11–15, 16–19, 20–29, 30–39, 40–49
Has———ever had any serious accidents in which he/she suffered prolonged unconsciousness or injury to his/her brain or spinal cord? Pass=No Fail=Yes	25–29, 36–47, 48–59	6–10, 11–15, 16–19, 20–29, 30–39, 40–49
Does———have any trouble walking? Pass=No Fail=Yes	30–35, 36–47, 48–59, 60–72	6–10, 11–15, 16–19, 20–29, 30–39, 40–49
Does———have any trouble seeing? Pass=No Fail=Yes	30–35, 36–47, 48–59	6–10, 11–15, 16–19, 20–29, 30–39, 40–49

	Age in Months	*Age in Years*
Does———have any trouble feeding him/herself? Pass=No Fail=Yes	30–35, 36–47, 60–72	6–10, 11–15, 16–19, 20–29, 30–39, 40–49
Does———have any trouble hearing? Pass=No Fail=Yes	48–59, 60–72	6–10, 11–15, 16–19, 20–29, 30–39, 40–49
Does———have any trouble dressing him/herself? Pass=No Fail=Yes		6–10, 11–15, 16–19, 20–29, 30–39, 40–49
Did illness interfere with———'s being able to finish high school? Pass=No Fail=Yes		16–19, 20–29, 30–39, 40–49
Is———currently unemployed due to illness? Pass=No Fail=Yes		16–19, 20–29, 30–39, 40–49
Did———receive special training for the physically handicapped while in school? Pass=No Fail=Yes		16–19, 20–29, 30–39, 40–49
Has———ever been a patient in a hospital for the mentally retarded or mentally ill? Pass=No Fail=Yes		16–19, 20–29, 30–39, 40–49

BIBLIOGRAPHY

Altus, W. D. 1949. The American Mexican: The survival of a culture. *Journal of Social Psychology,* 29: 211–220.

Arthur, G. 1947. Pseudo-feeblemindedness. *American Journal of Mental Deficiency,* 52: 137–142.

Arthur, G. 1950. Some factors contributing to errors in the diagnosis of feeblemindedness. *American Journal of Mental Deficiency,* 54: 495–501.

Bazelan, D. L., and Boggs, E. M. 1963. *Report of the Task Force on Law.* President's Panel on Mental Retardation, p. 26.

Becker Howard S. 1963. *Outsiders: studies in the sociology of deviance.* Glencoe, Ill.: Free Press.

Becker, Howard S., ed. 1964. *The other side: perspectives on deviance.* Glencoe, Ill.: Free Press.

Benda, C. E. 1954. Psychology of childhood. In *Manual of child psychology,* ed. L. Carmichael, pp. 1–115. 2nd ed. New York: Wiley.

Binet, A., and Simon, T. 1905. Sur la necessité d'éstablir un diagnostic scientifique des états inferieurs de l'intelligence. *Année Psychologique,* 11: 1–28.

Boring, E. G. 1923. Intelligence as the tests test it. *New Republic,* 35: 35–37.

Bremer, J. 1951. A social psychiatric investigation of a small community of Northern Norway. *Acta Psychiatrica et Neurologic.* Supplement 62, Ejinar Munksgaard, Copenhagen.

Brockopp, G. 1958. The significance of selected variables on the prevalence of suspected-mental retardates in the public schools of Indiana. Unpublished doctoral dissertation, Indiana University.

Brown, J., Jr., and Boyd, J. 1922. *History of San Bernardino and Riverside Counties.* Chicago: Lewis Publishing Co.

Buros, O. I., ed. 1965. *The sixth mental measurements yearbook.* Highland Park, N.J.: Gryphon Press.

California State Department of Education. 1967. *Racial and ethnic survey of California public schools.* Part I: Distribution of Pupils, Fall, 1966. Sacramento.

Cassel, R. H. 1949. Notes on pseudo-feeblemindedness. *Training School Bulletin,* 46: 119–127.

Cicourel, Aaron V., and Kitsuse, John, 1963. *The educational decision makers.* Bobbs-Merrill.

Clarke, A. M., and Clarke, A. D. B. 1958. *Mental deficiency: the changing outlook.* Glencoe, Ill.: Free Press.

Darcy, N. T. 1953. A review of the literature on the effects of bilingualism upon the measurement of intelligence. *Journal of Genetic Psychology,* 82: 21–57.

Davitz, J. R.; Davitz, L. J.; and Lorge, I. 1964. *Terminology and concepts in mental retardation.* New York: Bureau of Publications, Teachers College, Columbia University.

Deutsch, A. 1949. *The mentally ill in America.* New York: Columbia University Press.

Dexter, Lewis A. 1960. Research on problems of subnormality. *American Journal of Mental Deficiency,* 64: 835–838.

——— 1964. *The tyranny of schooling.* New York: Basic Books, Inc.

Doll, E. A. 1941. The essentials of an inclusive concept of mental deficiency. *American Journal of Mental Deficiency,* 46: 214–219.

——— 1965. *Vineland Social Maturity Scale, condensed.* Rev. ed. Manual of Direction. Minneapolis: American Guidance Service, Inc.

Eaton, J. W., and Weil, R. J. 1955. *Culture and mental disorders.* Glencoe, Ill.: Free Press.

Edgerton R. B. 1967. *The cloak of competence.* Berkeley and Los Angeles: University of California Press.

Eells, K. et al. 1951. *Intelligence and cultural differences.* University of Chicago Press.

The English Mental Deficiency Act of 1927, Section I, Paragraph 2.

Erickson, Kai T. 1964. Notes on the sociology of deviance. In *The other side: perspectives on deviance,* ed. Howard S. Becker. Glencoe, Ill.: Free Press.

Eron, L. D., and Walder, L. O. 1961. Test burning: II. *American Psychologist.* 16: 237–244.

Essen-Moller, E. 1956. *Acta Psychiatrica Scandinavia.* Supplement 100.

Ferguson, R. G. 1956. *A study of the problem of mental retardation in the city of Philadelphia.* Report of the Philadelphia Commission on the Mentally Retarded. City Hall Annex, Philadelphia.

Gesell, A. L. 1948*a. The first five years of life.* New York: Harper & Bros.

———. 1948 *b. Studies in child development.* New York: Harper & Bros.

———. 1956. *Youth: the years from ten to sixteen.* New York: Harper & Bros.

Gibson, W. A. 1966. Three multivariate models. In *Readings in mathematical social science,* ed. P. Lazarsfeld and N. Henry. Chicago: Science Research Associates, Inc.

Gordon, M. M. 1964. *Assimilation in American life.* New York: Oxford University Press, Pp. 72–76.

Group for the Advancement of Psychiatry. 1959. *Basic considerations in mental retardation: a preliminary report.* Report No. 43, p. 7.

The growth and economic structure of San Bernardino and Riverside Counties. 1960. Research Department, Security First National Bank, Riverside, California.

Gruenberg, E. 1955. A special census of suspected referred mental retardation in Onondaga County. *Technical report of the Mental Health Research Unit.* New York: New York State Department of Mental Hygiene.

Guenther, R. 1956. *Final report of the Michigan Demonstration Research Project for the Severely Mentally Retarded.* Hastings, Michigan.

Guertin, W. H. 1950. Differential characteristics of the pseudo-feebleminded. *American Journal of Mental Deficiency,* 54: 394–398.

Hayakawa, S. I. 1957. *Language in action.* Harcourt, Brace and Co., Pp. 115–116.

Heber, R. F. 1961. A manual on terminology and classification in mental retardation. *American Journal of Mental Deficiency,* 64. Monograph Supplement. 2nd ed.

Hyman, H. 1955. *Survey design and analysis.* Glencoe, Ill.: Free Press.

Jastak, J. F.; MacPhee, H. M.; and Whiteman, M. 1963. *Mental retardation: its nature and incidence.* Newark Del.: University of Delaware Press.

Jenkins, R. L., and Brown, A. L. 1935. The geographical distribution of mental deficiency in the Chicago area. *American Journal of Mental Deficiency,* 40: 291–308.

Jervis, G. A. 1954. Factors in mental retardation. *Children,* 1: 207–211.

Kanner, L. 1949 *a. A miniature textbook of feeblemindedness.* Child Care Monograph, No. 1. New York: Child Care Publications.

———. 1949*b*. Feeblemindedness: absolute, relative, and apparent. *Nervous Child,* 7: 365–397.

———. 1957. *Child Psychiatry.* 3rd ed. Springfield, Ill.: Charles C. Thomas, pp. 70–71.

———. 1964. *A history of the care and study of the mentally retarded.* Springfield, Ill.: Charles C. Thomas.

Kennedy, R. J. 1948. *The social adjustment of morons in a Connecticut city.* Willport, Conn.: Commission to Study the Human Resources of the State of Connecticut.

Kirk, S. A. 1957. *Public school provisions for severely retarded children.* Albany, N. Y.: Report to the New York State Interdepartmental Health Resources Board.

Kitsuse, John I. 1964. Societal reaction to deviant behavior: problems of theory and method. In *The other side: perspectives on deviance,* ed. Howard S. Becker. Glencoe, Ill.: Free Press.

Klapp, Orrin E. 1949. The fool as a social type. *American Journal of Sociology,* 55: 157–162.

Knobloch, H., and Pasamanick, B. 1959 Distribution of intellectual potential in an infant population. In *Epidemiology of mental disorder,* ed. B. Pasamanick, pp. 249–272. Washington, D.C.: American Association for the Advancement of Science.

Larsson, T., and Sjorgren, T. 1954. *A methodological and psychiatric study of a large Swedish rural population.* Department of Psychiatry, Karolinska Instituted Medical School, University of Stockholm, Sweden.

Lazarsfeld, P. F. 1959. Latent structure analysis. In *Psychology: a study of a science,* ed. S. Koch. New York: McGraw-Hill, 1959.

Leighton, D. C.; Arding, J. S.; Macklin, D. B.; Macmillan, A. M.; and Leighton, A. H. 1963. *The character of danger.* Vol. III. The Stirling County Study of Psychiatric Disorder and Sociocultural Environment. New York: Basic Books.

Leland, H.; Nihira, K.; Foster, R.; Shellhaas, M.; and Kagin, E., eds. 1966. Conference on measurement of adaptive behavior: II. Parsons State Hospital and Training Center. Parsons, Kansas.

Lemkau, P.; Tietze, C.; and Cooper, M. 1941. Mental-hygiene problems in an urban district. *Mental Hygiene,* 25: 624–646.

———. 1942. *Ibid.,* 26: 100–119, 275–288.

Levinson, E. J. 1962. *Retarded children in Maine: a survey and analysis.* University of Maine Studies, Second Series, No. 77, Orono, Me.: University of Maine Press.

Lewis, E. O. 1929. Parts I, II, and IV of the *Report of the mental deficiency committee,* a Joint Committee of the Board of Education and Board of Control. London: H. M. Stationery Office.

———. 1933. Types of mental deficiency and their significance. *Journal of Mental Science,* 79: 298–304.

Lilienfeld, A. M. 1957. Epidemiological methods and inferences in studies of noninfectious diseases. *Public health reports.* U.S. Department of Health, Education, and Welfare, Public Health Service, 72 (1) : 51–60.

Lin, T. 1953. Studies of the incidence of mental disorders in Chinese and other cultures. *Psychiatry,* 16: 313–336.

Lindman, F. T., and McIntyre, D. M., Jr., eds. 1961. California Code Ann., Deering, W. I., 5250, 1952; Nebraska Rev. Stat., 83–219, 1958; South Dakota Code, 30.0402, 1939; Washington Rev. Code, 72.33.020, 1958. *The mentally disabled and the law.* Chicago: University of Chicago Press.

McCarthy, Philip J. 1969. *Pseudo-replication: further evaluation and applications of the balanced half-sample technique.* Public Health Service Publication No. 1000, Series 2, Number 31, Washington, D.C.: U.S. Government Printing Office.

McCartin, Sister Rose Amata; Dingman, Harvey F.; Meyers, C. Edward; and Mercer, Jane R. 1966. Identification and disposition of the mentally handicapped in the parochial school system. *American Journal of Mental Deficiency,* 71 (2) : 202–206.

McCulloch, T. L. 1947. Reformulation of the problem of mental deficiency. *American Journal of Mental Deficiency,* 52: 130–136.

Masland, R. L.; Sarason, S. B.; and Gladwin, T. 1958. *Mental subnormality.* New York: Basic Books.

Mental Health Act of 1959, Section 4, Paragraph 2.

The Mentally Subnormal Child. 1954. *World Health Organization technical report series.* No. 75.

Mercer, Jane R. 1965. Social system perspective and clinical perspective: frames of reference for understanding career patterns of persons labelled as mentally retarded. *Social Problems,* 13 (1) : 18–34.

———. 1970. Sociological perspectives on mild mental retardation. In *Social-Cultural Aspects of Mental Retardation: Proceedings of the Peabody NIMH Conference,* ed. H. C. Haywood, pp. 378–391. New York: Appleton-Century-Crofts.

———. 1971. The meaning of mental retardation. In *The mentally retarded child and his family: A multidisciplinary handbook,* ed. Richard Koch and James Dobson. New York: Brunner/Mazel, Inc.

———. 1972. Who is normal? Two perspectives on mild mental retardation. In *Patients, physicians and illness,* ed. E. G. Jaco. Rev. ed. Glencoe, Ill.: Free Press.

Mercer, Jane R., and Butler, E. W. 1967. Disengagement of the aged population and response differentials in survey research. *Social Forces,* 46 (1) : 89–96.

Mercer, Jane R.; Butler, E. W.; and Dingman, H. F. 1964. The relationship between social-developmental performance and mental ability. *American Journal of Mental Deficiency,* 69: 195–205.

Meyers, C. E.; Orpet, R.; Attwell, S.; and Dingman, H. F. 1962. Primary abilities at mental age six. *Monographs of the Society for Research in Child Development,* 27 (1) . 40 pages.

Meyers, C. E.; Dingman, H. F.; Orpet, R. E.; Sitkei, E. G.; and Watts, C. A. 1964. Four ability-factor hypotheses at three preliterate levels in normal and retarded children. *Monographs of the Society for Research in Child Development,* 29 (5) . 80 pages.

Meyers, C. E.; Attwell, Arthur A.; and Orpet, Russell E. 1968. Prediction of fifth grade achievement from kindergarten test and rating data. *Educational and Psychological Measurement,* 28: 457–463.

Miller, C.; Eyman, R.; and Dingman, H. F. 1961. Factor analysis, latent structure analysis, and mental typology. *British Journal of Statistical Psychology,* 14: 29–34.

Minnesota Department of Public Welfare. 1964. Individual and family characteristics of Anoka County's mentally retarded population. *Report to the Anoka County Association for Retarded Children.* Unpublished.

Mullen, F. A., and Nee, M. M. 1949. Distribution of mental retardation in an urban school population. *American Journal of Mental Deficiency,* 56: 291–308.

National Center for Health Statistics, Public Health Service, Department of Health, Education, and Welfare. 1965. *Health interview responses compared with medical records.* Series 2, No. 7. Washington, D.C.: Public Health Service Publication.

National Center for Health Statistics. 1967. *Interview data on chronic conditions compared with information derived from medical records.* Series 2, No. 23. U. S. Department of Health, Education, and Welfare.

New Jersey. Committee to Study the Education of Handicapped Children. 1955. *Found. A report. The first complete survey of handicapped children in the State of New Jersey.* Trenton.

New York State, Department of Mental Hygiene. Interdepartmental Health Resources Board. 1956. Census of severely retarded children in New York State. Albany.

Nickell, V. L. 1954. *Report on study projects for trainable mentally handicapped children.* Illinois Council for Mentally Retarded Children.

Nihira, Kazuo; Foster, Ray; Shellhaas, Max; and Leland, Henry. 1969. *Adaptive behavior scale.* Adaptive Behavior Project, Parsons State Hospital and Training Center. American Association on Mental Deficiency.

Pasamanick, B., and Knobloch, H. 1958. The contributions of some organic factors to school retardation in Negro children. *Journal of Negro Education,* 27: 4–9.

Perry, Stewart E. 1965. The middle class and mental retardation in America. *Psychiatry,* 28: 108–118.

Plunkett, R. J., and Gordon, J. E. 1960. *Epidemiology and mental illness.* New York: Basic Books.

President's Committee on Mental Retardation and Bureau of Education of the Handicapped. 1969. *The six-hour retarded child.* Report on a Conference on Problems of Education of Children in the Inner City, August 10–12, 1969. Washington, D.C.

President's Panel on Mental Retardation. 1962. *Report to the President: A proposed program for national action to combat mental retardation.* Washington, D.C.

Primrose, Edward J. R. 1962. *Psychological illness: a community study.* Springfield, Ill.: Charles C. Thomas.

Reid, D. D. 1960. Epidemiological methods in the study of mental disorders. *Public Health Papers.* World Health Organization. No. 2, pp. 27–29.

Reiss, A. J., Jr. 1961. *Occupations and social status.* Glencoe, Ill.: Free Press.

Richardson, W. P.; Higgins, A. C.; and Ames, R. G. 1965. *The handicapped children of Alamance County, North Carolina: a medical and sociological study.* Wilmington, Del.: Nemours Foundation.

Robbins, R. C.; Mercer, Jane R.; and Meyers, C. E. 1967. The school as a selecting-labeling system. *Journal of School Psychology,* 5 (4) : 270–279.

Robinson, W. S. 1950. Ecological correlations and the behavior of individuals. *American Sociological Review,* 15: 351–357.

Roth, W. F., and Luton, F. H. 1943. The mental health program in Tennessee. *American Journal of Psychiatry,* 99: 662–675.

Saenger, G. 1957. *The adjustment of severely retarded adults in the community.* Albany, N.Y.: A Report to the New York State Interdepartmental Health Resources Board.

Scheff, Thomas J. 1966. *Being mentally ill: a sociological theory.* Chicago: Aldine Publishing Company.

Scottish Council for Research in Education, 1949. 1953. *The trend in Scottish intelligence and social implications of the 1947 Scottish mental survey.* London: University of London Press.

Selltiz, C.; Jahoda, M.; Deutsch, M.; and Cook, S. W. 1965. *Research methods in social relations.* Rev. one-volume ed. New York: Holt, Rinehart and Winston.

Sewell, W. H. 1949. Field techniques in social psychological study in a rural community. *American Sociological Review,* 14: 718–726.

Sheerenberger, R. C. 1965. Presentation to the Division of Special Studies of the American Association on Mental Deficiency, September, 1965.

Sloan, W., and Birch, J. W. 1955. A rationale for degrees of retardation. *American Journal of Mental Deficiency,* 60: 258–264.

Stern, W. L. 1912. Uber de psychologischen methoden der intelligenzprufund.

Ber V. Kongress exp. Psycho., Pp. 48ff.

Terman, L. M. 1932. Trails in psychology. In *A history of psychology in autobiography,* ed C. Murchinson. Worchester, Mass.: Clark University Press.

Terman, L. M., and Merrill, M. A. 1960. *Stanford-Binet Intelligence Scale.* Boston: Houghton Mifflin.

Tizard, J. 1964. *Community services for the mentally handicapped.* New York: Oxford University Press.

———. 1968. The role of social institutions in the causation, prevention and alleviation of mental retardation. Paper delivered at the Inaugural Peabody NIMH Conference in Socio-Cultural Aspects of Mental Retardation. Nashville, Tenn., June 9–12, 1968.

Tredgold, A. F., and Soddy, K. 1956. *A textbook of mental deficiency.* 9th ed. Baltimore: Williams & Wilkins.

Tuddenham, Reed D. 1962. The nature and measurement of intelligence. In *Psychology in the making,* ed. L. Postman, pp. 469–525. New York: Alfred A. Knopf.

U.S. censuses of population and housing: 1960. 1962. Final report PHC (1) – 135, census tracts, San Bernardino-Riverside-Ontario, California, standard metropolitan statistical area. Washington, D.C.: U.S. Government Printing Office.

U.S. Department of Health, Education, and Welfare. 1962. *International index of diseases.* Public Health Service Publication 719, Vols. 1 and 2. Washington, D.C.: U.S. Printing Office.

Waskowitz, C. H. 1948. The psychologist's contribution to the recognition of pseudo-feeblemindedness. *Nervous Child,* 7: 398–406.

Watts, C. A.; Sitkei, E. G.; and Meyers, C. E. 1969. A methodological report on household psychometric screening for retardation. *Community Mental Health Journal,* 5 (1) : 88–94.

Wechsler, D. 1958. *The measurement and appraisal of adult intelligence.* 4th ed. Baltimore: Williams & Wilkins.

Windle, C. 1962. Prognosis of mental subnormals. *Monograph Supplement to American Journal of Mental Deficiency,* 66 (5) .

Woolf, B. 1957. Log-Likelihood Ratio Test (The G-Test) : Methods and tables for a test of heterogeneity in contingency tables. *Annals of Human Genetics,* 21 (4) : 397–409.

World Health Organization. 1954. *The mentally subnormal child, technical report series #5,* Geneva.

Zigler, E. 1967. Familial mental retardation: a continuing dilemma. *Science,* 155: 292–298.

INDEX

AAMD. *See* American Association on Mental Deficiency
Adaptive behavior: subnormal, 131; description, 132–33; working construct, 133–37; multivariate analysis, 163–64; and IQ, 168–70; sociocultural component, 249–51
Adaptive Behavior Scales: in Riverside study, 144–51; scoring, 153; those failing, 155–64; in follow-up interviews, 225; pluralistic norms, 251–52; limitations, 269–70; analyzed, 281–82
Adults: minorities not labeled, 82; not rated by family, 84; role expectations, 136
Adults, retarded: on clinical register, 74–5; sex differences in adaptive behavior, 156–57; physically disabled, 157–58; socioeconomic level and adaptive behavior, 158–59; characteristics, 178–81; case histories, 215–16; Anglo, 220; "borderline," 219, 221
Age: labeling by organizations, 56; on clinical register, 73–75; ethnic groups, 79–80
Alvord School District, 260–61
American Association on Mental Deficiency: definition of mental retardation, 5, 128, 185; classification, 10, 14, 145; and adaptive behavior, 132–33
—criterion: developmental period, 137; chronicity, 139; effect on prevalence rates, 190; ethnic differences, 207; borderline retardates, 220; one-dimensional, 222; and Adaptive Behavior Scales, 282
Angiocentrism: of mental tests, 13–14; in labeling retardates, 120–23
Anglos, retarded: characteristics, 91, 220, 229, 240–41; sex difference, 154; prevalence rates, 190–91, 207, 254
Anglos in Riverside, 46–47

Bandini, Juan, 39
Behavioral maladjustment: compared with retardation, 173–74; interpersonal relations, 177; reclassification, 262; rating by parents, 266
Binet, Alfred, 12, 197
Biological impairment, 137–39, 140
Black children: in school, 82, 101, 106, 111, 114, 117; sociocultural modality, 245–47; interview with mother, 268
Blacks, retarded: 91, 175–76, 190–91, 207; labeled by organizations, 57; age, 79–80; socioeconomic status, 79; adaptive behavior, 160; IQ scores, 167–68; sociocultural factors, 229, 238–41, 242–43
Blacks in Riverside, 42–43, 47
Borderline retardates, 209–12; physical disability, 214–20; Mexican American, 247
Brain, defective development, 137

Cain-Levine Social Competency Scale, 145*n*
California. Department of Mental Hygiene: IQ in hospitals, 24; models used for labeling, 59, 61–62, 66; and situational retardates, 93–94; patients in Riverside study, 286
California State School for the Deaf, 70
Case histories, 193–195, 212–20, 268–69
Catholic schools. *See* Schools, Catholic
Census, U.S., 276–77
Child, pre-school: immune to labeling, 82; adaptive behavior, 135
—school age: overrepresented on clinical register, 74–75; adaptive behavior, 135–36; role performance, 175
Chronicity, 139–40
Clinical epidemiology, 128
Clinical perspective: defined, 2, 256; and social system perspective, 36–37, 257–60; 266–69
Colony Association, 39–41
Community Research Project. *See* Riverside mental retardation study
Conclusions, 271–72
Convergence of systems, 266–69
Core culture, 12–13
Criteria for mental retardation: com-

pared, 197–221. *See also* American Association on Mental Deficiency criterion; Traditional criterion
Cultural differences, 8–9
Cultural groups, tolerance of deviance, 27–31*n*

De Anza, Juan Bautista, 39
Deaf, 70
"Defect theorists," 226
Defense mechanism, mental retardation as, 30
Denial of official label, 16
Developmental period, appearance of symptoms, 137
Deviance: coping with, 25–26; tolerance of, 27–31*n*
Diagnosis, clinical, 11
Dingman, Harvey F., ix
Divorce, 227–28
Duncan Socioeconomic Index, 45*n*, 88, 158, 171, 227, 229, 230; Mexican-Americans, 240; sociocultural modality and, 244

Educable mentally retarded classes reevaluated, 260–65
Education of family of retardates, 173–74
Eligibility *vs.* labeling, 198–200
English language. *See* Language
English Mental Deficiency Act of 1927, 128, 137, 138
Epidemiologies: compared, 201–204; methods in Social System Epidemiology, 284
Epidemiology of Mental Retardation. *See* Riverside mental retardation study
Ethnic groups: nominations by organizations, 57; socioeconomic levels, 78; compared as to age, IQ, and physical disability, 80–81; socioeconomic level and adaptive behavior, 159–163; IQ scores, 167–68; two-dimensional definition, 190–92; criteria and, 208; sociocultural factors, 237–38; rates of retardation, 253
Ethnocentrism. *See* Anglocentrism
Etiology: emphasis in research, 11

Familial-genetics, 223, 226
Family: as nominators, 83–86; norms, 88; background, 171–75; size, 242
"Fear of appearing stupid," 29*n*
Feeblemindedness, 136
"Fool-making," 33

Genetic theory, 226
Genotype, 235, 258
Gesell Development Scales, 145–48, 269
Gifted: special classes, 104; referrals, 110; Anglos, 114
Group for the Advancement of Psychiatry, 128–29; on chronicity, 139

Head of household, 240–42
Housing: value of homes of retarded, 76, 91; effects of low status, 117; overcrowding, 241; unit defined, 276; in Riverside study, 277*n*

IQ: as criterion, 5–6, 130–31, 222; Catholic schools, 24; labeled by organizations, 59; clinically diagnosed, 68–69; and physical disability, 71, 165–66; community opinion, 86; family opinion, 88; of situationally retarded, 90; in schools, 114; and socioeconomic level, 166, 168–70; sociocultural factors, 235–41, 245; pluralistic norms, 248–49
Incurability, 18, 139–40
Infant, adaptive behavior, 134–35
Intelligence *vs.* adaptive behavior, 186–87
Intelligence tests: proliferation of, 12; criticized, 13, 37; labeling of minorities, 115; selected for Riverside study, 144; those failing, 165–70; logic behind, 236; Spanish, 283; validity, 284
International Index of Diseases, 10
Interviewers: described, 152, 277–79; ethnic distribution, 152, 278; falsification, 279*n*
Interviews: screening, 152–53; follow-up, 225

Jastak, Joseph F., 147, 202–203

Kuhlman-Binet test, 69, 144

Labeling: "labeled retardate," 28; legitimate, 33–35; *vs.* eligibility, 198–200
Language spoken: Spanish, 109, 162, 173, 194, 208, 217, 219–20, 230; by interviewers, 152, 278, 279; Spanish language intelligence test, 283; English, 228, 229, 241–42
Latent class analysis, 227–34

Law: mental disability, 15; psychological testing, 111–13; definitions of retardation, 132; as criteria, 209
Law enforcement agencies, 61–64
Lorge-Thorndike test, 284

Marriage laws, 15
Medical doctors: diagnosis of mental retardation, 66, 68–69
Medical model. *See* Pathological model
Mental Health Act of 1959, 128–29, 137, 138
Mental Measurements Yearbook, Sixth, 12
Mental retardates: background characteristics, 208; reclassification 261–65
Mental retadation: as syndrome, 7; suprasocietal, 8; diagnostic nomenclature, 14; social system definition, 27; as abstraction, 30, 256; definitions, 127–140; *vs.* mental deficiency, 138; clinical, 222, 252
Mental Retardation Abstracts, 11
Mental Retardation in a Community, ix*n*. *See also* Riverside mental retardation study
Mexican-American children: in public schools, 101; referred for special class, 106, 111, 114, 115, 117; retained, 108–109; sociocultural modality, 239, 241–42, 244–47
Mexican-Americans: modal configurations, 47; labeled by organizations, 57–58; age of labeled, 79–80; and public schools, 82; situationally retarded, 91; adaptive behavior scales, 159–63; IQ scores, 167–68, 238–41; clinically retarded, 175–76; prevalence rate, 190–91, 207, 254; in the U.S. population, 205; eligibility *vs.* labeling, 198–200; adult retardates, 216–18; sociocultural factors, 229, 238–41; heads of households, 230; mislabeled, 233; rates for clinical retardation, 254
Mexicans: in early Riverside, 41–42, 45; school attendance, 150
Multiple nominations, 200–201

NORC (National Opinion Research Center) scale, 45*n*
National Institute of Mental Health, ix, x, xi
Neighborhood problems, 177
Neighbors as nominators, 83–84, 86–87
Nonretarded, 143–44
Normality: defined, 2–5; example, 6; in a social system, 22; return to by retardate, 118–19; normals compared with retardates, 174
Norms: of behavior in a social system, 23–25; tolerance of deviation from, 25

Occupations: role expectancy, 150–51; family of the retarded, 171; of retarded adults, 178–81, 231–32
"One-dimensional retardates," 142
One-dimensional taxonomy, 222
Organic involvement: in retardation, 138–39; "organics," 223, 226, 230; in taxonomy, 233
Organizations: contacted for study, 52, 53*n*, 284–86; as nominators 55–66; joint nominations, 65; as labelers, 93
Overcrowding, 241

Pacific State Hospital, ix, 151
Parents rating of children, 88–89, 266–68
Parsons' Adaptive Behavior Scale, 145*n*, 269
Pathological model: defined, 2–3; *vs.* statistical model, 5, 71, 122–23, 256; suprasocietal, 8; cause-and-effect, 9–11; biological emphasis, 10; impact on terminology, 17; inadequacy, 20–21, 259
Pathological norm, 59, 61
Pathology, 7
Phenotype, 235, 258
Physical disability: clinical register, 70–71; deviance, 77; ethnic groups, 81–82; neighbors and, 87; situationally retarded, 90–91; questions on, 151; scales, 153; adaptive behavior, 157, 187; role performance, 212–15; "organics," 227–33
Pluralistic evaluation, 259–66
Pluralistic Intelligence Test Norms, 270
Pomona pilot study, 273–75
President's Panel on Mental Retardation, 15, 20, 128–30
Prevalence of mental retardation: social system factors, 32, 36; in Riverside, 188–89; compared, 202–204; in population, 205; nonwhite, 205, 252–54; choice of criteria, 206–209; dependence on perspective, 257
Principal, school, 109–11, 114
"Problem profiles," 61
Professionals: diagnostic function, 15; as

labelers, 34–35, 67; compared with family and neighbors, 85–86
Programs needed, 270–71
Pseudoretardation, 12, 18, 139, 185–86
Psychological testing law, 111–13
Psychologist, school, 96–97, 113–14, 261
Psychometrists, 284
Pupil Personnel Department: explained, 96–98; referrals to, 104, 110–11; Riverside and Alvord Unified school districts, 260–61

Quasi-retarded: defined, 142–43, 188; *vs.* pseudoretardation, 185–86; role performance, 192–95; in taxonomy, 233; and reclassification, 262, 265
Questions: asked in study, 83*n*; in household interview, 149

Referrals: by teacher, 104, 114; ethnic distribution, 106; by principal, 110–11, 114
Refusals, 281
Religious organizations, 65–66
Retained students, 104, 107–109
"Retardate roster," 97
Retardation. *See* Mental retardation
Riverside, California: selection for study, x; description, 38–39, 43–50; history, 39–43; as typical, 48–50; census tracts, 152
Riverside epidemiology, 269
Riverside Field Study, 275–81
Riverside mental retardation study: background, ix–x; personnel, xi–xiii; a clinical epidemiology, 19; definition of mental retardation, 140; three-group taxonomy, 223–24; geographic boundaries, 286
Riverside Unified School District: mentioned, 96; children tested, 237; Pupil Personnel Department, 260–61
Role, social: defined, 21–22; expectations for the retarded, 33, 89; in the classroom, 104; fulfillment as a test item, 149–51; performance, 212

Sample: size, 270; design for screened sample, 276–78
Scheff, Thomas J., 12
Schools, Catholic: retarded in, 24, 98, 102; attendance of, 97; ethnic groups, 101; transfer to, 116; intelligence testing, 283
Schools, private, 97–98
Schools, public: as labelers, 60–61, 64–66, 93–123; enrollment in, 97; achieving status of retarded, 99–100; rates of referral compared, 110–11; risk of being labeled, 112; retardation a "school specific," 177
Sex: in organizational labeling, 56; clinical register, 72; retained students, 108; and IQ in school, 114; adaptive behavior scales, 155–57
Situationally retarded: defined, 33, 89; characteristics, 90–92
"Six-hour retarded child," 89, 94
Social incompetence. *See* Adaptive behavior
Social role. *See* Role, social
Social status. *See* Status, social
Social system perspective: defined, 2, 256; *vs.* clinical perspective, 36–37; convergence with clinical perspective, 257–60, 266–69
Socio-Behavioral Study Center for Mental Retardation, x*n*
Sociocultural factors: and IQ, 168–70; and adaptive behavior, 168–70; in retardation, 224–34, 265; modality, 233–35, 243–44
Socioeconomic status: persons on clinical register, 75; adaptive behavior and, 158
Sources of information, 280
Southerners, 228–30
Spanish language. *See* Language
Special education class: placement in, 104, 115; Anglo females and, 116; students, 117; reevaluation of EMR classes, 260–65
Speech, 70
Stanford-Binet: LM form, 5, 98, 130–31, 144; norms, 13*n*; and clinical register, 69; in Catholic schools, 98; selected for Riverside study, 144; Spanish language, 283
Statistical model: defined, 3–7; *vs.* pathological model, 5, 71, 122–23, 256
Statistical norm, 59, 61
Status, social: defined, 21; latent and active, 30–31; of retardates, 32–33; factor in organizational labeling, 56
Sterilization laws, 15
Student: status, 150; interviewers, 277

Tarjan, George, ix
Taxonomy: one-dimensional, 222; two-

group, 225; three-group, 226; four-group, 233
Teacher: role in identifying retardates, 103–107; and special class placement, 114; teacher-principal team, 114
Terminology, influence of medical concepts, 17
Traditional criterion, 221
Two-dimensional definition: and prevalence, 187–92; justified, 196
Typology of mental retardation, 141–44

Vacating status of retardate, 118–19
Variables dichotomized, 236
Vineland Social Maturity Scale, 145–49, 269

Wechsler Adult Intelligence Scale, 13*n*, 69
Wechsler-Bellevue I, 13*n*
Wechsler Intelligence Scale for Children: and sociocultural modality, 239, 241–43, 244; in pluralistic evaluation, 261; validity, 284; mentioned, 69, 130, 131, 237
Wechsler Intelligence Scales, 5
Welfare organizations as labelers, 59, 62–64
White, Anglo-Saxon Protestants, 13
World Health Organization, 138

Zigler, E, 223, 226, 228, 259